LWW's
VISUAL
ATLAS
OF MEDICAL ASSISTING
SKILLS

DEBORAH J. BEDFORD, AAS, CMA

Program Coordinator/Instructor, Medical Assisting (Retired)
North Seattle Community College
Seattle, Washington

MICHAELANN MARIE ALLEN, MAEd, CMA

Program Director/Instructor, Medical Assisting
North Seattle Community College
Seattle, Washington

 Wolters Kluwer | Lippincott Williams & Wilkins
Health

Philadelphia · Baltimore · New York · London
Buenos Aires · Hong Kong · Sydney · Tokyo

Executive Editor: John Goucher
Senior Managing Editor: Rebecca Kerins
Marketing Manager: Nancy Bradshaw

Associate Production Manager: Kevin Johnson
Designer: Risa Clow
Compositor: Hearthside Publishing Services
Printed in China

9 8 7 6 5 4 3 2 1

Library of Congress Cataloging-in-Publication Data
Bedford, Deborah J.
LWW's visual atlas of medical assisting skills / Deborah J. Bedford, Michaelann Marie Allen.
p. ; cm.
Includes index.
ISBN-13: 978-0-7817-6202-1 (alk. paper)
ISBN-10: 0-7817-6202-2 (alk. paper)
1. Medical assistants--Atlases. I. Allen, Michaelann Marie. II. Lippincott Williams & Wilkins. III. Title.
   IV. Title: Visual atlas of medical assisting skills.
[DNLM: 1. Delivery of Health Care—Atlases. 2. Allied Health Personnel—education—Atlases. W 17 B411L 2008]
R728.8.B444 2008
610.73'70690222—dc22
2007035035

DISCLAIMER

Care has been taken to confirm the accuracy of the information present and to describe generally accepted practices. However, the authors, editors, and publisher are not responsible for errors or omissions or for any consequences from application of the information in this book and make no warranty, expressed or implied, with respect to the currency, completeness, or accuracy of the contents of the publication. Application of this information in a particular situation remains the professional responsibility of the practitioner; the clinical treatments described and recommended may not be considered absolute and universal recommendations.

The authors, editors, and publisher have exerted every effort to ensure that drug selection and dosage set forth in this text are in accordance with the current recommendations and practice at the time of publication. However, in view of ongoing research, changes in government regulations, and the constant flow of information relating to drug therapy and drug reactions, the reader is urged to check the package insert for each drug for any change in indications and dosage and for added warnings and precautions. This is particularly important when the recommended agent is a new or infrequently employed drug.

Some drugs and medical devices presented in this publication have Food and Drug Administration (FDA) clearance for limited use in restricted research settings. It is the responsibility of the health care provider to ascertain the FDA status of each drug or device planned for use in their clinical practice.

To purchase additional copies of this book, call our customer service department at **(800) 638-3030** or fax orders to **(301) 223-2320**. International customers should call **(301) 223-2300**.

Visit Lippincott Williams & Wilkins on the Internet: http://www.lww.com. Lippincott Williams & Wilkins customer service representatives are available from 8:30 am to 6:00 pm, EST.

I dedicate my work on this book to my granddaughter, Millie, who brightens my life. I also want to thank those close to me whose love and support I treasure (and who have put up with a lot over the years!): my children Ryan and Lea Bedford and Kristin and Michael Bruington; the rest of my family and friends; Sharon and Doug Holliker; Jack Arnold; Scott, AJ, and Nate Holliker; Traci Holliker; Brianna Lyon; Ron and Jan Fagot; Bill and Janis McCarty; and to Bill in Scotland. In loving memory of Dwight, Lucille, Edna, and Mark—you are still with me.

Deborah J. Bedford

I wish to dedicate my part in this book to my son, Mo, a true survivor of the reality of life; I wish I had more than this page to tell the world how proud I am of him!

Michaelann Marie Allen

Preface

Medical assisting is an exciting, challenging, and fulfilling field, and it requires accuracy, efficiency, critical thinking, and flexibility. Medical assistants are known as the most versatile allied health professionals, which means a medical assistant must be knowledgeable and competent in a wide variety of areas. Years ago, medical assistants learned on the job, usually working for a physician and performing both administrative and clinical duties. Today, the medical assistant's job has greatly expanded, the complexity of tasks has increased, the expected level of performance is higher, and numerous legal requirements and ethical issues affect the medical assistant's responsibilities. The need for well educated, competent, and people-oriented medical assistants is tremendous.

LWW's Visual Atlas of Medical Assisting Skills is designed to provide medical assisting students with step-by-step instruction on the administrative, clinical, and general tasks they must master to pass an accredited program to qualify to sit for the national exam to become either a Certified Medical Assistant or a Registered Medical Assistant. Intended to supplement any core medical assisting text, this resource assists students in reviewing and practicing a wide variety of medical assisting skills, and the photographic approach will appeal especially to visual learners. With the use of this atlas, students can maximize lab time and practice their skills independently instead of relying solely on classroom demonstration or one-on-one assistance from instructors.

ORGANIZATION

LWW's Visual Atlas of Medical Assisting Skills is divided into three major areas of performance: administrative, clinical, and general. The 11 chapters correspond to the major headings outlined by the 2003 *Standards and Guidelines for Medical Assisting Educational Programs* by the Commission on the Accreditation of Allied Health Education Programs (CAAHEP), and the related procedures included within each chapter address the 61 competencies as required by CAAHEP. Although the organization of this book is based on CAAHEP's competencies, the competencies required by the Accrediting Bureau of Health Education Schools (ABHES) are addressed as well, either in the text itself or in the accompanying instructor resource materials.

Part 1, Administrative Competencies, covers procedures related to performing clerical functions, performing bookkeeping procedures, and processing insurance claims.

Part 2, Clinical Competencies, covers fundamental procedures, specimen collection, diagnostic testing, and patient care.

Part 3, General Competencies, covers professional communications, legal concepts, patient instruction, and operational functions.

FEATURES

Each chapter presents a variety of medical assisting procedures in a step-by-step fashion. Each step is accompanied by a photograph, and the explanatory text is written in concise, straightforward, and easy-to-understand language to facilitate learning. In addition to this visual, step-by-step approach, the following features are included:

Tips accompany many of the individual steps and provide students with additional information to help them understand and execute the procedures.

WHY❓ Rationales are included where appropriate to provide students with the logic behind the various steps in the procedures and help to promote critical thinking.

LEGAL ALERT❗ Legal Alerts are included to highlight important legal issues that medical assistants need to know.

✎ Charting Examples are included at the end of procedures to show students how to correctly document what they have done in a patient's medical record.

In addition to the above features, the procedures are supplemented where appropriate by boxed content, tables, and anatomical art to aid in student learning.

TO THE STUDENT

LWW's Visual Atlas of Medical Assisting Skills is intended to work with, not to be used instead of, a core medical assisting textbook. Use of this valuable resource assumes that you learn the theory, the basics and supporting information of the assigned procedures, and the general knowledge about medical assisting by reading your core textbook and by following classroom instruction. This text, with its multitude of photographs, in addition to the step-by-step explanations of the included procedures, allows you to practice your skills when an instructor is not immediately available.

In addition to the text, the following free supplemental materials are available for students on thePoint (refer to the inside cover of this book for information on how to access the site):

• **A complete set of Competency Evaluation Forms.** Print and use these forms to practice the medical assisting procedures you will need to master. Practice on your own and practice with a partner so you'll be ready when it's time to demonstrate your skills for your instructor!
• **A selection of video clips.** Watch the video clips to see select medical assisting procedures demonstrated by professionals.

TO THE INSTRUCTOR

LWW's Visual Atlas of Medical Assisting Skills was created to fill a void in existing medical assisting texts. Existing core textbooks never seemed to include enough photographs and other visual aids, so we set out to create a resource that includes a thorough collection of realistic visuals to help students in the practice of performing the procedures, since many people learn best when they can easily see the steps as they perform them. As an instructor, this text and its accompanying ancillaries can help you in the following ways:

• The Atlas can assist you in the lab setting when you can't immediately help all students.
• The accompanying Competency Evaluation Forms allow you to set your own evaluation criteria, while recommending the critical steps for passing performance of the procedure.
• The text and Competency Evaluation Forms together can prove extremely useful in meeting and documenting accreditation requirements, whether CAAHEP or ABHES.
• The Atlas will hopefully give you new ideas, make your lab time more productive for students, and enhance your limited time in assisting individual students.

In addition to the text, an **Instructor's Resource CD-ROM** includes the following valuable resources:

• A vast library of **Competency Evaluation Forms**. The forms cover all CAAHEP and ABHES competencies and are customizable to help you optimize your teaching.
• A **Competency Correlation Grid**. This tool clearly matches the CAAHEP and ABHES competencies with the Competency Evaluation Forms provided for easy reference.
• A selection of **video clips** demonstrating a variety of medical assisting procedures.

Instructor resources are also available on thePoint; refer to the inside cover of this book for information on how to access the site.

Acknowledgments

First, I would like to thank everyone at Lippincott Williams & Wilkins for believing in my idea and giving us this opportunity. Next, my appreciation goes to Michaelann Allen for the many hours and amount of work she put into this book. And, of course, I thank the students and instructors who were my inspiration for this project. I hope this book will be helpful and will contribute to the quality of medical assisting. I thank you all sincerely.

Deborah J. Bedford

There are so many people who helped with the creation of this textbook that it is hard to name them all. First, I wish to thank my great friend and fellow instructor, Meredith Crichton, for all her help with the administrative procedures. An immense amount of credit also goes to the staff of Lippincott Williams & Wilkins, who supported us throughout many delays and complications and still kept their faith in the final product; they always worked to find solutions as well as modeled when needed. What can I say about the photographers; I will never forget you guys. To the students and others in Philadelphia who helped us with the final shoot; you were amazing, fun, and kept the energy going! On a personal note, I wish to thank my friends and family who supported me through the long hours and absences, especially my two sons, Mabruk and Farouk, who sacrificed as much time and effort as I did. And last but not least, to my students who posed for the initial photos, you rock!

Michaelann Marie Allen

Reviewers

The following individuals provided feedback on the proposal or draft manuscript for book chapters. Their helpful feedback has resulted in a stronger book.

Michelle Buchman, RN, BSN, BC
Educational Support Services, LLC
St. John's Marian Center
Springfield, Missouri

Robyn Gohsman, AAS
Medical Careers Institute
Newport News, Virginia

Joanna Holly, RN, RS, MS
Midstate College
Peoria, Illinois

Geri Kale-Smith, MS, CMA
Medical Office Administration Programs
William Rainey Harper College
Palatine, Illinois

Julayne Masterman, MA, BSBA, CMA
Ivy Tech State College
Muncie, Indiana

Pat Moeck, PhD, MBA, CMA
El Centro College,
Dallas, Texas

Nina Thierer, BS
Ivy Tech Community College
Fort Wayne, Indiana

Contents

Expanded Contents

PART

ONE

Administrative Competencies

CHAPTER 1

Perform Clerical Functions

INTRODUCTION

Scheduling patient appointments and procedures and keeping medical records organized are some of the most important duties performed by a medical assistant. By understanding the administrative functions of a medical office and effectively managing these tasks, the medical assistant ensures a smooth work flow and creates an atmosphere of calm professionalism that makes patients feel comfortable and secure throughout the medical visit.

PROCEDURES

1-1 Develop Appointment Matrix

1-2 Check in Patients

1-3 Schedule Appointments

1-4 Cancel or Reschedule Appointments

1-5 Schedule Inpatient and Outpatient Procedures

1-6 Organize a Patient's Medical Record

1-7 File Medical Records

Procedure 1-1

Develop Appointment Matrix

PURPOSE

An appointment matrix helps manage daily workflow by allowing efficient scheduling of patient appointments, provider time, and office facilities.

EQUIPMENT/SUPPLIES

- appointment book
- computer
- pen
- pencil
- highlighters

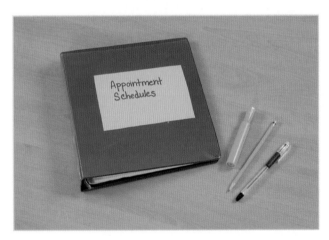

1. Gather all supplies.

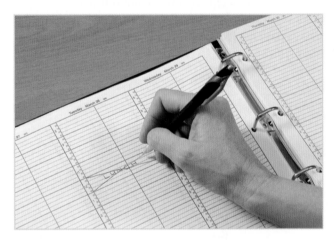

2. Block off non-patient (closed) times by marking X through the time slots.

WHY? *Blocking off parts of the schedule ensures that appointments are not made during times when providers are unavailable. An organized schedule serves the greatest number of patients in a limited amount of time, thus meeting the needs of patients as well as the business.*

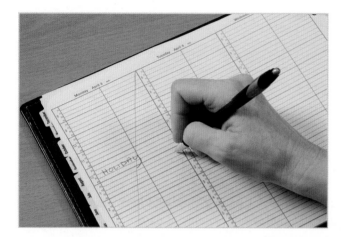

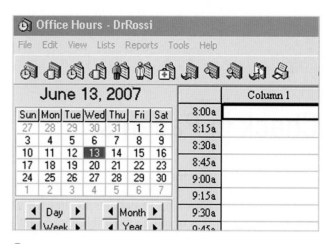

3. Write in all holidays and other office closures.

3. Variation.

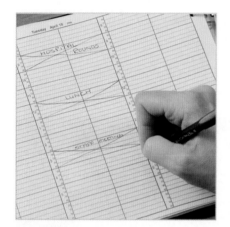

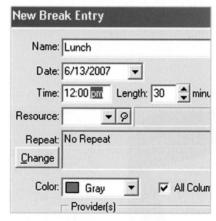

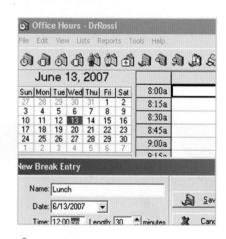

4. Write in all meetings, hospital rounds, conferences, vacations, etc.

4. Variation.

WHY? *This information shows the provider's activities or locations during certain times or days.*

4. Variation.

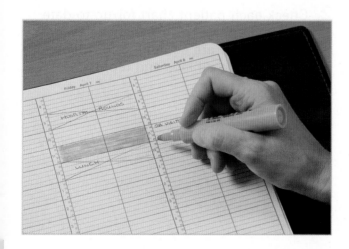

5. Highlight specialty times, such as acute visits, OB visits, well child visits, etc.

WHY? *Different types of visits require specific time allotments and use of certain medical office facilities. Knowing in advance what is needed for each type of visit allows efficient use of staff and office resources.*

TIP Specialty visits will depend on the type of medical office in which you work.

TIP If you are using computerized scheduling, the software program will set up the appointment matrix after you enter the information once.

Procedure 1-2

Check in Patients

PURPOSE

Checking in patients as they arrive promotes efficient patient flow and keeps the medical office running smoothly. A pleasant greeting also helps put patients at ease.

EQUIPMENT/SUPPLIES

- appointment book
- patient charts
- computer
- pen
- pencil
- highlighter

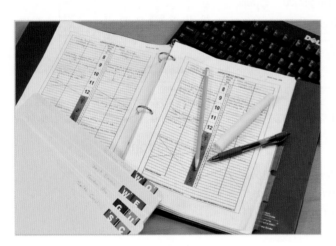

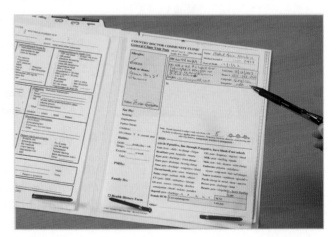

1. Gather all supplies.

TIP▶ The day before, pull all scheduled patient charts for the next day, print or copy appointment lists as needed for providers and medical personnel, and make patient reminder calls if required.

2. Check each patient chart for up-to-date information. Make sure that charts for patients who are coming in for follow-up visits include all labs and reports.

TIP▶ The back office medical assistant may be responsible for this task.

WHY? The provider needs current and accurate information to ensure appropriate patient care.

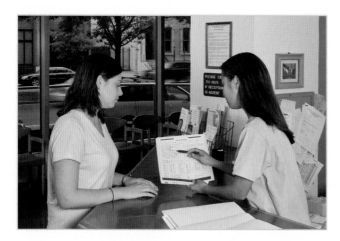

3. As patients arrive, greet them appropriately and confirm demographic information such as insurance, address, telephone number, referral needs, etc.

WHY❓ *Always be pleasant and helpful, as the medical assistant is the patient's first office contact. Confirming demographic information ensures that the chart contains correct patient data.*

TIP▶ Always preserve confidentiality as per HIPAA compliance.

TIP▶ If a patient has a new insurance card, photocopy the front and back of it, and place it in the chart.

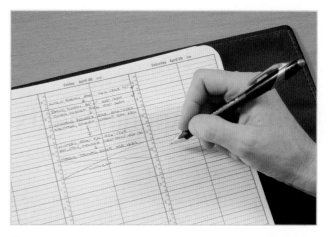

4. Check off the names on the master schedule as patients arrive per your office policy.

WHY❓ *Noting patient arrivals helps maintain control of the appointment schedule and allows the medical assistant to identify potential problems, such as late patients or no-shows.*

TIP▶ Some offices highlight patients' names as they come in; others make a mark of some sort. With computer scheduling software, names are marked automatically as the patient checks in. Be sure to mark all cancellations and no-shows appropriately on the schedule and in the patient chart.

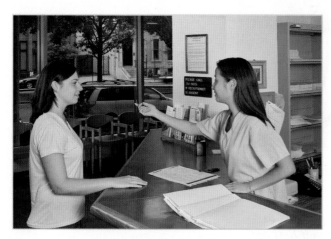

5. Ask the patient to be seated.

WHY❓ *Polite behavior helps the patient feel comfortable in the medical office.*

TIP▶ You may need to ask a patient to leave a sample, use the restroom, or provide necessary forms for special visits, etc.

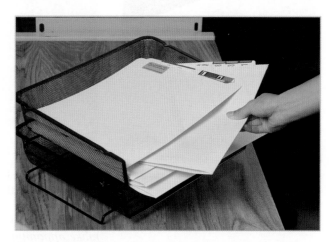

6. Place the chart in a rack or other appropriate place and notify the back office personnel that the patient is ready as per office policy.

WHY❓ *This promotes efficient patient flow and keeps the medical office running smoothly.*

Procedure 1-3

Schedule Appointments

PURPOSE

Appointments serve patient care needs and allow the medical assistant to manage the office schedule effectively.

EQUIPMENT/SUPPLIES

- appointment book
- patient charts
- computer
- telephone
- pen
- pencil
- highlighters
- appointment cards

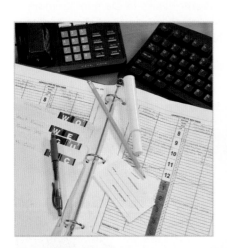

1. Gather all supplies.

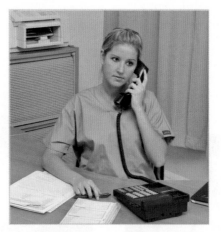

2. Offer the patient several appointment options.

WHY? *Allowing patients to make appointments that best fit their schedules helps improve compliance.*

TIP When making patient appointments, always be polite, friendly, and helpful.

2. Variation.

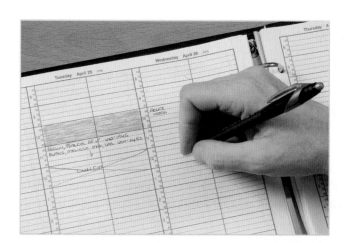

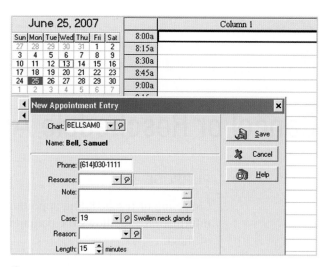

3. Write in the appointment book, or enter into the computer, the patient's name and other pertinent information, including telephone number, reason for visit, and insurance information if this is a new patient or per office policy.

WHY❓ Documenting essential patient information helps maintain accurate records. Recording each patient appointment properly helps avoid overbooking.

TIP➤ Give the patient directions to the medical office if necessary.

3. Variation.

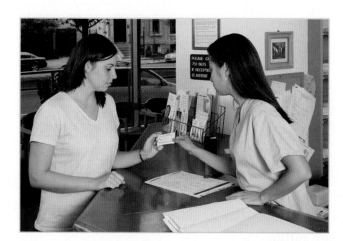

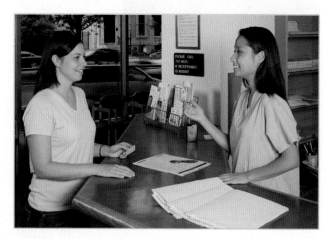

4. If the patient is scheduling in person, provide an appointment card. If the patient is scheduling by phone, restate the appointment time and date at the end of the conversation.

WHY❓ Reminders promote clear communication and help avoid missed appointments.

5. Thank the patient.

WHY❓ It is important to be professional and polite when communicating with patients.

TIP➤ If you are speaking on the phone, always let the patient hang up first.

Procedure 1-4

Cancel or Reschedule Appointments

PURPOSE

Canceling or rescheduling appointments ensures that the schedule contains the most up-to-date information and allows the patient to see the provider at a new time that is convenient for both of them.

EQUIPMENT/SUPPLIES

- appointment book
- patient charts
- computer
- telephone
- message pad
- pen
- pencil
- highlighters
- appointment cards

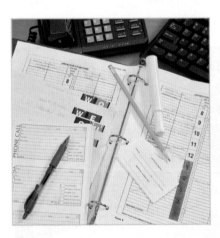

1. Gather all supplies.

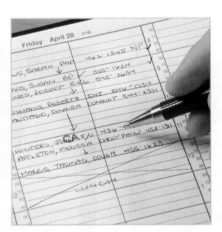

2. When a patient cancels an appointment, either erase the name, mark cancelled (CA) or rescheduled (RS), or enter the change in the computer as per office policy. Also mark this in the patient's chart if applicable.

2. Variation.

WHY? *Erasing the patient's appointment or deleting it from the computer avoids scheduling errors and keeps the office running smoothly.*

LEGAL ALERT! Documentation of no-shows is often done by many offices for risk management purposes.

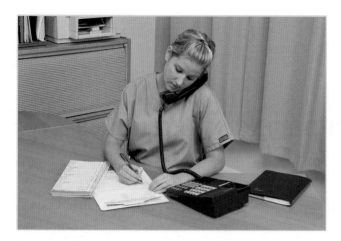

3. If rescheduling, give the patient several appointment options.

WHY? *Offering the patient convenient times will help ensure that the appointment is kept.*

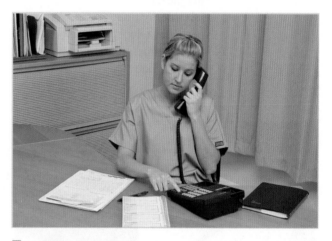

3. Variation.

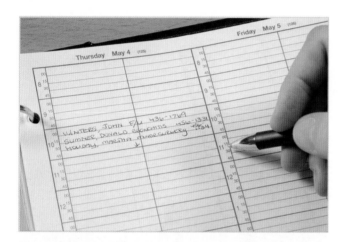

4. Write the new appointment time in the appointment book or enter it into the computer if rescheduling.

WHY? *Maintaining an accurate appointment schedule avoids wasting time for patients, providers, and staff.*

TIP If the patient is rescheduling in person, provide a new appointment card.

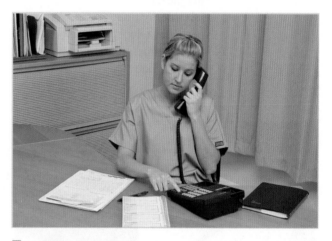

5. Thank the patient.

WHY? *It is important to be professional and polite when communicating with patients.*

TIP If you are speaking on the phone, always let the patient hang up first.

Procedure 1-5

Schedule Inpatient and Outpatient Procedures

PURPOSE

Scheduling inpatient or outpatient procedures ensures that patients receive appropriate medical care and timely diagnosis.

EQUIPMENT/SUPPLIES

- patient chart
- computer
- telephone
- pen
- diagnosis
- lab information
- pertinent telephone numbers
- patient time preferences
- fax machine

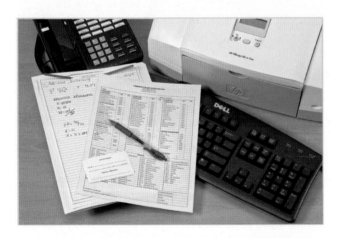

1. Gather all supplies.

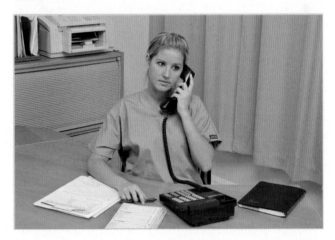

2. Call the hospital, stating your name, the clinic or doctor you are representing, and the name of the procedure you are trying to schedule.

ᴡʜʏ❓ *Providing essential information promotes good communication.*

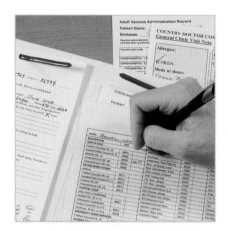

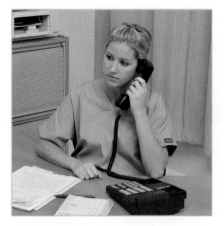

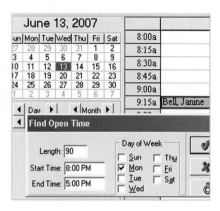

3. Give the patient's name, details of diagnosis, and other pertinent information.

WHY? *The hospital needs this information to best serve the patient's needs.*

4. Confirm the date and time for the procedure, type of patient preparation that may be required, and any other special instructions.

WHY? *Confirming key information avoids miscommunication.*

4. Variation.

TIP The date and time for the procedure may depend on physician availability; for example, some surgeons perform certain procedures only on set days of the week.

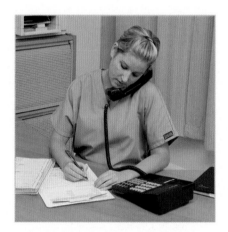

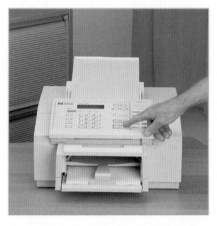

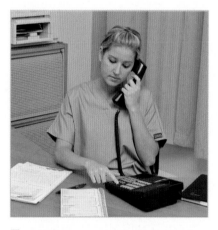

5. Call the patient's insurance company for preauthorization if necessary.

WHY? *Some insurance companies have strict requirements for preauthorization that must be followed.*

TIP See chapter 3 for referrals.

6. Fax any labs, chart notes, and insurance, or patient information as necessary.

WHY? *Having all pertinent information available ensures the hospital will provide appropriate patient care.*

TIP Be sure to follow HIPAA guidelines for faxing.

7. Call to inform the patient of the date, time, and any preparation needed for the procedure.

WHY? *The patient needs this information in order to arrange his or her schedule and to carry out the required preparations.*

TIP Some hospitals or inpatient service institutions require the patient to call them directly for preparation steps; determine if this is the case when scheduling procedures, and be sure to inform the patient.

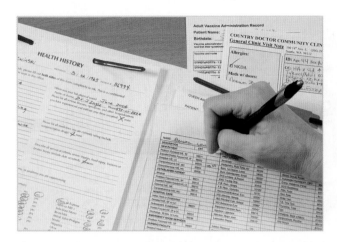

8. Document the information and inform the provider.

WHY❓ *Proper documentation and good communication are vital to providing quality patient care.*

✎ *Charting Example*

8/12/06 10:45 a.m. Pt. scheduled for tubal ligation @ Swedish Downtown with Dr. Mark Jones, 11/20/06. Pre-op instructions given. _____ M. Allen, CMA

✎ *Charting Example*

8/22/06 11:15 a.m. Pt. scheduled for colonoscopy with Dr. Mark Jones. 12/12/06. Procedure prep given.
_____ A. Ware, CMA

Procedure **1-6**

Organize a Patient's Medical Record

PURPOSE

The medical record is a legal document. Great care must be taken to ensure accuracy, provide proper documentation, and allow easy retrieval of information for providers and staff.

EQUIPMENT/SUPPLIES

- patient chart
- patient records
- labs
- correspondence
- notes

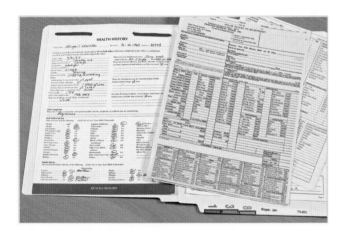

1. Gather all supplies.

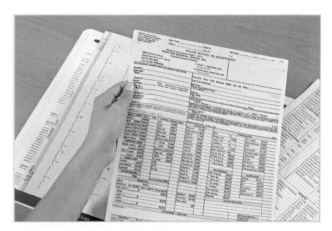

2. Determine which information goes where.

ᴡʜʏ❓ *Each office uses different types of medical record filing, such as POMR, SOMR, SOAP notes, and report types. The medical assistant needs to ensure that all patient records adhere to the practice's preferred organizational system.*

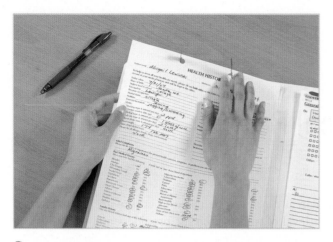

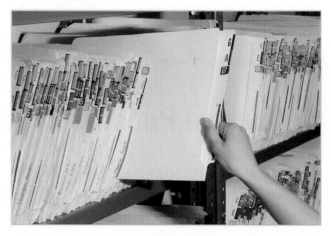

3. File information into correct area in chart.

WHY? *It is important to maintain consistent organization within patient charts, as this promotes easy retrieval of information.*

4. File chart or place in proper area to be filed.

WHY? *This ensures that patient information is stored where it can be easily obtained when needed.*

TIP Computerized medical records file the patient record automatically within the database.

TIP See procedure 1-7.

Procedure 1-7

File Medical Records

PURPOSE

Filing medical records correctly is crucial for quick and accurate retrieval of patient charts.

EQUIPMENT/SUPPLIES

• patient charts

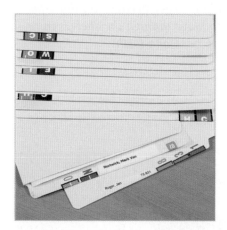

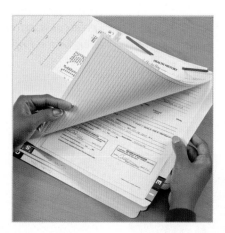

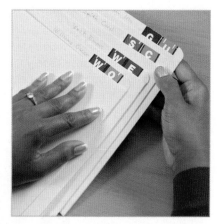

1. Gather charts to be filed.

2. Inspect the charts for accuracy of organization and no loose papers.

WHY❓ *By keeping charts organized, the medical assistant helps prevent errors in patient information, which aids patient care.*

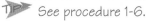 See procedure 1-6.

3. Properly index the chart or identify its index to determine how the chart will be located.

WHY❓ *This helps avoid filing errors and allows for easy retrieval.*

TIP▶ Indexing units are how a chart is identified and separated into smaller subunits for filing. This is done most often by using the patient's legal name, last name first. It may also be numerical. See your textbook to learn the rules for indexing.

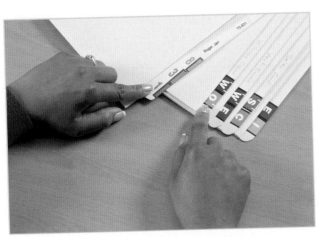

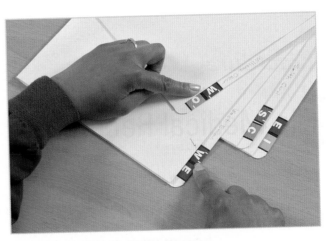

4. Code the chart or identify its code to determine where to file it.

WHY❓ *Proper coding prevents filing errors.*

TIP▶ If a charting system is strictly alphabetical, then file alphabetically; if it is a color coded system, identify the proper color coding; if numerical, determine the proper sequence. See your textbook for how to use Tab-Alpha, Numerical, Colorscan, or other color coded systems.

5. Sort the charts for filing.

WHY❓ *Some filing systems can be quite large. Sorting charts into either alphabetical or numerical order first makes filing easier because it allows the medical assistant to move through the shelves in order, instead of going back and forth.*

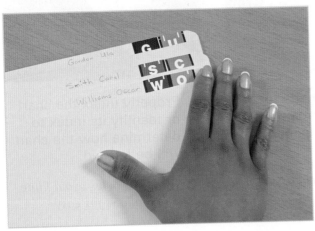

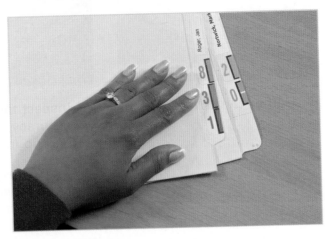

6. File charts in alphabetical order (left) or numerical order (right), per office policy.

WHY❓ *Charts need to be stored in appropriate order so they can be readily retrieved when needed.*

Quick Reference on Filing Rules

Box 1·1

Filing Procedures

To ensure efficient and speedy filing and document retrieval, follow these four steps:

1. *Condition.* Prepare items by removing loose pieces of tape or paper clips. Make sure each sheet of paper includes the patient's name in case a second page gets separated from the first page.
2. *Index.* Separate business records from patient records.
3. *Sort.* Put each group of records in proper order to be filed on shelves, either alphabetic or numeric. This makes actual filing go much faster because you are not moving up and down and back and forth to find the proper letter area; you will just move down in order.
4. *Store.* Place each record in the proper storage area for active, inactive, or closed records.

From Molle EA, Kronenberger J, Durham LS, West-Stack C. Lippincott Williams & Wilkins' Comprehensive Medical Assisting. 2nd ed. Baltimore: Lippincott Williams & Wilkins, 2005.

Box 1·2

Indexing Rules for Alphabetic Filing

When filing records alphabetically, use these indexing rules to help you decide the placement of each record. Indexing rules apply whether you use the title of the record's contents or a person's name.

* File by name according to last name, first name, and middle initial, and treat each letter in the name as a separate unit. For example, Jamey L. Crowell should be filed as Crowell, Jamey L. and should come before Crowell, Jamie L.
* Make sure professionals initials are placed after a full name. John P. Bonnet, D.O., should be filed as Bonnet, John P., D.O.
* Treat hyphenated names as one unit. Bernadette M. Ryan-Nardone should be filed as Ryan-Nardone, Bernadette M., not as Nardone, Bernadette M. Ryan.
* File abbreviated names as if they were spelled out. Finnigan, Wm. Should be filed as Finnigan, William, and St. James should be filed as Saint James.
* File last names beginning with Mac and Mc in regular order or grouped together, depending on your preference, but be consistent with either approach.
* File a married woman's record by using her own first name. Helen Johnston (Mrs. Kevin Johnston) should be filed as Johnston, Helen, not as Johnston, Kevin Mrs.
* Jr. and Sr. should be used in indexing and labeling the record. Many times a father and son are patients at the same facility.
* When names are identical, use the next unit, such as birth dates or the mother's maiden name. Use Durham, Iran (2-4-94) and Durham, Iran (4-5-45).
* Disregard apostrophes.
* Disregard articles (a, the), conjunctions (and, or), and prepositions (in, of) in filing. File *The Cat in the Hat* under Cat in Hat.
* Treat letters in a company name as separate units. For ASM, Inc., "A" is the first unit, "S" is the second unit, and "M" is the third unit.

From Molle EA, Kronenberger J, Durham LS, West-Stack C. Lippincott Williams & Wilkins' Comprehensive Medical Assisting. 2nd ed. Baltimore: Lippincott Williams & Wilkins, 2005.

Filing Examples

Alphabetic Filing Examples

The following patient records are to be filed alphabetically:

> Mary P. Martin
> Floyd Pigg, Sr.
> Susan Bailey
> Ellen Eisel-Parrish
> Anita Putrosky
> Susan R. Hill
> Sister Mary Catherine
> Cher
> Stephen Dorsky, MD
> Mrs. John Moser (Donna)

The proper order is:

> Susan Bailey
> Cher
> Stephen Dorsky
> Ellen Eisel-Parrish
> Susan R. Hill
> Mary P. Martin
> Donna Moser
> Floyd D. Pigg
> Anita Putrosky
> Sister Mary Catherine

Numeric Filing Examples

The following patient records are to be filed numerically:

> LeRoy Flora   213456
> Ramsey Curtis   334387
> Sharon Moore   979779
> Cathy King   321138

In straight digit filing, the proper order is:

> 213456
> 321138
> 334387
> 979779

In terminal digit filing, the proper order is:

> 321138
> 213456
> 979779
> 334387

With files in which one or two groups of numbers are the same numbers, you refer to the second or third group of numbers. For example, in straight digit filing (reading from left to right), the number 003491 comes before 004592. The first group of numbers (00) is the same for both files, so you determine the order of filing by the second group of numbers; in this case, 34 comes before 45.

In terminal digit filing (reading from right to left), 456128 would come before 926128. The first two groups of numbers (28 and 61) are the same for both files, so you go to the third group of numbers; in this case, 45 comes before 92.

From Molle EA, Kronenberger J, Durham LS, West-Stack C. Lippincott Williams & Wilkins' Comprehensive Medical Assisting. 2nd ed. Baltimore: Lippincott Williams & Wilkins, 2005.

CHAPTER 2

Perform Bookkeeping Procedures

INTRODUCTION

Sound financial practices are essential to the smooth functioning of any medical office. By handling office finances skillfully, medical assistants perform one of the most vital administrative roles. For example, careful records of income and expenses are needed for tax and legal purposes. Neatness, accuracy, and good math skills are required for correct financial documentation. Timeliness is also important because prompt billing keeps the accounts receivable flowing so bills and salaries can be paid, and patients will know what charges and fees to expect.

PROCEDURES

2-1 Prepare a Bank Deposit

2-2 Post Entries on a Day Sheet

2-3 Perform Accounts Receivable Procedures

2-4 Balance a Day Sheet

2-5 Perform Billing and Collection Procedures

2-6 Post Adjustments

2-7 Process a Credit Balance

2-8 Process Refunds

2-9 Post NSF Checks

2-10 Post Collection Agency Payments

2-11 Reconcile a Bank Statement

2-12 Balance Petty Cash

Procedure 2-1

Prepare a Bank Deposit

PURPOSE

Maintaining bank accounts is one of the medical assistant's financial duties. Daily bank deposits serve as proof of posting and ensure that adequate funds are available to the practice.

EQUIPMENT/SUPPLIES

- copy machine
- checks
- credit card receipts
- adding machine
- deposit slip
- cash box
- cash
- pen
- deposit bag

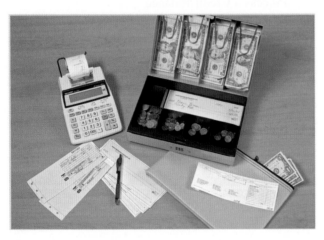

1. Gather all supplies.

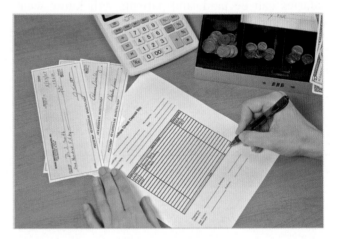

2. Endorse all of the checks, then add them to the deposit slip in the appropriate place.

   TIP Avoid using blank endorsements, such as a signature only, in case the check is lost or stolen. Always put "for deposit only" as this prevents others from cashing the checks. Most offices have a rubber stamp endorsement with the practice name and address and "for deposit only" on it for expediency.

   TIP Be sure to include name of payer, check number or bank number, and total.

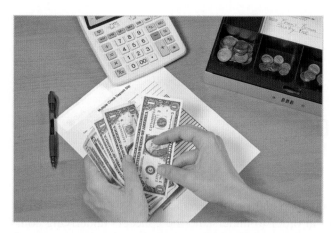

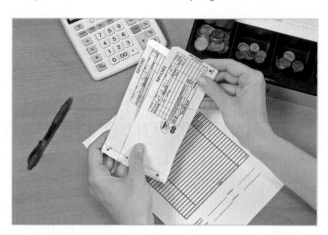

3. Count cash and add total to deposit slip in appropriate place.

4. Add credit card totals to deposit slip in appropriate place.

TIP This varies; at some offices, you would not include credit card totals on the deposit slip.

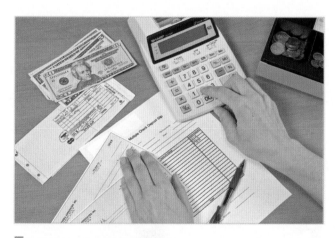

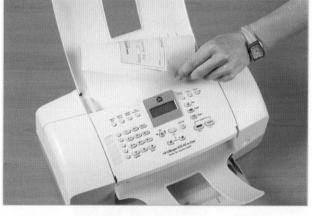

5. Total all amounts.

WHY? *Accuracy and attention to detail are critical when completing financial tasks.*

6. Photocopy all checks.

WHY? *Keeping a record of checks for liability purposes is good office practice. Some offices photocopy all cash serial numbers as well.*

TIP Keep all credit card slip copies.

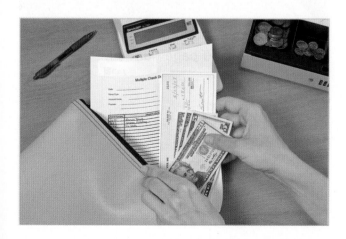

7. Place checks, cash, and deposit slip into bank security deposit bag or take to bank for deposit.

WHY? *This ensures the money goes into the practice's account.*

TIP Many offices have routine pick-ups for bank deposits from a bank employee, while others have office personnel make the deposits.

Procedure 2-2

Post Entries on a Day Sheet

PURPOSE

Although many offices use computerized financial programs, medical assistants must know how to use the manual pegboard system in order to understand the concepts underlying computerized systems. Posting entries on a day sheet documents each patient's account information, ensuring the provider receives payment for services rendered. The pegboard system is part of accounts receivable; it keeps track of the debt owed *to* the practice.

EQUIPMENT/SUPPLIES

- day sheet
- ledger cards
- receipts
- day's schedule
- computer
- pen
- pegboard
- patient charts

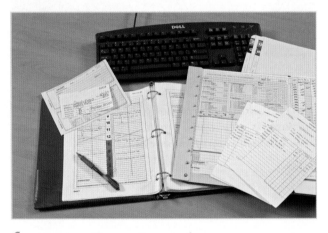

1. Gather all supplies.

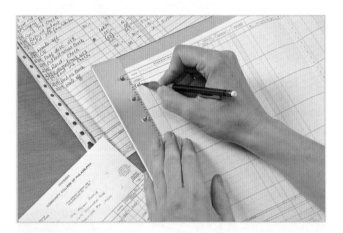

2. Fill in date and page number.

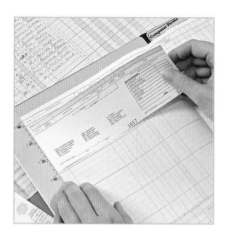

3. Align new day sheet and blank charge slips on pegboard.

ᴡʜʏ❓ *Proper alignment ensures that information recorded will be legible and correctly placed. Carbon and carbonless forms are used.*

🖅 The pegboard system is considered a "write it once" system, with forms working together to simplify record keeping and avoid costly mistakes.

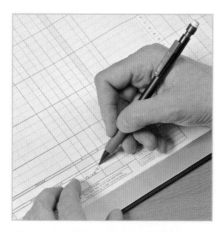

4. Carefully enter all balances forwarded from previous day's sheet (page) in the appropriate section.

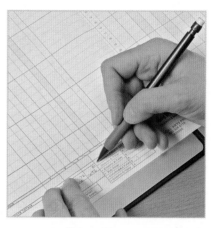

5. Carefully enter balances from columns A–D from previous page in correct box.

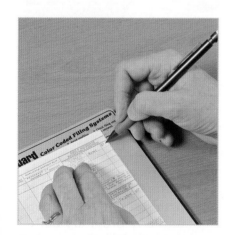

6. Enter "previous day's total" in accounts receivable box.

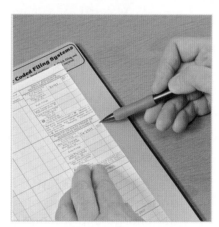

7. Enter "accounts receivable 1st of month" in accounts receivable proof box.

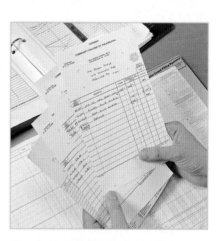

8. Arrange ledger cards in order of patient appointment times at the front desk.

ᴡʜʏ❓ *Organizing ledger cards this way saves time and allows for easy retrieval.*

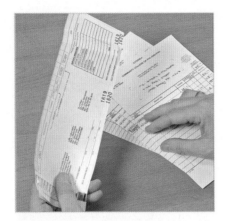

9. Keep receipt forms handy.

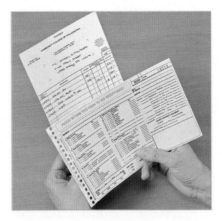

10. When each patient arrives, pull his or her ledger card. Generate a super bill if using a computer; if not, write the patient's name on the super bill.

WHY❓ Patients' financial records are kept on ledger cards. The super bill lists procedures and diagnostic codes for various types of medical office charges.

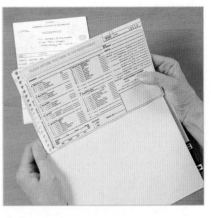

11. Attach the super bill to the patient's chart.

WHY❓ The provider will fill out the super bill after seeing the patient.

TIP▶ If the patient has a co-pay, collect this and write a receipt at this time, and note this on the super bill.

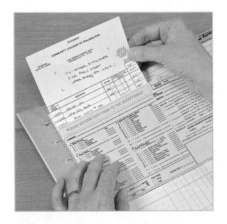

12. When the super bill is returned after the patient's visit with the provider, put the ledger on the pegboard and carefully align with the patient's name on the day sheet.

WHY❓ Proper alignment prevents errors and ensures legibility.

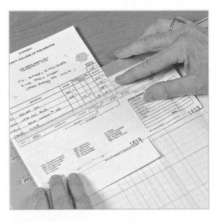

13. Insert the ledger card under the last page of the charge slip (receipt), being sure to align the first blank line of the ledger with the entry strip on the charge slip.

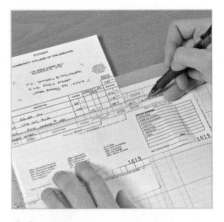

14. Write the date, name of insured, patient name, and any previous balance on the charge slip in the correct space.

WHY❓ This allows the patient's current balance to be calculated.

TIP▶ Most patients do not pay for medical services in cash up front; patients usually have some type of medical insurance that pays for their care. Consequently, many patients have a balance that is owed after insurance is billed.

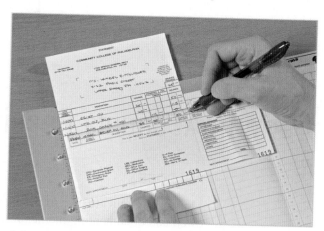

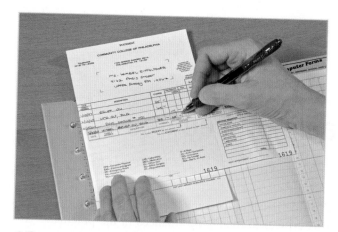

15. Enter the total charge and any payment (such as a co-pay) in the correct column.

WHY? *Correct placement of information ensures accurate financial records.*

16. Determine the final balance by adding any previous balance, that day's charge and subtracting any payments. Enter the final balance on the day sheet/ledger.

WHY? *Careful math calculations help prevent errors and ensure accurate financial records.*

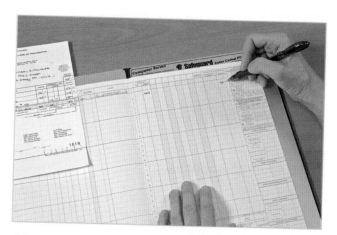

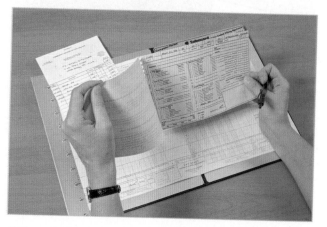

17. If a payment is made and if a receipt is given to patient, enter the receipt number and method of payment in the appropriate column on the right.

18. When posting is complete, file the first copy of the superbill by date of service. If you have a computer, enter codes into the computer when the day is complete. Give the patient the second copy.

WHY? *It is vital to keep accurate records of patient accounts. Patients may need a copy of the super bill to file insurance claims and claims for reimbursement from medical savings accounts.*

TIP Most offices save all receipts and do a batch at the end of the day or when there is time. Batching is when the day's receipts are matched to the day sheet totals and super bills. Super bills, which are attached to a copy of the day's schedule, are also entered into the computer at the end of the day. This info is used to generate the CMS 1500 forms that are sent to insurance companies by mail.

Procedure 2-3

Perform Accounts Receivable Procedures

PURPOSE

Money that patients owe to the medical office is called accounts receivable. Tracking monies owed and documenting monies received is critical to managing finances in the practice.

EQUIPMENT/SUPPLIES

- day sheet
- ledger cards
- receipts
- day's schedule
- adding machine or calculator
- computer
- pen

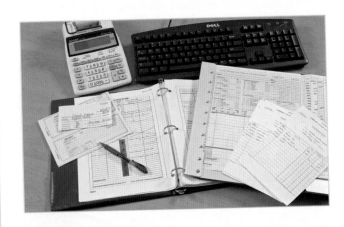

1. Gather all supplies.

If payment is in person:

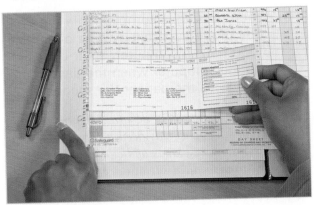

2. Place receipt form on pegboard instead of charge slip, being sure to align correctly and carefully.

ᏮᕼᎽ❓ *Careful alignment prevents errors.*

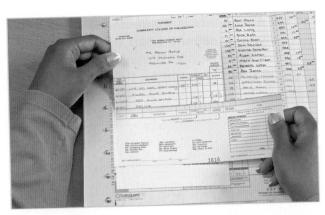

3. Pull patient ledger card and place under receipt form with 1st blank line of ledger card under carbon slip of receipt form.

4. Enter the date, reference (patient name), description, payment, and previous balance on top of the receipt in the proper space.

WHY❓ *The receipt provides the patient with a record of services rendered and payments made to the practice. It must contain full and accurate information.*

▷ Accounts receivable may take the form of co-payments, insurance payments, or patient deductibles as well as the patient's percentage owed after the insurance company has made a payment. Accounts receivable requiring a receipt usually take the form of co-payments only.

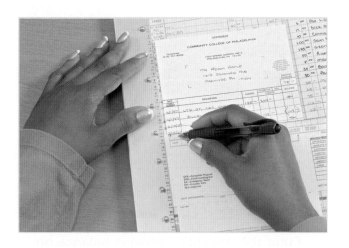

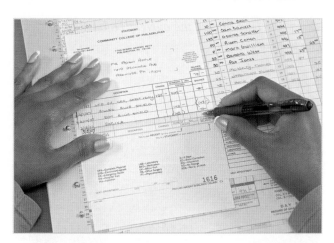

5. Calculate new balance by subtracting payment from previous balance and enter in appropriate space.

WHY❓ *Accuracy in data entry helps keep the books balanced.*

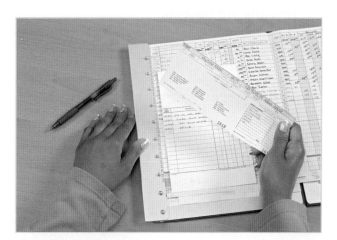

6. Give the receipt to the patient.

If payment is by mail (from patient or insurance company):

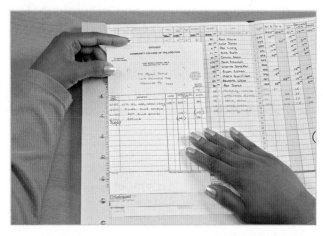

7. Pull patient ledger card and place directly on day sheet in place of charge slip; no receipts are needed.

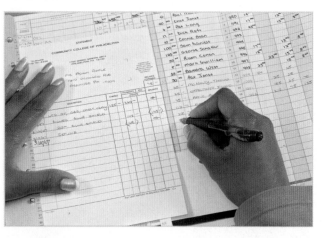

8. Enter the patient's previous balance on the day sheet.

✐*WHY?* *This allows the current balance to be calculated.*

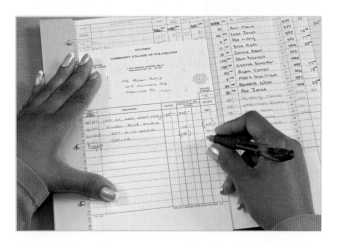

9. Post (write) directly on ledger card the date, reference description (received on account, ROA or check number), and payment amount.

✐*WHY?* *The ledger card contains the patient's financial information, so accurate documentation is vital.*

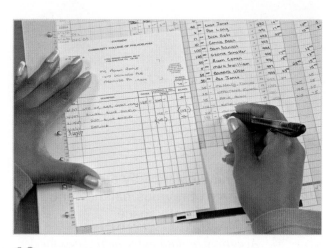

10. Calculate the new balance and enter in appropriate space on the ledger.

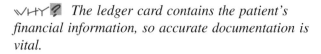

Procedure 2-4

Balance a Day Sheet

PURPOSE

Although not a directly listed competency, balancing a day sheet is critical for complete and accurate record keeping associated with Procedures 2-1, 2-2, and 2-3.

EQUIPMENT/SUPPLIES

- day sheet from previous day
- new day sheet
- calculator
- ledger
- receipts
- pen

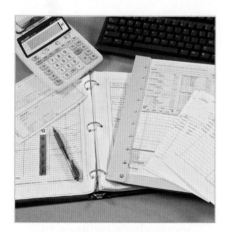

1. Gather all supplies.

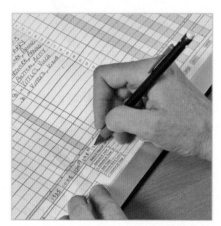

2. Total all columns: A, B, C, D, and E; enter totals in the boxes marked "totals this page."

📑 Write totals in pencil first, then in ink after totals are verified.

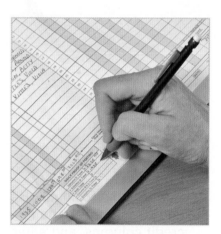

3. Use "proof of posting" box to verify correct entries and accuracy.

📑 All numbers entered here are taken from the "totals this page" column boxes.

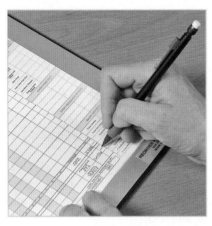

4. Add column totals to figures entered in the "previous page" column boxes to arrive at "month-to-date" totals.

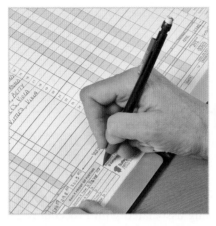

5. Enter today's column E, showing sum of all previous balances.

TIP You are still in the proof of posting section when doing this.

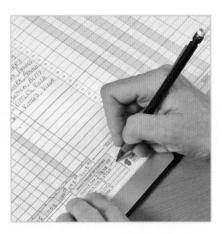

6. Enter column A totals of charges of the day.

TIP This will be a subtotal.

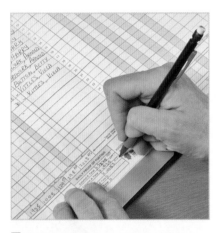

7. Add together columns B and C, as they are both credit columns, and enter into box labeled "less columns B and C."

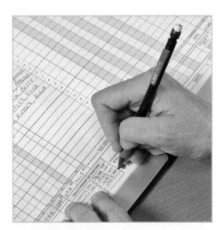

8. Subtract total credits from subtotal in column A.

TIP If correct, result will equal column D and you have balance. If the results don't balance, go back and recheck all totals until you find the mistake.

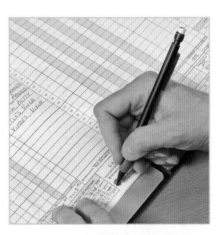

9. Use "accounts receivable control box" to add previous day's balance to current day's business totals.

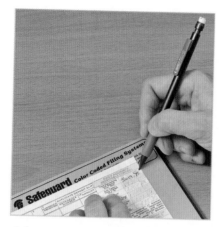

10. Carry column A and B totals straight across from "proof of posting" box to corresponding spaces in "accounts receivable control box."

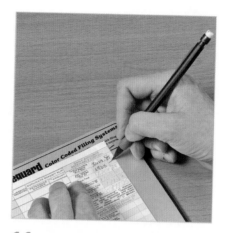

11. Add amount from previous day's total space to column A amount to get a subtotal.

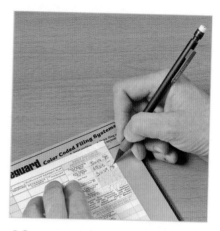

12. Subtract amount from (lines B and C) "less columns B and C" box to get new balance and enter into appropriate space.

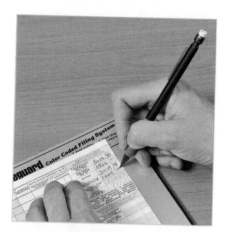

13. Use accounts receivable "proof" to verify accounts receivable balance in accounts receivable control box.

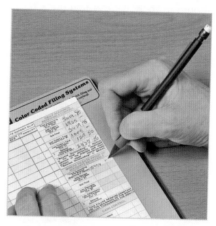

14. Enter number from column A in appropriate space.

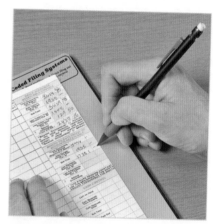

15. Add column A to the "accounts receivable 1st of month" figure and enter sum in subtotal space.

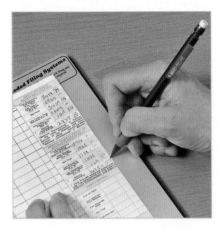

16. Enter B and C month-to-date amounts and subtract from subtotal; then enter in "total accounts receivable" space.

▶ *Accounts receivable control total accounts receivable. A/R control and A/R proof will match if the math is correct. If these do not match, double check your math calculations until you find the mistake.*

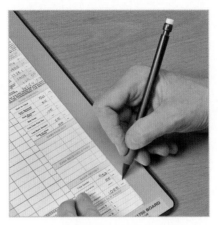

17. Verify deposit by totaling columns in section 2 and entering sum in space marked "total deposit."

▶ *Total deposit and total payments received in Column B should match, with a few noted exceptions.*

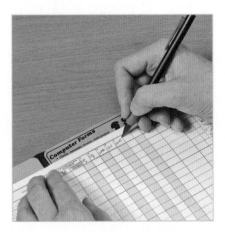

18. Total each column in the summary section of the "Business Analysis Summary" per office policy.

▶ *Some offices use this space, others do not; be sure to follow your office's procedure.*

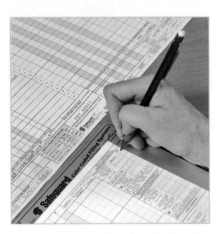

19. Remove day sheet and replace with a new one, then transfer all balances to new day sheet by entering month-to-date column totals from previous page columns onto the new sheet.

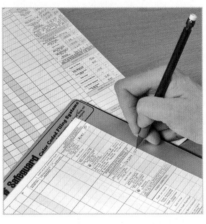

20. Enter total accounts receivable amount in "previous day's total" space of accounts receivable control box on new sheet.

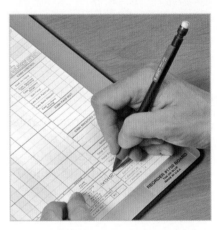

21. Enter accounts receivable 1st of month in "accounts receivable proof" box on new sheet.

▶ *There are many types of pegboard systems, using various lettering systems such as A, B, C, D and E, or A, B1, B2, C and D. Be sure your columns are the correct ones by reading the descriptions.*

Procedure 2-5

Perform Billing and Collection Procedures

PURPOSE

The financial status of a practice is dependent on accurate and timely billing and collection processes. To ensure prompt reimbursement, the medical assistant must understand the payment policies of various insurance companies and keep accurate financial records.

EQUIPMENT/SUPPLIES

- computer
- patient ledger cards
- envelopes
- stamps or postage meter
- adding machine

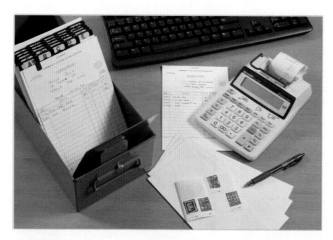

1. Gather all supplies.

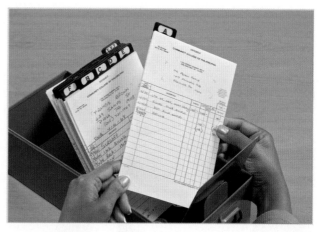

2. Determine which system is used, monthly or cycle billing.

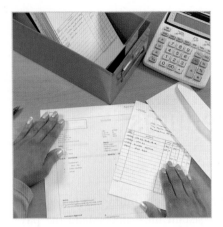

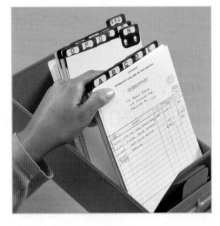

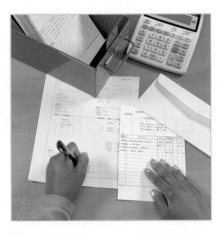

3. If monthly billing is used, prepare all statements and send out by the 25th of each month.

TIP► *Computerized systems can be set up to automatically produce billing statements when needed.*

4. If cycle billing is used, divide alphabet into sections and send out patient bills accordingly.

TIP► *Do half the alphabet at a time for cycle billing (first half on the first of the month and second half on the 15th of the month).*

5. Print or copy statements, making sure all pertinent information is included.

TIP► *Statements include patient name and address, insurance information, date of service, description of service, balance owed, clinic name and address, and a statement saying "if paid, disregard." Computerized systems do this automatically.*

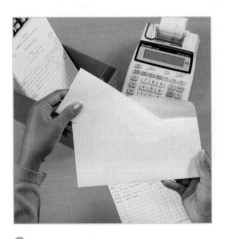

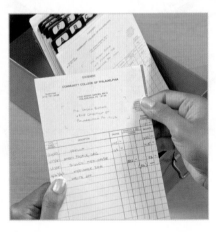

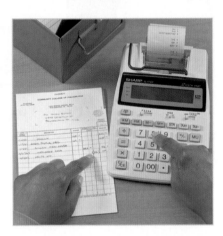

6. Mail statements.

7. If an account is past due, age the account.

TIP► *Use written codes in the pegboard system, color coded by the amount of time overdue. Computer programs for billing will do this automatically when you run a report for overdue balances. Run this report monthly.*

8. Determine the accounts receivable ratio as per office policy. Use collection techniques if necessary.

TIP► *The ratio is*

$$\frac{payments}{charges} + adjustments.$$

The goal is 90%.

If using collection techniques:

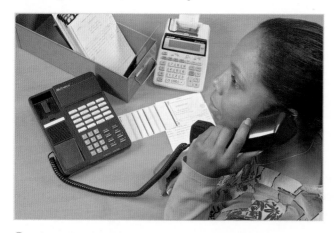

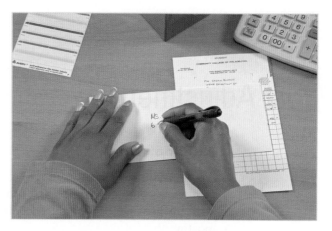

9. Make a telephone call to the patient or insurance company (whichever is delinquent).

WHY? *Timely patient notification of delinquency helps keep collection ratios in the 90th percentile.*

TIP Follow legal and ethical guidelines per the Fair Debt Collection Practices Act. If an insurance company is delinquent, the next step is to write a letter; if still not satisfied, contact the state insurance commission.

10. If payment is not received from the patient, send a collection letter.

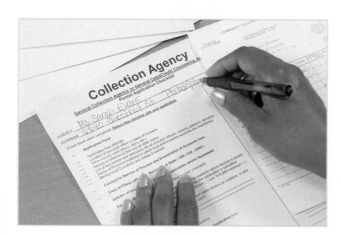

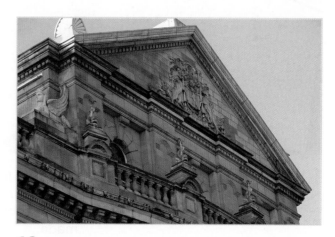

11. Use an outside collection agency if steps 9 and 10 do not produce results.

TIP A collection agency is better for large amounts only; small amounts may just have to be written off by the office. Some collection agencies may charge high fees for their services. Each office has its own policy regarding outside collection agencies. The physician should review the patient's chart prior to the claim being sent to a collection agency.

12. Last, use small claims court per office policy.

TIP Be aware of the statute of limitations, bankruptcy rules, skips (patient leaving town), and estate laws.

Procedure 2-6

Post Adjustments

PURPOSE

Posting adjustments onto a day sheet are required in order to change the patient's balance. Adjustments commonly reflect the provider's allowance for fees below the usual and customary amount because of insurance contracts or patient need. They may also reflect an error in posting.

EQUIPMENT/SUPPLIES

- ledger cards
- pegboard
- insurance payment amount
- pen

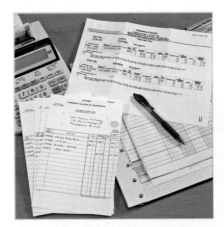

1. Gather all supplies.

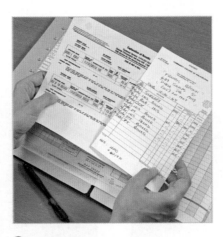

2. Obtain ledger card of the patient for whom the adjustment is being made.

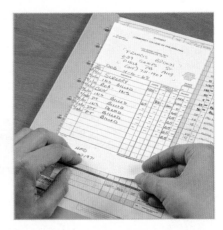

3. Place ledger card on the pegboard, being careful to align correctly.

WHY? *Proper alignment ensures legibility and correct placement of written information.*

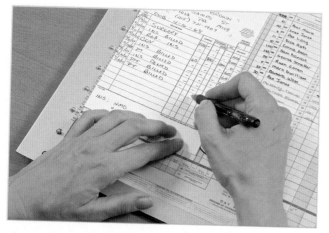

4. Enter insurance payment for the patient in the appropriate column.

WHY❓ *Accuracy is vital for financial record keeping.*

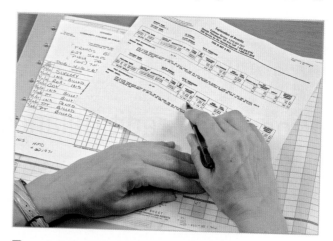

5. Determine amount of adjustment.

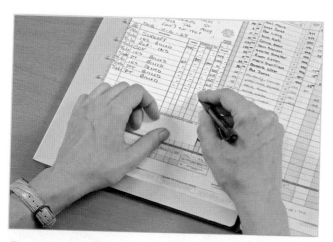

6. Enter amount of adjustment in adjustment column on the ledger card.

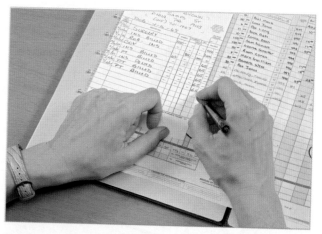

7. Subtract the adjustment amount (credit) and insurance payment from previous patient balance to arrive at new balance.

TIP▶ Adjustments may occur when a provider accepts assignment for insurances such as Medicare and Medicaid, Blue Cross/Blue Shield, most Preferred Provider Organizations, and Health Maintenance Organizations.

Procedure 2-7

Process a Credit Balance

PURPOSE

Credit balances need to be processed to correct errors in patient payment or insurance over-payment.

EQUIPMENT/SUPPLIES

- ledger cards
- pegboard
- insurance payment amount
- checkbook
- envelope
- stamps or postage meter
- pen

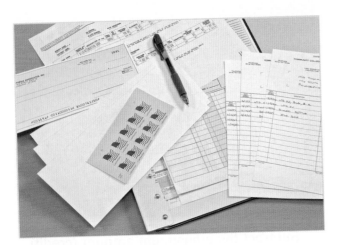

1. Gather all supplies.

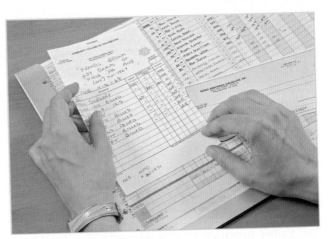

2. Obtain ledger card for patient whose account requires an adjustment.

TIP If you are using the computer, run a credit balance report monthly or more often; if you are using the pegboard, pull ledgers with credit balances monthly or more often.

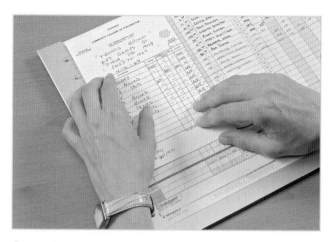

3. Place ledger card on the pegboard being careful to align correctly.

WHY? *Proper alignment ensures legibility and correct placement of written information.*

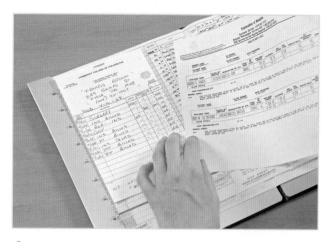

4. Determine amount of credit balance.

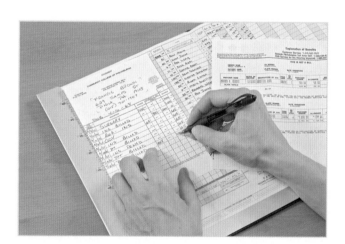

5. Enter amount of credit balance in the payment column on the ledger card, putting it in brackets to indicate a negative. When you add up the payments column at the end of the day, subtract this amount instead of adding it.

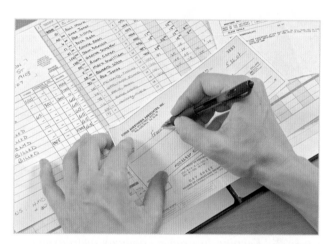

7. Subtract the adjustment amount (credit) from previous patient balance to arrive at the new balance. The amount is entered on the Day Sheet and the ledger card.

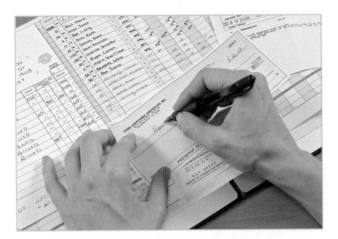

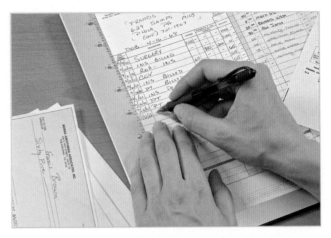

7. Write a check for the refund amount to the patient or insurance company (or to whomever the balance is owed).

TIP If you are sending a check to an insurance company, be sure to include a letter and a copy of the explanation of benefits.

8. Document on the patient ledger card and in the office checkbook.

WHY? *Proper documentation ensures accurate financial record keeping.*

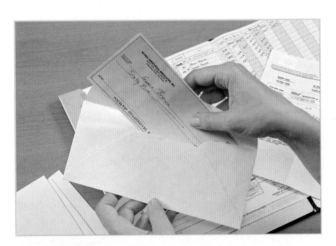

9. Mail refund.

WHY? *Keeping insurance company overpayments is illegal and unethical.*

TIP With patient overpayments, some practices either mail a refund to the patient or keep the over-payment as a credit on the patient's account (depending on the amount and the practice).

Procedure 2-8

Process Refunds

PURPOSE

Processing refunds is the final aspect of processing a credit balance. Making sure all payments received are documented correctly and refunds are distributed when overpayment is made is both an ethical and a legal issue. Timeliness and accuracy in this area ensure trust in the medical office's financial practices and keep the relationship between the office and the patient or insurance company in good standing.

EQUIPMENT/SUPPLIES

- ledger cards
- pegboard
- overpayment amount
- checkbook
- envelope
- stamps or postage meter
- pen

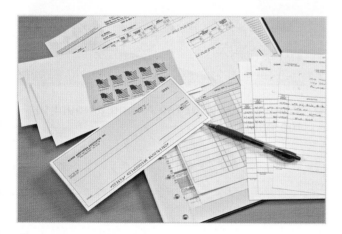

1. Gather all supplies.

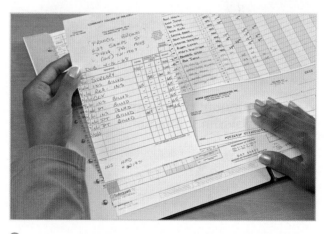

2. Obtain ledger card for patient whose account requires an adjustment.

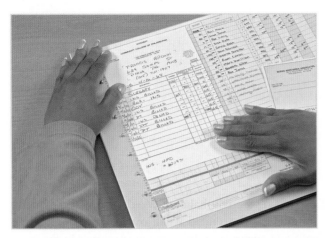

3. Place ledger card on the pegboard, being careful to align correctly.

WHY❓ *Proper alignment ensures correct data entry.*

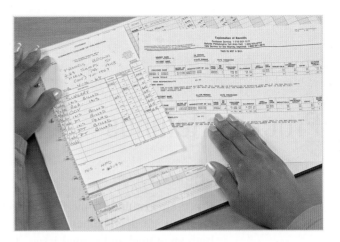

4. Determine the amount of adjustment.

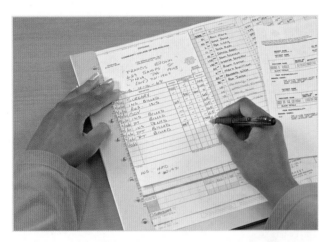

5. Enter amount of adjustment in adjustment column in brackets.

TIP▶ If you are using a computer, run the report on credit balances, review the patient ledger, and be sure refund is correct.

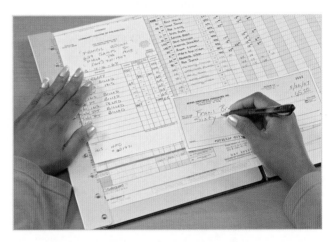

6. Write a check for the refund amount to the patient.

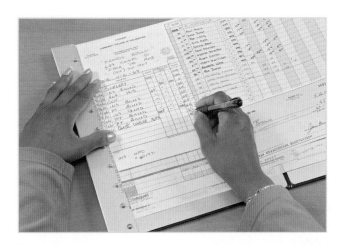

7. Document on the patient ledger card and pegboard, and in the office checkbook.

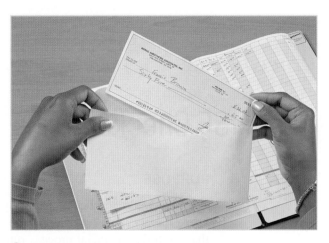

8. Mail refund.

Procedure 2-9

Post NSF Checks

PURPOSE

Tracking returned checks promptly and accurately, and documenting this process properly, keeps the accounts receivable ratio in the medical office within acceptable limits and ensures that the office financial process runs smoothly.

EQUIPMENT/SUPPLIES

- ledger card
- checkbook
- bank telephone numbers
- telephone
- deposit slip
- pen

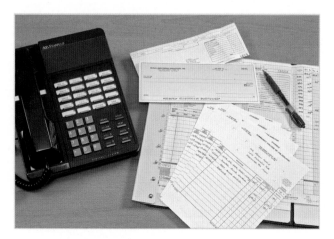

1. Gather all supplies.

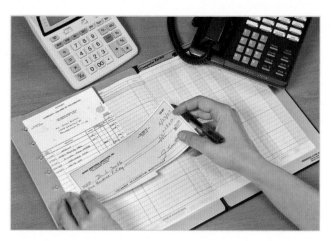

2. Obtain the ledger card for the patient whose check has been returned.

TIP▶ Checks often are returned to the medical office marked NSF or "non-sufficient funds." This may be due to a miscalculation on the patient's part, a bank or employer error, or more seriously, patients who fail to pay for services received.

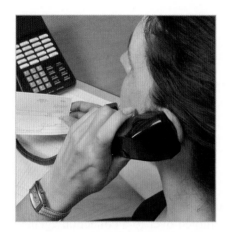

3. Call the bank that returned the check (the bank the check is written from) and verify availability of funds.

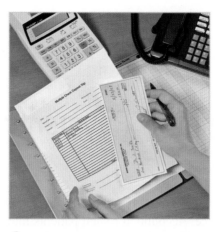

4. Redeposit check if funds are available.

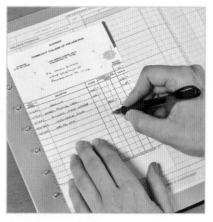

5. If funds are not available, add the amount of the check and any applicable fees to the patient's account.

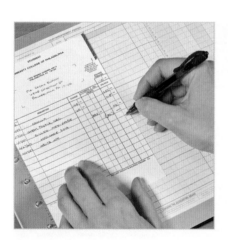

6. Adjust the balance accordingly.

TIP The patient's current balance will be higher than before by the amount of the NSF check and the returned check fee.

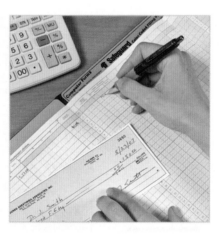

7. Adjust the office checking account balance as necessary.

TIP This is a very important step to remember! You need to know how much money is in the account so that you do not overdraw it and accrue additional fees.

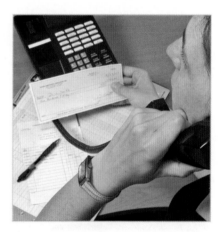

8. Follow office procedure for notifying the patient.

WHY? *It is important to follow all legal and ethical collection procedures when contacting patients regarding monies owed as well as bad checks written.*

Procedure 2-10

Post Collection Agency Payments

PURPOSE

Some patients may have extremely delinquent accounts, but collecting fees owed is important to the medical practice. Accounts for such patients may be turned over to a collection agency. In large medical facilities, this may occur for any severely delinquent amount; in smaller practices, this is usually done only for larger amounts.

EQUIPMENT/SUPPLIES

- ledger card
- day sheet
- collection agency payment amount
- envelope
- pen

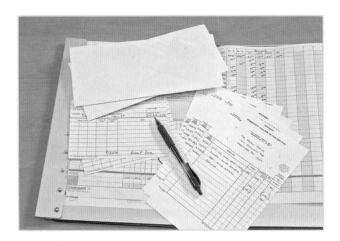

1. Gather all supplies.

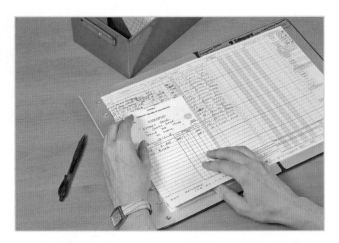

2. Pull patient ledger card and place it directly on the day sheet in place of a charge slip; no receipts are needed.

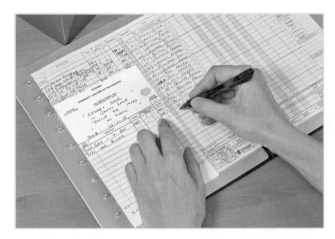

3. Enter the patient's previous balance on the day sheet.

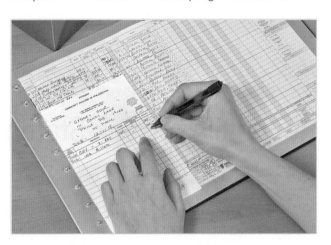

4. Post (write) directly on the ledger card the date, reference description (ROA), and payment amount.

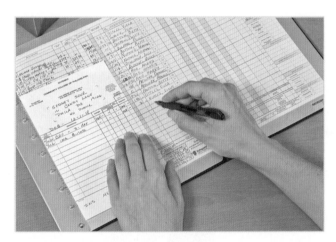

5. Calculate the new balance and enter it in the appropriate space on the day sheet.

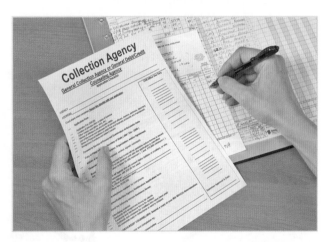

6. Write off amount not paid in the adjustment column. The patient's current balance will be zero.

TIP▶ The expense of using a collection agency may not justify the amount that is delinquent; the agency receives a percentage of the owed amount (sometimes as much as 50%) and reimbursement is less this fee. Each office sets its own policy for using outside collection agencies. Many offices do not use collection agencies in order to maintain "good will."

TIP▶ You have removed the debt from the accounts receivable. Make a note on the ledger, the collection list, and the chart. If the patient will be "fired" (terminated) by the practice for nonpayment, review the chart with the physician and write the letter using guidelines from your liability company.

Procedure **2-11**

Reconcile a Bank Statement

PURPOSE

Although not a directly listed competency, reconciling the monthly bank statement helps the medical assistant monitor office finances and prevent errors or overdrawn accounts.

EQUIPMENT/SUPPLIES

- checkbook
- bank statement
- adding machine
- pen

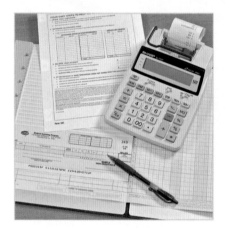

1. Gather all supplies.

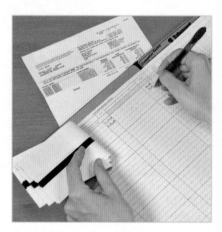

2. Make sure balance in checkbook is current by determining that all checks and deposits have been entered.

WHY? *A correct balance ensures that you do not bounce checks.*

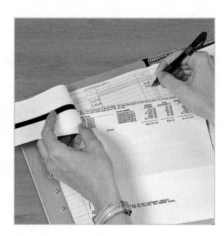

3. Subtract any service charges from last balance.

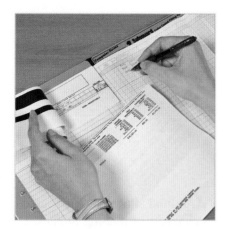

4. Mark off all checks in the checkbook that are listed in the bank statement.

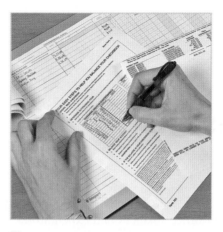

5. Mark off each deposit in the checkbook that is listed in the bank statement.

WHY❓ Double-checking all amounts ensures proper math and correct accounting of the funds in the account.

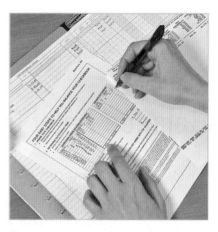

6. Using the back of statement worksheet, copy the ending balance to the proper area.

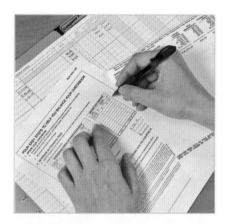

7. List all check stubs on the back that have not cleared and any deposits not shown on bank statement.

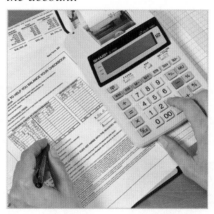

8. Total all checks that have not cleared.

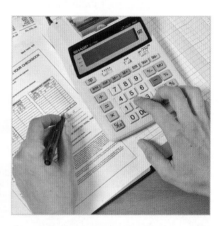

9. Total all non-listed deposits.

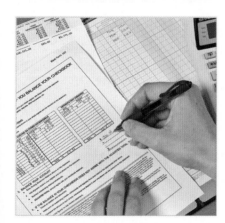

10. Add statement balance and total deposits not credited.

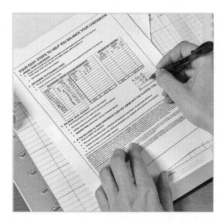

11. Subtract total of checks not cleared.

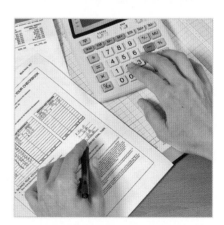

12. Verify for accuracy.

WHY❓ It is best practice to double-check all math.

Procedure 2-12

Balance Petty Cash Fund

PURPOSE

Although not a directly listed competency, balancing a petty cash fund allows the medical assistant to track minor office finances and expenditures and catch errors or missing monies.

EQUIPMENT/SUPPLIES

- cash
- receipts
- vouchers
- checkbook
- cash box
- adding machine
- pen

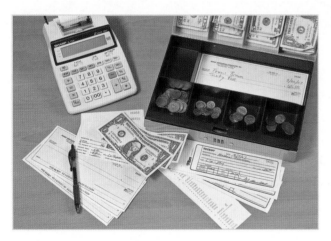

1. Gather all supplies.

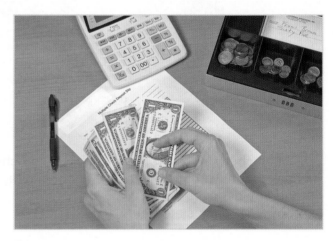

2. Count money in cash box.

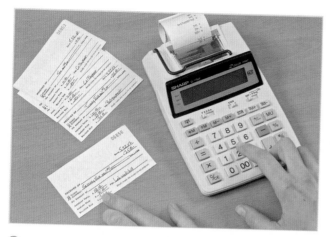

3. Total all vouchers.

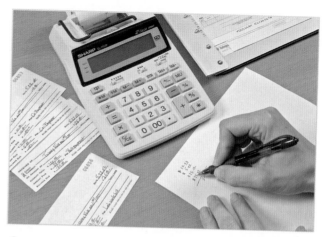

4. Subtract amount of receipts from original amount in petty cash.

TIP➤ This total should equal the amount of cash remaining.

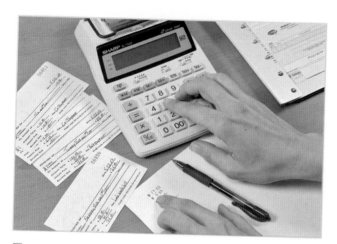

5. Verify for accuracy.

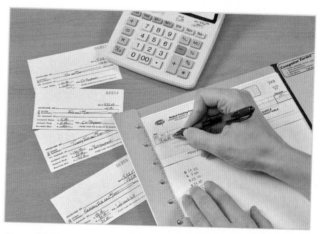

6. When cash is balanced against receipts, write a check to be cashed for the amount that was used.

WHY? *This will bring back the dollar amount to the original amount.*

CHAPTER 3

Process Insurance Claims

INTRODUCTION

Patients seen in the medical office will have varied types of health insurance plans. Medical assistants need to understand each plan's requirements in order to help patients determine their coverage and obtain referrals. Medical assistants also must know how to perform diagnostic and procedural coding. By submitting properly coded insurance claims, the medical assistant helps ensure timely and efficient reimbursement for the medical practice.

PROCEDURES

3-1 Apply Managed Care Policies and Procedures

3-2 Apply Third Party Guidelines by Correctly Interpreting a Patient's Insurance Card

3-3 Perform Procedural Coding

3-4 Perform Diagnostic Coding

3-5 Complete Insurance Claim Forms

Procedure 3-1

Apply Managed Care Policies and Procedures

PURPOSE

By obtaining referrals, the medical assistant helps patients get the specialty care or diagnostic services they need while avoiding undue charges.

EQUIPMENT/SUPPLIES

- patient chart
- insurance information
- referral form
- diagnosis
- ICD-9 book

- specialist name
- telephone or Computer
- fax machine
- pen

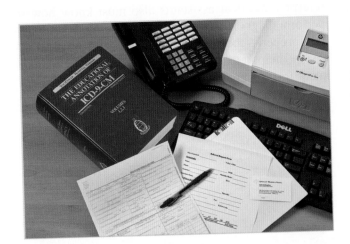

1. Gather all supplies.

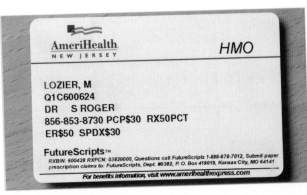

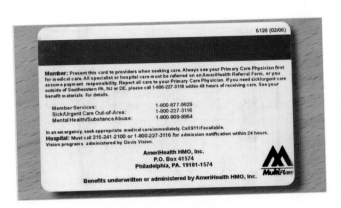

2. Locate the insurance card information, patient ID number, and insurance company's customer service number (usually found on the back of the insurance card).

WHY？ *This information is necessary to obtain the referral.*

TIP The patient ID number is usually the social security number.

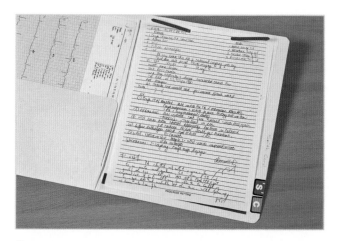

3. Determine the diagnosis using information supplied by the doctor or from the patient's chart.

WHY❓ *The patient's insurance company and the specialist will need this information.*

▷ It is helpful to the specialist if you leave the diagnosis open, if possible, or as general as acceptable (e.g., *leg pain* instead of *meniscal tear*).

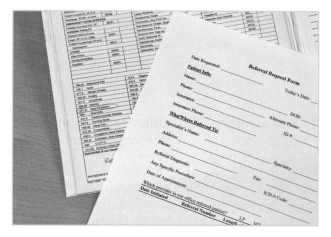

4. Determine which type of specialist the doctor wants the patient to see.

WHY❓ *This information is necessary to complete the referral.*

▷ Some offices require patients to find out which specialists participate in their health plan and how many visits they are allowed. Be prepared to help patients who have urgent referral needs or do not understand the insurance requirements.

5. Call the insurance company after filling out the referral form with the above information and get an authorization code, if required. If an authorization code is not needed, document this in the patient's chart or on the form, and file in chart.

WHY❓ *Proper documentation verifies what information the medical assistant received from the insurance company. It is also essential for appropriate patient care and record keeping.*

▷ Try to leave the referral open for a year if possible, so the patient can have follow-up visits without needing a new referral. Be sure to include all necessary services.

▷ Some insurance companies allow referrals to be processed online via their Web site.

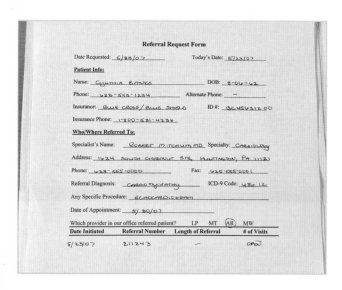

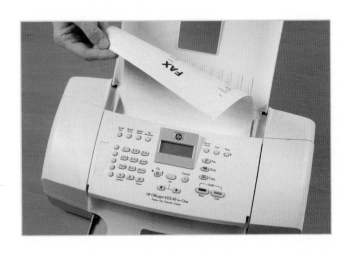

6. Fax a copy of the authorization number to the specialist with any pertinent chart notes or labs.

WHY❓ *The specialist will need this information to provide appropriate care for the patient and to ensure that insurance payment will be made.*

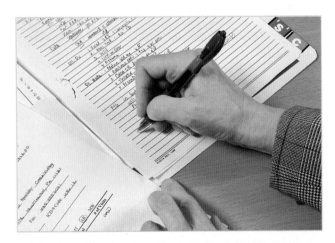

7. Document in chart.

WHY❓ *Proper documentation helps ensure quality patient care. Be sure to document this per HIPAA.*

TIP▶ Some insurance companies have special forms. Many offices have created their own forms.

TIP▶ Be aware that some insurance companies require only a written prescription or a note in the chart stating the referral, rather than a preauthorization. If in doubt, ask the customer service representative when you call the insurance company. Determine if preauthorization is needed when ordering expensive tests, such as MRI. Remember that Labor & Industries (L&I) is different; everything must be pre-approved.

Charting Example

12/12/07 10:30 a.m. Called pts insurance for preauthorization to see neurologist. Ben from Aetna stated no preauthorization required. _____ M. Nguyen, CMA

Procedure **3-2**

Apply Third Party Guidelines by Correctly Interpreting a Patient's Insurance Card

PURPOSE

This procedure can be combined with Procedure 3-1. Obtaining a referral can also cover applying third party guidelines. Third party refers to insurance coverage: the patient and the provider are the first and second parties. Other aspects of third party guidelines may be second opinions, drug formularies, managing chronic illness, understanding the wide variety of insurance coverage, and being able to determine which is the parent company on a patient's insurance card, or which company covers what service. For example, a patient card may say AETNA, yet Ethix manages the plan, and drug coverage may be provided from yet another group, such as Express Scripts. To help medical assisting students better understand third party, the instructor may choose to show them a variety of insurance cards or a variety of insurance plan drug formularies.

EQUIPMENT/SUPPLIES

• patient insurance card
• photocopy machine

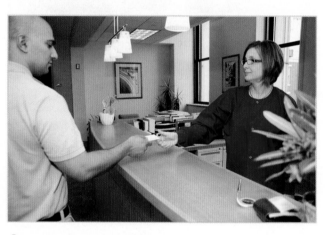

1. Look at the patient's insurance card.

Be sure that the card is current and that it pertains to that particular patient rather than a family member.

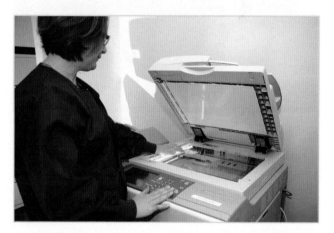

2. Copy the front and back of the insurance card.

Be sure that the copy is legible.

WHY? *It is always good to keep a copy for reference in the patient chart.*

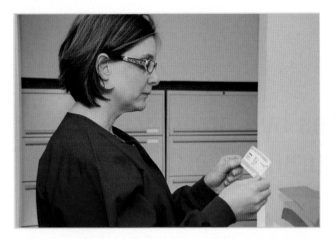

3. Check the front of the card for type of plan: PPO or HMO.

Make sure your provider participates in the plan; some plans allow for out-of-network care. If it is an HMO, see Procedure 3-1 for preauthorization procedure.

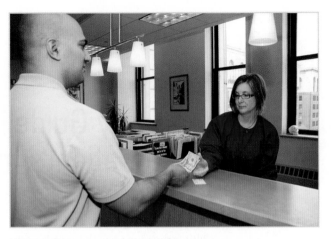

4. Determine whether the patient has a co-pay, and if so, collect it.

WHY? *Avoid billing costs by collecting co-payments at the time of service.*

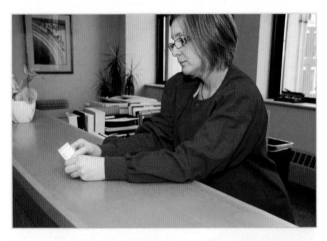

5. Check the back of the card for the insurance company address. This is where you will send the claim.

Many insurance cards state which company administers the plan on the back of the card, and the vast majority have a number to call for questions.

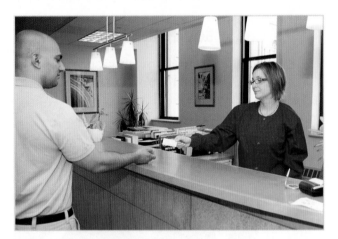

6. Return the card to the patient.

Procedure 3-3

Perform Procedural Coding

PURPOSE

Procedural coding is used when billing health insurance companies for services provided. By coding correctly, the medical assistant can avoid rejected claims and obtain prompt reimbursement for the medical practice.

EQUIPMENT/SUPPLIES

- patient chart
- superbill or encounter form
- CPT book
- pen

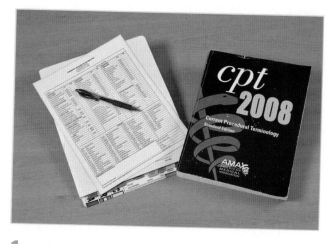

1. Gather all supplies.

☞ The superbill may also be called the fee slip or encounter form.

☞ Be sure to use the most current CPT book.

WHY? Using up-to-date information ensures accurate coding.

2. From the CPT book, elect the name of the procedure or service that accurately identifies the service performed. Be sure that the procedures and diagnoses match.

WHY? It is important to avoid errors because inaccurate coding can result in denied claims.

....24640	Attended, Manual 97032
....24155	Unattended 97014
....24105	
....24102	**Electro-Hydraulic**
24000, 24101	**Procedure** 52325
	Electro-Oculography 92270
..24620-24635	
..24586-24587	**Electroanalgesia**
	See Application, Neurostimulation
age 23930	
	Electrocardiography
....24164	24 Hour Monitoring 93224-93237
....24000	Evaluation 93000, 93010, 93014
	Patient-Demand Recording
....24220	Transmission and Evaluation 93270
Imaging (MRI) ...73221	Patient-Demand Transmission and Evaluation
....24300	Transmission and Evaluation
	Interpretation 93272
sue and Bone	Monitoring 93271
re Release 24149	Rhythm
	Evaluation 93042
24000, 24101, 24200-24201	Microvolt T-wave Alternans 93025
	93041
	Tracing 93040

Electrolysis	
Electromyog	
See Electromyog	
Electromyog	
Anorectal with B	
Fine Wire	
Dynamic ...	
Needle	
Extremities	
Extremity ..	
Face and Ne	
Guidance	
for Chemo	
Hemidiaphra	
Larynx ...	
Ocular ...	
Other than T	
Single Fiber	
Thoracic Pa	
Sphincter Musc	
Anus	
Needle	

3. Look in the alphabetic index for the procedures.

WHY?　*It is not possible for the medical assistant to memorize every code number in the book, so checking the alphabetic index is the first step.*

therectomy;	code for primary procedure)
"therapeutic	(Use 92998 in conjunction with 92997)
oplasty or	
see 92984,	**Cardiography**
	(For echocardiography, see 93303-93350)
ion delivery	**93000** Electrocardiogram, routine ECG with at least 12 leads;
rapy, use	with interpretation and report
	93005 tracing only, without interpretation and report
see 77781-	**93010** interpretation and report only
	(For ECG monitoring, see 99354-99360)
n angioplasty;	**93012** Telephonic transmission of post-symptom
in addition to	electrocardiogram rhythm strip(s), 24-hour attended
	monitoring, per 30 day period of time; tracing only
82, 92995)	**93014** physician review with interpretation and report only
of angioplasty	**93015** Cardiovascular stress test using maximal or submaximal
	treadmill or bicycle exercise, continuous

4. Confirm by finding that number in the tabular list and reading the description. Always code to the greatest specificity, including any modifiers as necessary.

WHY?　*Assigning the proper code is vital for reimbursement.*

LEGAL ALERT!　Do not unbundle services, such as charging for a pre-op or post-op visit when these are included in the surgery charge. Doing so is illegal.

TIP　Coding is a way to turn what providers do and why they do it into a numeric sequence that the insurance company can understand. It is a method of communication. It is not medical care; it only describes medical care.

Procedure 3-4

Perform Diagnostic Coding

PURPOSE

Diagnostic coding is used when billing health insurance companies for services provided. By coding correctly, the medical assistant can avoid rejected claims and obtain prompt reimbursement for the medical practice.

EQUIPMENT/SUPPLIES

- patient chart
- superbill or encounter form
- ICD-9 book
- pen

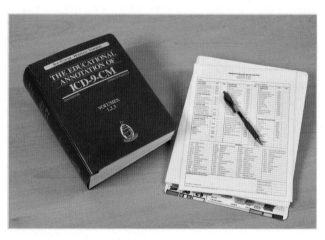

DIAGNOSIS			
722.6	Degenerative Disc Disease	242.90 Hyperthyroidism	V70.3
276.5	Dehydration	244.9 Hypothyroidism	486
296.20	Depression	703.0 Ingrown Toenail	V22.
250.00	Diabetes	780.52 Insomnia	256.
692.9	Eczema/Dermatitis	564.1 Irritable Bowel Syndrome	601.
782.3	Edema	785.6 Lymphadenopathy	473.
780.79	Fatigue	626.9 Menstrual Disorder	780.
780.6	Fever	346.90 Migraine	465.
610.1	Fibrocystic Breast Disease	848.9 Muscle Strain	599.
558.9	Gastroenteritis	728.85 Muscle Spasms	616.
274.9	Gout	733.00 Osteoporosis	780.
784.0	Headache	382.9 Otitis Media	078.
785.3	Heart Murmur	V72.3 Pelvic Exam	
272.0	Hypercholesterolemia	533.90 Peptic Ulcer Disease	
272.4	Hyperlipidemia	462 Pharyngitis, Acute	
401.9	Hypertension	V70.0 Physical Exam, General	
			PREVIOUS

1. Gather all supplies.

▷ Be sure to always use the most current ICD-9 book.

WHY? *Using up-to-date information ensures accurate coding.*

2. Find the diagnosis in the ICD-9 book, using information provided by the doctor.

WHY? *Only doctors can diagnose. Correct diagnoses ensure correct and prompt reimbursement.*

LEGAL ALERT! If the doctor has not provided an exact code, look at the description of services, find a code, and check with the doctor. Do not code greater than the information provided; if the diagnosis is "suspected," code by the symptoms.

art syndrome   746.7
evelopment)   783.40
.1
31

chemicals
Dextraposition, aorta   747.21
   with ventricular septal defect, pulmonary stenosis
     or atresia, and hypertrophy of right ventricle
     745.2

essive   315.32
NEC   315.2

   in tetralogy of Fallot   745.2
Dextratransposition, aorta   745.11
Dextrinosis, limit (debrancher enzyme deficiency)
   271.0

5.4

Dextrocardia (corrected) (false) (isolated)
   (secondary) (true)   746.87

315.2
ming   315.8

   with
     complete transposition of viscera   759.3
     situs inversus   759.3

kinesia   314.1
9

Dextroversion, kidney (left)   753.3
Dhobie itch   110.3
Diabetes, diabetic (brittle) (congenital) (familial)
   (mellitus) (poorly controlled) (severe) (slight)
   (without complication)   250.0

5.2
re also Anomaly

n)   764.9
orn)   764.9
f pregnancy   656.5

Note — Use the following fifth-digit
subclassification with category 250:
* 0 type II or unspecified type, not stated as*
*   uncontrolled*
* Fifth-digit 0 is for use for type II patients,*
*   even if the patient requires insulin.*
* 1 type I [juvenile type], not stated as*
*   uncontrolled*

- see Hypoplasia
3.9
259.1

[581.81]
iritis   250.5 [36-
ketosis, ketoacido-
Kimmelstiel (-Wi
   (intercapillar
   [581.81]
Lancereaux's (dia
   emaciation)
latent (chemical)
   complicating pr
     puerperiun
lipoidosis   250.8
macular edema
maternal
   with manifest d
     affecting fetus
microaneurysms,
mononeuropathy
neonatal, transien
nephropathy   25(
nephrosis (syndro
neuralgia   250.6
neuritis   250.6 [
neurogenic arthro
neuropathy   250.
nonclinical   790.
osteomyelitis   25
peripheral autono

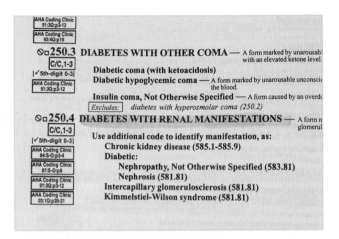

3. Look in the alphabetic index for the key words in the diagnosis.

WHY❓ *It is not possible for the medical assistant to memorize every code number in the book, so checking the alphabetic index is the first step.*

4. Confirm by finding that number in the tabular list and reading the description.

WHY❓ *This helps avoid errors.*

TIP▶ Be as specific as possible. Do not forget any 4th or 5th digit that may be needed. A code is invalid if it has not been coded to the full number of digits required for that code.

TIP▶ Correct codes are less likely to be rejected by the insurance company, saving employee time and avoiding rebilling issues. Coding correctly also helps avoid audits. Remember that procedures must always match the diagnosis. For example, if a patient is seen for a sore throat and you code for an x-ray for a prior injury, you must code for that prior injury as well.

Procedure 3-5

Complete Insurance Claim Forms

PURPOSE

Insurance forms that are filled out correctly ensure prompt reimbursement, saving time and money for the medical office.

EQUIPMENT/SUPPLIES

- patient chart
- superbill or encounter form
- ICD-9 book
- CPT book
- pen
- computer or envelopes
- CMS-1500 form

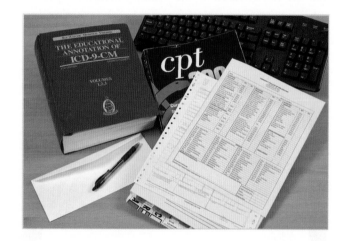

1. Gather all supplies.

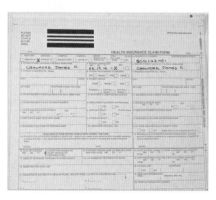

2. Fill in the numbered boxes in the CMS-1500 form in order, making sure to complete each box as necessary.

WHY？ *Attention to detail avoids errors; insurance companies will not process incomplete claim forms.*

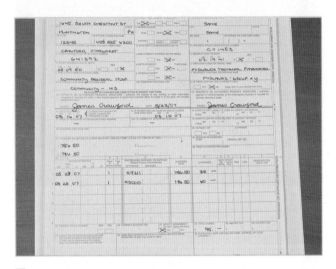

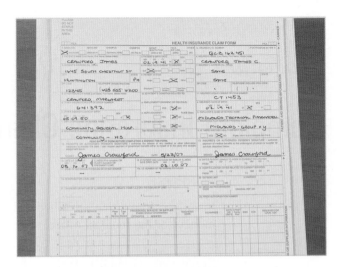

3. Make sure any secondary insurance information is filled in, if applicable.

WHY? *If a patient is covered by more than one insurance plan, the secondary plan may pay benefits that are not covered by the primary insurance plan.*

4. Make sure the form is signed, if necessary.

WHY? *Claims will not be processed if required information is missing.*

TIP Signature on file can be used.

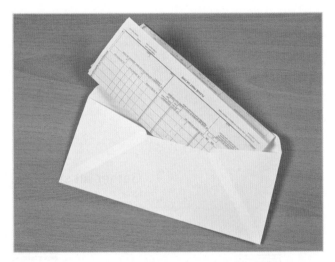

5. Make sure diagnosis codes match procedure codes by entering the correct codes in order of priority.

WHY? *Inaccurate coding can result in denied claims.*

6. Send the form via mail or electronic filing, whichever your office uses.

WHY? *It is important to follow office policy when submitting insurance claim forms.*

TWO

Clinical Competencies

CHAPTER 4

Fundamental Principles

INTRODUCTION

Asepsis means free from infection or free from pathogenic organisms. Every healthcare professional needs to understand how to prevent the spread of disease by using aseptic techniques in daily tasks. The most important way to prevent the spread of infection is appropriate handwashing. Asepsis also includes preventing infection by disinfecting and sterilizing instruments and equipment used in the office or clinic. Every aspect of daily clinic routine requires understanding the chain of infection in order to determine the appropriate action needed to prevent the spread of pathogens. It should become second nature to know what is contaminated and what is clean or sterile so that you can rapidly make decisions and act correctly. Patient safety, as well as your own and other staff, depends on appropriate aseptic techniques. A critical part of safety, and an OSHA mandate, is the observance of Standard Precautions. Observing Standard Precautions means to treat all body fluids as potentially infectious and requires the use of barriers such as gloves, gowns, and masks.

PROCEDURES

4-1 Perform Handwashing: Medically Aseptic Handwashing

4-2 Wrap Items for Autoclaving: Wrap Two Sheets Together

4-3 Wrap Items for Autoclaving: Wrap Each Sheet Separately

4-4 Wrap Items for Autoclaving: Use a Sterilization Pouch

4-5 Perform Sterilization Techniques: Sterilize by Autoclave

4-6 Perform Sterilization Techniques: Sterilize by Cold Chemical Sterilization

4-7 Dispose of Biohazardous Materials

4-8 Practice Standard Precautions: Wear Appropriate Personal Protective Equipment (PPE)

Procedure 4-1

Perform Handwashing: Medically Aseptic Handwashing

PURPOSE

Appropriate handwashing is the number one way to prevent the spread of infection, and the medical assistant should conscientiously practice this daily. Removing as much of the debris and microorganisms on your hands as possible before working with the patients provides them as well as you and your colleagues with the best infection control possible. This is an area that cannot be compromised, and appropriate handwashing will become second nature. The usual handwash is the medically aseptic handwash, which you will perform numerous times daily.

EQUIPMENT/SUPPLIES

- sink
- soap
- water
- water-based lotion
- hand or nail brush
- orangewood stick or nail instrument
- paper towels

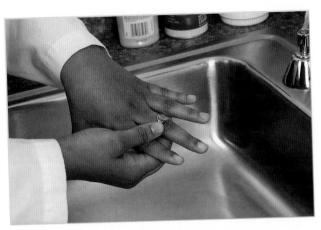

1. Remove all jewelry, although a plain wedding band may be acceptable.

WHY? *Items such as rings or bracelets can harbor microorganisms that are not removed by handwashing.*

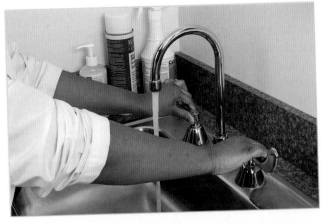

2. Stand near to the sink without touching clothing to the edge of sink and turn on and adjust water. You may be expected to turn on the faucet with a paper towel to avoid the pathogens there, or it may be felt that handwashing will remove any pathogens from the faucet. Do as your office policy dictates.

WHY? *Microorganisms on the counter and edge of sink can be transferred to your clothing.*

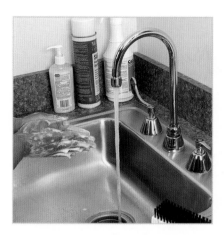

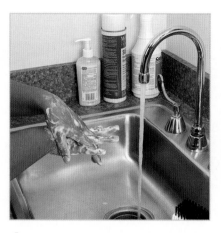

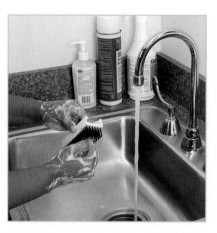

3. Adjust the water to warm, not hot, and wet hands. Apply soap and rub hands together to work up a lather. Your employer may provide one-time use sponges or brushes that are imbedded with soap.

WHY❓ *Hot water will dry hands more than warm and cannot be hot enough to destroy pathogens anyway.*

4. Use friction to briskly rub the palm (anterior) of each hand, then the back (posterior) of each. Scrub between each finger and the thumb. Work on the creases of the palm.

WHY❓ *Friction is the most effective way to physically scrub away debris and microorganisms.*

5. If this is the first hand-wash of the day or if you have just participated in a procedure involving body fluids or pathogens, you should clean under and around the nails as well. Use either a brush or a nail stick or the appropriate implement your employer provides.

WHY❓ *Nails can harbor microorganisms just as jewelry can. They must be cleaned daily at least.*

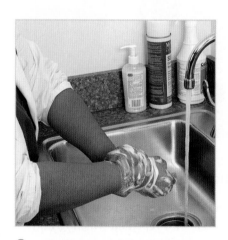

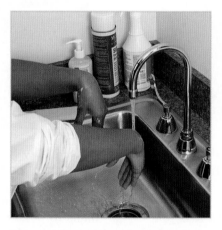

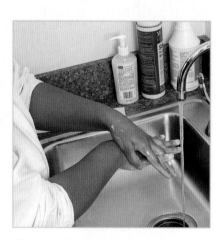

6. Wash to approximately 2–3 inches above the wrist. This should take about 2–3 minutes.

7. Rinse hands thoroughly, keeping them downward. Remove all soap residue.

WHY❓ *Keeping hands downward while rinsing directs the flow to the tips of the fingers and away. Soap residue will attract and adhere to pathogens as will dampness.*

8. If your hands were extremely soiled, repeat the procedure.

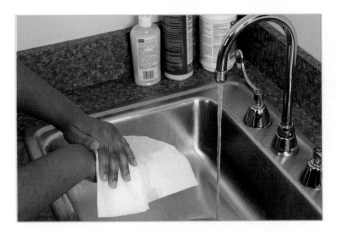

9. Use a disposable paper towel to thoroughly dry hands by blotting. Be careful not to touch the dispenser but only the towel.

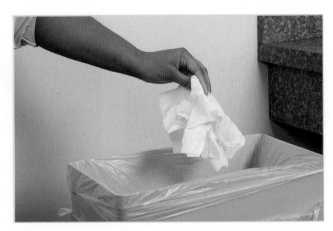

10. Dispose of paper towels in the appropriate receptacle. Usually it is regular trash unless there are visible body fluids or known contamination.

WHY? *It is important to avoid filling the biohazard trash with non-biohazardous items. It is expensive to dispose of this kind of trash, and damp paper towels from a handwash would not usually be put here. Follow your employer's guidelines.*

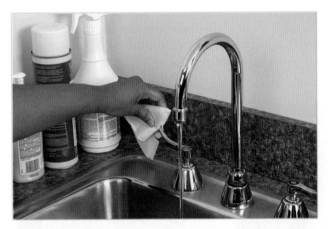

11. If the faucet is not foot or elbow operated, turn off the water with a new, dry paper towel.

WHY? *Do not use the same paper towels you used to dry your hands. If they are wet or even just damp, the microorganisms will be transferred to them and to your hands by "wicking."*

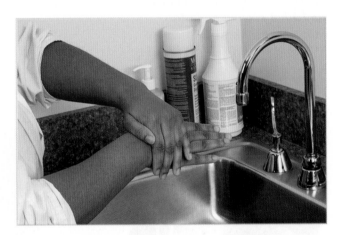

12. Apply lotion to prevent chapping and dryness that can cause broken skin.

WHY? *It is important to keep skin on hands as intact as possible, even with repeated washing daily, because breaks in the skin may lead to infection.*

Procedure **4-2**

Wrap Items for Autoclaving: Wrap Two Sheets Together

PURPOSE

Before instruments can be used in the medical office, pathogens and their spores must be destroyed to provide infection control to the patient. There are basic ways to wrap and prepare packages to ensure sterility is reached during autoclaving. Using two sheets of autoclave wrap is one such method.

EQUIPMENT/SUPPLIES

- sanitized instruments
- autoclave wrap
- sterilization indicators
- gauze
- wrapping tape
- permanent marker or pen

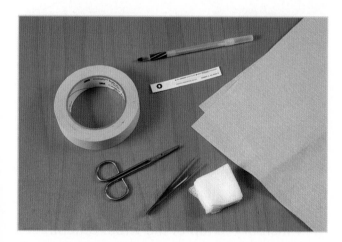

1. Determine method and gather supplies needed for various packs and group instruments as needed. Always use two layers of wrap, utilizing either the double wrap or the two single wrap methods.

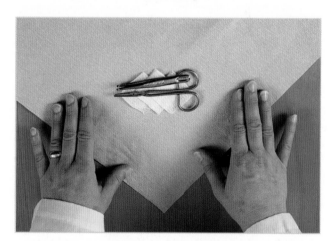

2. Prepare the correct size of wrap, whether cloth or paper, laying on the counter in a diamond fashion—the bottom point should be pointing at you.

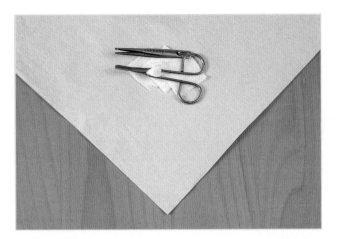

3. Place the instruments just below the middle of the paper, placing them lengthwise (from side to side).

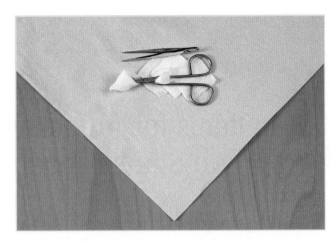

4. Place gauze over the tips of sharp instruments to prevent dulling; place gauze between handles to prevent hinged instruments from closing while autoclaving.

WHY? *Instruments when closed may retain pathogens that cannot be reached by the steam and heat. It is also advisable to include extra gauze in the packs.*

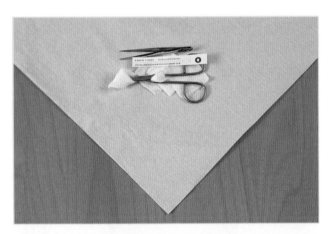

5. Place the sterilization indicator in with the instruments.

WHY? *This will show that the steam and heat reached as far into the package as the instruments, thus indicating they are, in fact, sterile. You will not know the results until the package is opened, usually when needed, so you may also place an indicator within the folds, leaving a portion showing to allow reading immediately.*

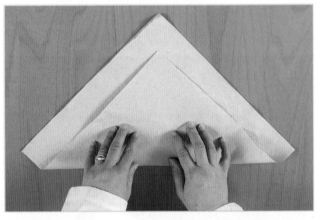

6. Using both sheets together, fold the bottom of the sheets up to within about 1 inch of the top of the wrap. Smooth out edges.

TIP Remember, there is a one-inch border at the outer edge of the sterile field.

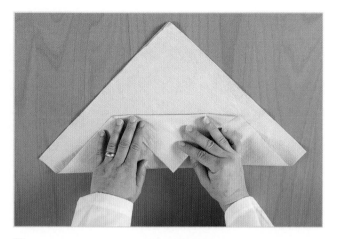

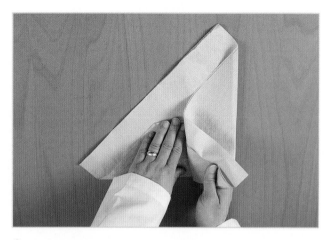

7. Feel for the top of the items inside and fold the bottom flap downward, using an accordion-style fold to ensure that the corner tip is pointing downward (toward you) but is not outside of the package.

WHY? *The tips need to be outward to facilitate opening the pack later without contaminating the contents.*

8. Fold the right side flap inward using the same technique. The tip must be pointing outward.

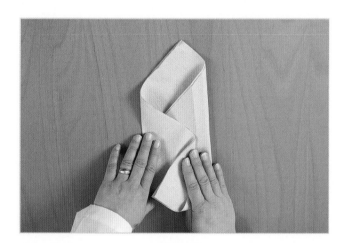

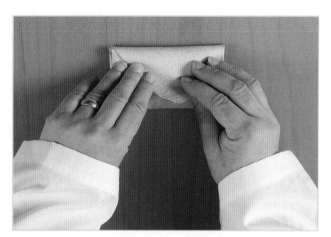

9. Fold in the left side flap inward as stated above.

10. Fold the top down and around the package until you have the tip pointing downward.

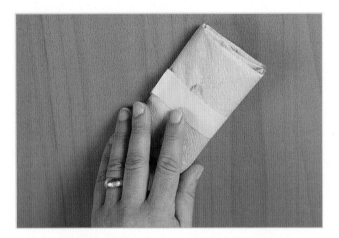

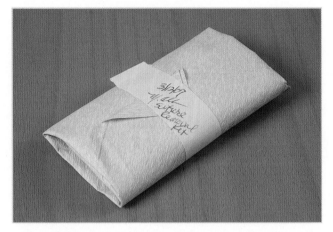

11. Apply tape to secure the package together.

WHY❓ *There is not one certain way to tape packages, but they need to be secure to avoid contamination while stored. Also consider the ease of opening the pack later. Sometimes it helps to put tape on the tip of the final flap; this can then be folded over and taped to the bottom of the surgical tray to keep it in place (when using the wrap as the sterile field).*

12. Write on the tape: your initials, the contents of the package, and the date you autoclaved them.

WHY❓ *Wrapped items that were autoclaved and not opened or contaminated in any way can be stored for up to 30 days. At that time, if not used, they must be opened and cleaned and autoclaved again, as if they were soiled. It is vital to record the date to ensure all staff can tell if the package is still sterile.*

Procedure 4-3

Wrap Items for Autoclaving: Wrap Each Sheet Separately

PURPOSE

Before instruments can be used in the medical office, pathogens and their spores must be destroyed to provide infection control to the patient. There are basic ways to wrap and prepare packages to ensure sterility is reached during autoclaving. Wrapping each sheet of autoclave wrap separately is one such method.

EQUIPMENT/SUPPLIES

- sanitized instruments
- autoclave wrap
- sterilization indicators
- gauze
- wrapping tape
- permanent marker or pen

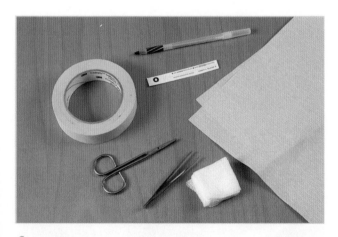

1. Determine method and gather supplies needed for various packs and group instruments as needed. Always use two layers of wrap, utilizing either the double wrap or the two single wrap methods.

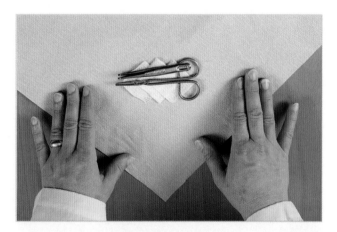

2. Prepare the correct size of wrap, whether cloth or paper, laying on the counter in a diamond fashion—the bottom point should be pointing at you.

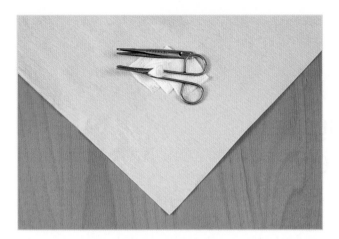

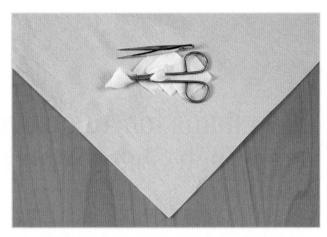

3. Place the instruments just below the middle of the paper, placing them lengthwise (from side to side).

4. Place gauze over the tips of sharp instruments to prevent dulling; place gauze between handles to prevent hinged instruments from closing while autoclaving.

WHY? *Instruments when closed may retain pathogens that cannot be reached by the steam and heat. It is also advisable to include extra gauze in the packs.*

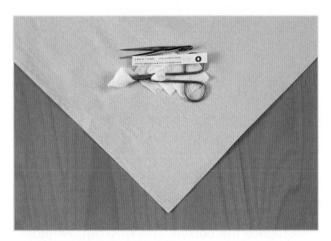

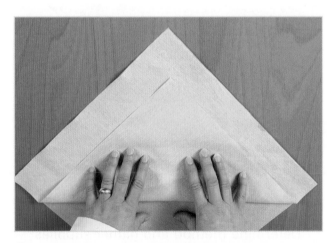

5. Place the sterilization indicator in with the instruments.

WHY? *This will show that the steam and heat reached as far into the package as the instruments, thus indicating they are, in fact, sterile. You will not know the results until the package is opened, usually when needed, so you may also place an indicator within the folds, leaving a portion showing to allow reading immediately.*

6. Using only the inner sheet, fold the bottom of the sheets up to within about 1 inch of the top of the wrap. Smooth out edges.

TIP Remember, there is a one-inch border at the outer edge of the sterile field.

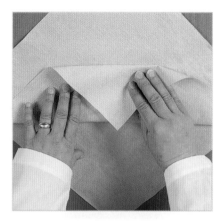

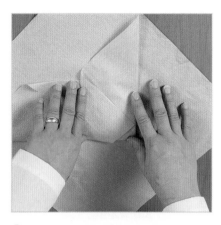

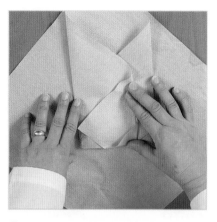

7. Feel for the top of the items inside and fold the bottom flap downward, then use an accordion-style fold to ensure that the corner tip is pointing downward (toward you) but is not outside of the package.

WHY? *All four tips of the wrapping paper need to point outward to facilitate opening the pack later without contaminating the contents.*

8. Fold the right side flap inward using the same technique. The tip must be pointing outward.

9. Fold the left side flap inward as shown above.

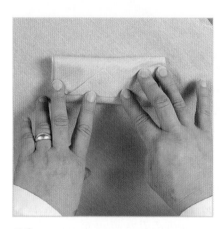

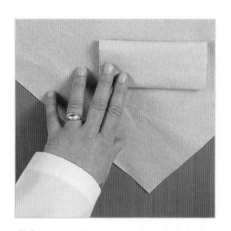

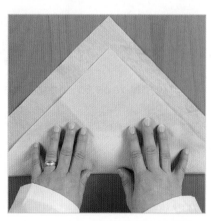

10. Fold the top down and around the package until you have the tip pointing downward and this last flap is on top of the pack.

11. Do NOT apply tape at this time but continue wrapping. Lay the wrapped pack side-to-side as instruments would be placed on the second sheet.

WHY? *You will be dropping the inner wrapped pack onto a sterile field, so you will not want tape on this one.*

12. Wrap as above: fold the bottom flap up over the pack, feeling for the inner pack's top edge and folding accordion style to ensure tip points downward but will not be outside of the pack.

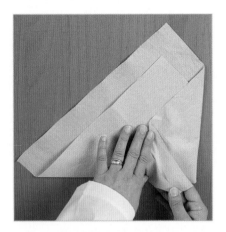

13. Fold right flap in the usual fashion.

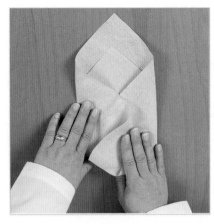

14. Fold left flap in the usual fashion.

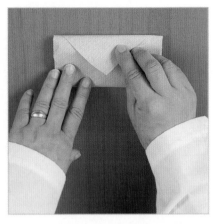

15. Fold the top flap downward and around the pack until you have the tip pointing downward.

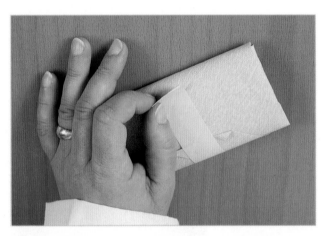

16. Apply tape to secure the package together.

WHY? *There is not one certain way to tape packages, but they need to be secure to avoid contamination while stored. Also consider the ease of opening the pack later. Sometimes it helps to put tape on the tip of the final flap; this can then be folded over and taped to the bottom of the surgical tray to keep it in place (when using the wrap as the sterile field).*

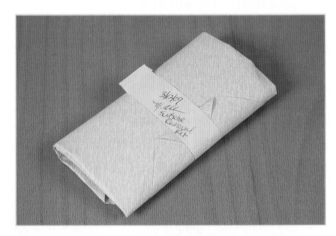

17. Write on the tape: your initials, the contents of the package, and the date you autoclaved them.

WHY? *Wrapped items that were autoclaved and not opened or contaminated in any way can be stored for up to 30 days. At that time, if not used, they must be opened and cleaned and autoclaved again, as if they were soiled. It is vital to record the date to ensure all staff can tell if the package is still sterile.*

Procedure **4-4**

Wrap Items for Autoclaving: Use a Sterilization Pouch

PURPOSE

Before instruments can be used in the medical office, pathogens and their spores must be destroyed to provide infection control to the patient. There are basic ways to wrap and prepare packages to ensure sterility is reached during autoclaving. Using a sterilization pouch is one such method.

EQUIPMENT/SUPPLIES

• sanitized instruments
• autoclave pouch
• gauze
• pen

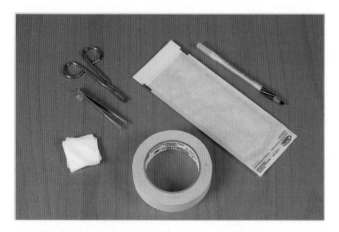

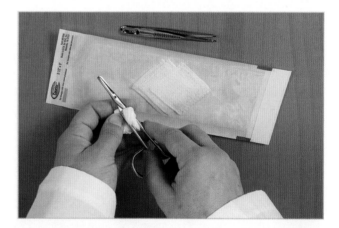

1. Gather all supplies.

2. Place gauze over the tips of sharp instruments to prevent dulling; place gauze between handles to prevent hinged instruments from closing while autoclaving.

ᐯᕼY❓ *Instruments when closed may retain pathogens that cannot be reached by the steam and heat. It is also advisable to include extra gauze in the packs.*

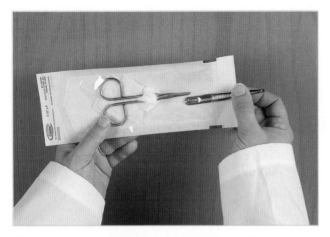

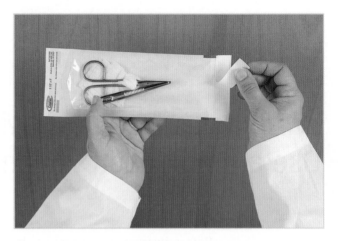

3. Put single instruments or groups of instruments into a self-sealing pouch with handles down.

WHY? *The pouch will be opened later from the other end and the handles must be at the top for the physician to take hold of instead of the tips.*

TIP Autoclave pouches have sterilization indicators built into them, so separate indicators are not used by most medical offices.

TIP Add extra gauze depending on the use of the instruments (e.g., suture removal).

4. Peel off the paper on the flap to expose the adhesive, fold over, and press in place, sealing the pouch.

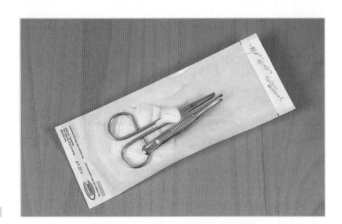

5. Write on the flap: your initials, the contents of the package, and the date you autoclaved them.

WHY? *Pouches that were autoclaved and not opened or contaminated in any way can be stored for up to 6 months if not compromised. At that time, if not used, pouches must be opened and instruments cleaned and autoclaved again, as if they were soiled. It is vital to record the date to ensure all staff can tell if the package is still sterile.*

Procedure 4-5

Perform Sterilization Techniques: Sterilize by Autoclave

PURPOSE

Any item that will make, touch, or enter an unnatural body opening must be sterile. The most common way to do this in ambulatory care is by countertop autoclave machine, which sterilizes by using steam under pressure. Operating an autoclave correctly ensures infection control.

EQUIPMENT/SUPPLIES

- instruments and packs to sterilize
- indicator strip
- autoclave
- distilled water

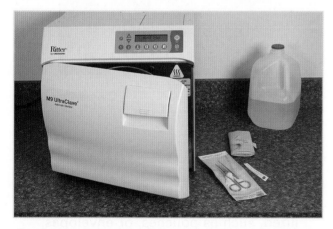

1. Gather all supplies and determine what, if any, trays are needed to ensure packs have room to allow steam to circulate. Prepare autoclave as needed and determine the time needed for the particular load's contents.

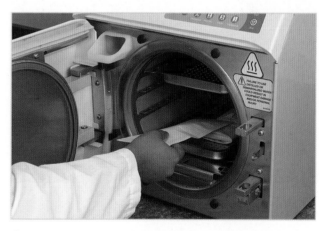

2. Load packs into chamber, standing packs on end or in a rack as possible.

✓WHY? *This allows steam to circulate in between the packages, ensuring that all instruments are sterilized properly.*

TIP Add sterilization indicator in the middle of wrapped packages.

TIP Although non-wrapped items can be autoclaved, wrapped items take a longer time so be sure to time correctly.

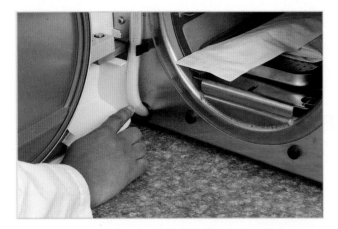

3. Check the water level of the autoclave.

WHY? *Enough water is needed to produce sufficient steam.*

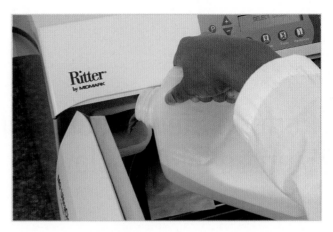

4. Add distilled water only as needed to ensure proper amount of water.

WHY? *Tap water causes mineral buildup that can be harmful to an autoclave. Distilled water is the only type that should be used.*

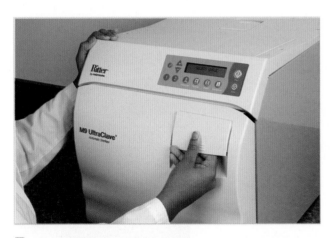

5. Secure the autoclave door.

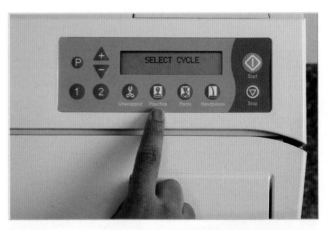

6. Select the type of instruments to be sterilized, such as pouches, or envelopes, etc., and push the appropriate button.

WHY? *By selecting the proper type of instrument preparation, the autoclave will automatically set itself for the correct amount of time and pressure for that particular type of wrapping, thus ensuring sterility.*

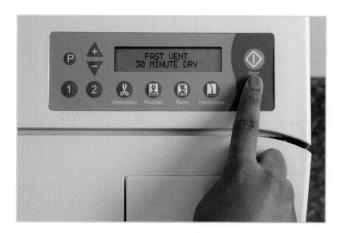

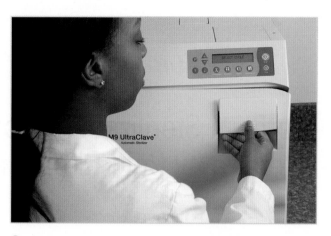

7. Push the "start" button.

TIP *The autoclave will automatically run the proper amount of time, depending on which instrument type was selected.*

8. Vent the door by opening slightly. The type of door varies with each machine, but open it only enough to allow heat and steam to escape or contents to air dry.

TIP *Many digital autoclaves will cool and dry the instruments as part of the cycle.*

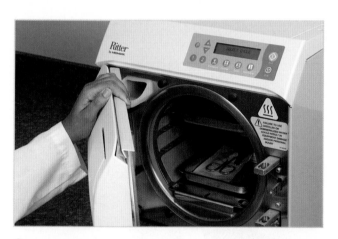

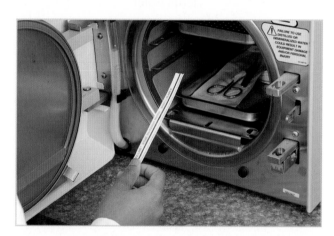

9. Allow packs to remain in the autoclave until completely dry.

WHY? *Moist packs will be considered contaminated because moisture draws microorganisms and debris to it.*

10. Remove packs and check to see that the autoclave tape has changed color. Store packs in appropriate place.

Procedure 4-6

Perform Sterilization Techniques: Sterilize by Cold Chemical Sterilization

PURPOSE

Because some instruments are too delicate or too vulnerable to be autoclaved, they must be sterilized by chemical means.

EQUIPMENT/SUPPLIES

- instruments to sterilize that cannot go in an autoclave
- covered soaking tray/container
- chemical sterilant
- sterile towels
- sterile water

- PPE
- pen
- forceps
- tape

STANDARD PRECAUTIONS

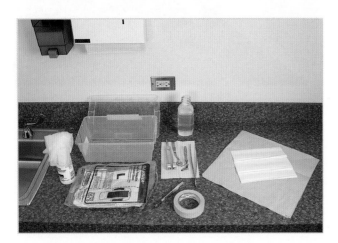

1. Gather supplies as well as clean and sanitized instruments that need to be sterilized. Apply appropriate PPE.

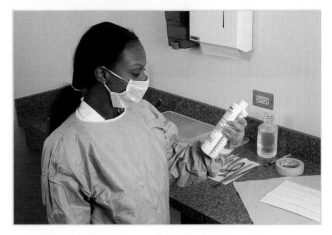

2. Read the label of the chemical sterilant to be used.

WHY? *It is imperative to follow the instructions carefully to ensure proper sterilization.*

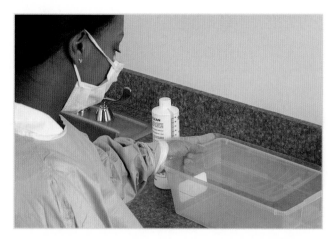

3. Choose appropriate container for the instruments' sizes and the chemical to be used. It must have a lid or cover and is typically a stainless steel container specially made for soaking instruments.

WHY? *The cleaner is caustic and can destroy the wrong type of container. The lid must be present so that it can be closed to prevent contaminants or microorganisms from entering the container.*

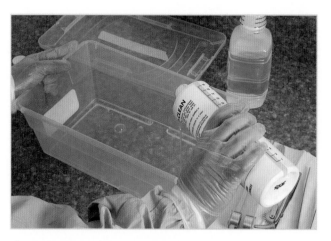

4. Prepare solution as needed or simply pour into the container.

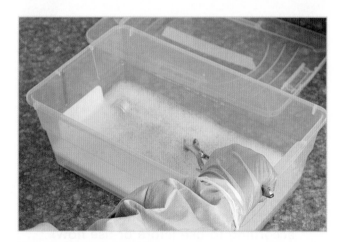

5. Place instruments carefully into the container, using forceps or pick ups to transfer the instruments and being careful not to splash the chemical.

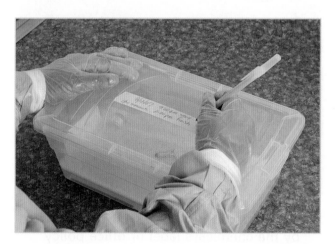

6. Using a strip of tape, label the container on the lid with your initials, the date, the solution, the instruments, the start time, and the end time.

WHY? *The end time must be noted so that others will not remove the instruments too soon.*

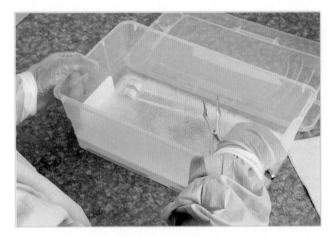

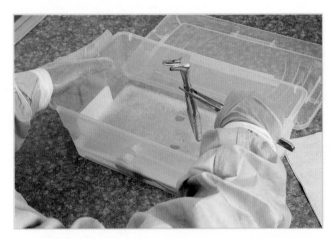

7. Leave the instruments until the end time has been reached. Remove the instruments with either sterile instruments or pick ups or by lifting the tray.

WHY❓ *If the items are not soaked for the full amount of time recommended by the solution's label, the items will not be considered sterile.*

8. Allow the excess fluid to drip off and then place items on a sterile towel to dry.

WHY❓ *This prevents the chemical sterilant from contaminating other areas, which is dangerous.*

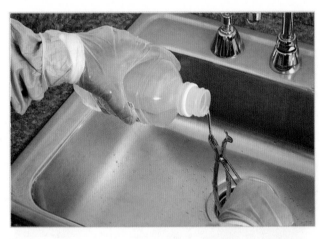

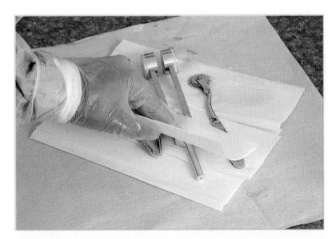

9. Rinse items with sterile water if instructed by the chemical's label or office policy.

10. Dry with sterile towel and prepare according to use (store or use now).

TIP➤ Items will have to be sealed in sterile packing or wrap to be stored.

Procedure **4-7**

Dispose of Biohazardous Materials

PURPOSE

Many waste items are contaminated with body fluids or tissues or other potentially pathogenic microorganisms. Properly disposing of biohazardous materials helps break the chain of infection and prevents the spread of pathogens.

EQUIPMENT/SUPPLIES

- biohazard waste container
- sharps container
- biohazard laundry bag
- biohazard waste: gauze, syringe/needle, gown, gloves, minor surgery tray set-up (tray with ring forceps for pickups, iris scissors, scalpel, suture tray)
- PPE

STANDARD PRECAUTIONS

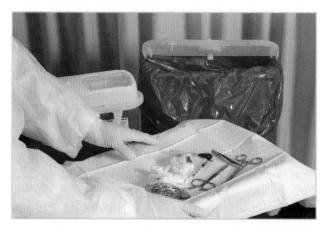

1. Apply PPE. Gather biohazardous items for disposal: soiled gauze, a syringe/needle, soiled gloves, scalpel, suture needle.

WHY? *Wearing PPE protects you from infectious material.*

TIP Always wear gloves when handling any potentially infectious material or items. It may also be necessary to wear a barrier gown to prevent contamination of your clothes, depending on what items you are disposing.

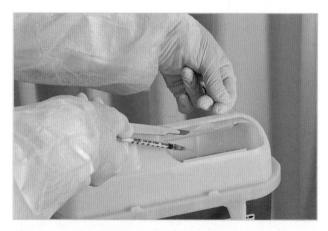

2. Place the scalpel, suture needle, and syringe/needle in the sharps container.

TIP This is typically a large counter-top red, puncture resistant container with a mechanism on the top to allow for disposal of syringes, blood tubes, slides, hematocrit tubes, sed rate containers, etc.

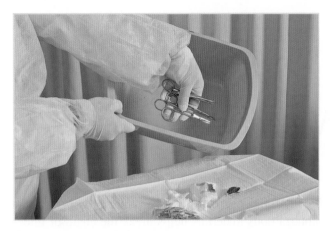

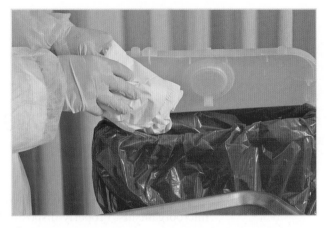

3. Place reusable instruments in tray to be cleaned, sanitized, and later autoclaved.

ᗯᕼᎽ❓ *It is important to place items in the correct containers.*

TIP▶ Many offices use retractable and disposable safety scalpels now to comply with OSHA guidelines. Always be careful when cleaning up a surgery tray and look for any sharps potentially covered by gauze or other materials so that you do not injure yourself.

4. Roll up and place soiled gloves, gauze, and sterile field material in the biohazard container. If there is a gown to be washed, place it in biohazard laundry.

ᗯᕼᎽ❓ *Biohazardous laundry is done in machines using water pipes that are separate from regular laundry. Sinks or toilets that are used to flush body fluids and tissues must have separate pipes to avoid contamination of general facilities and water resources.*

TIP▶ Laundry bags, like the plastic liners and outside of the sharps and other biohazardous containers, will have large lettering and the universal symbols for biohazardous waste on them.

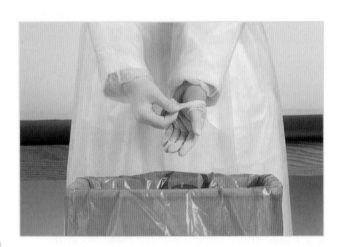

5. Remove gloves and wash hands.

LEGAL ALERT❗ Many local, state, and federal agencies strictly regulate the disposal of biohazardous waste. Any person who prepares biohazardous waste containers for disposal, seals and prepares containers for shipping and for pickup by a disposal company, and those who drive the trucks for the disposal company are examples of those who must complete specified training and are the ONLY ones allowed to perform those tasks.

TIP▶ All washable laundry may be considered biohazard laundry, as it is sent out in one wrapped load with a laundry service.

Procedure 4-8

Practice Standard Precautions: Wear Appropriate Personal Protective Equipment (PPE)

PURPOSE

Standard Precautions outline specific things healthcare workers can do to prevent exposure to biohazards and infections. Medical assistants must know how to apply personal protective equipment (PPE) such as gown, gloves, and masks to protect themselves from pathogens.

EQUIPMENT/SUPPLIES

- barrier gown
- non-sterile gloves
- mask, safety goggles or glasses, or face shield

STANDARD PRECAUTIONS

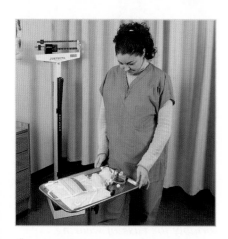

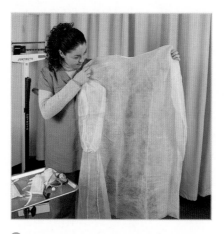

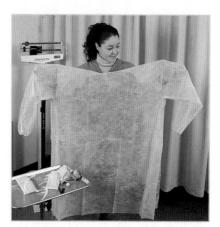

1. Gather all supplies and wash hands as usual.

WHY? *Proper handwashing removes microorganisms.*

2. Choose appropriate barrier gown to use.

WHY? *Wearing the appropriate gown ensures that you will be adequately protected.*

3. Apply the gown by holding gown with opening in the back.

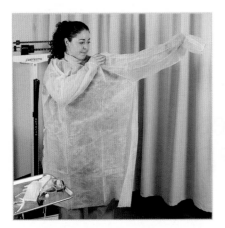

4. Slip your arms into sleeves.

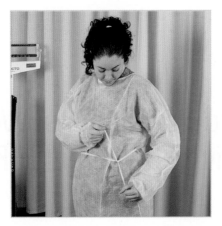

5. Tie or fasten the gown at the neck and the waist.

WHY❓ *Fastening the gown properly ensures that it will not come undone or slip off while you are performing a procedure requiring protection.*

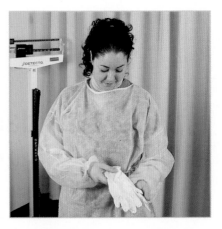

6. Obtain two non-sterile gloves in appropriate size.

WHY❓ *Do not choose gloves that are too big as the wrinkles caused by the extra material at the fingertips may adversely affect your sense of touch and dexterity.*

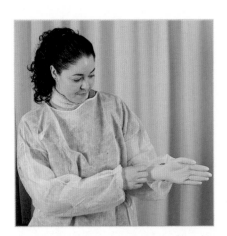

7. Grasp the top of one glove and slip it completely onto the other hand.

TIP➤ It does not matter which is first, or how they are held (as it does with sterile gloves).

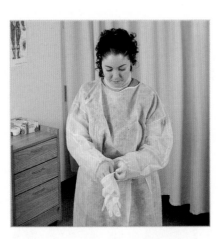

8. Grasp the top of the other glove and apply to the non-gloved hand.

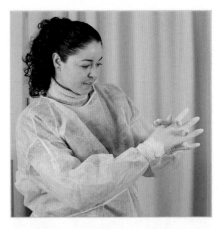

9. Adjust as needed to fit smoothly but not too tight.

WHY❓ *Gloves should fit comfortably for ease of wearing.*

TIP➤ If you have a sensitivity to latex, try vinyl or nitrile. Use non-powdered if that causes any discomfort or breathing difficulty.

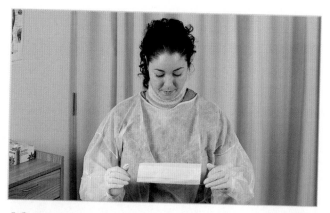

10. Choose a mask and goggles (or safety glasses) to use as appropriate.

TIP This is determined by the anticipated risk and type of exposure. If in doubt, more is better.

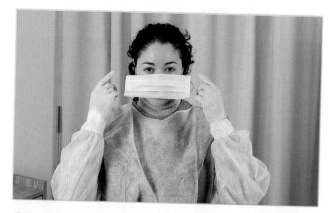

11. Apply mask over nose and mouth.

WHY? *The mask must cover both the nose and mouth in order to prevent pathogens from entering the body.*

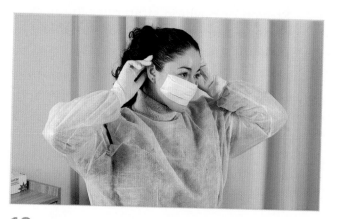

12. Secure mask in place by tying straps at the back of the neck and on the back of the head or by stretching elastic over ear auricles.

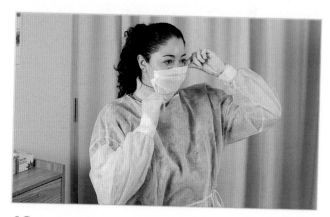

13. Adjust the mask over the bridge of the nose to avoid exhalations from escaping upward and drying the eyes.

WHY? *A properly fitting mask ensures that the wearer is protected.*

OR

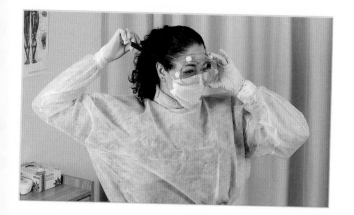

14. Slip on safety glasses as usual or goggles by putting strap over the back of the head.

TIP To maintain protection, make sure the glasses fit well enough to not slip down the nose when you lean forward.

OR

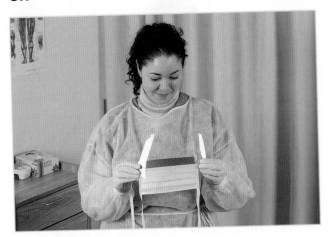

15. Choose a face shield to use.

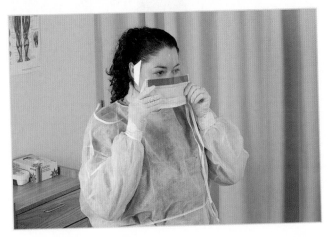

16. Hold shield to face in position.

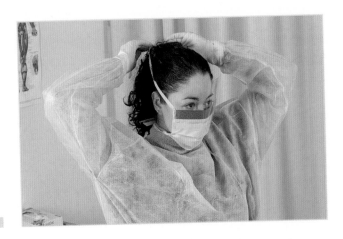

17. Stretch or position strap over the back of head and secure in a comfortable position.

ᴡʜʏ❓ *The face shield must be secured appropriately to ensure that the face is covered completely and the wearer is protected properly.*

ᴸᴱᴳᴬᴸ ᴬᴸᴱᴿᵀ❗ Your employer is required by law to provide you with the PPE you determine necessary even when beyond the employer-specific requirements. The employer also must provide hypo-allergenic PPE as needed.

CHAPTER 5

Specimen Collection

INTRODUCTION

Proper specimen collection is extremely important for the care and diagnosis of patient conditions. By understanding why this is done and performing the procedures correctly, the medical assistant fulfills an important role in the ambulatory care setting. Providers count on the medical assistant to collect and/or process specimens accurately so that patients can be treated accordingly. As the liaison between the provider and the patient, the medical assistant must be able to explain to the patient the reasons for the test, provide instructions on proper collection techniques, and answer any questions. Being comfortable when explaining procedures that involve personal bodily functions is crucial to ensuring patient comfort and cooperation.

PROCEDURES

5-1 Perform Venipuncture: Syringe Draw

5-2 Perform Venipuncture: Vacutainer Draw (Evacuated Tube)

5-3 Perform Venipuncture: Butterfly Draw

5-4 Perform Capillary Puncture

5-5 Obtain Specimens for Microbiological Testing: Throat Culture

5-6 Obtain Specimens for Microbiological Testing: Wound Culture

5-7 Instruct Patients in the Collection of a Clean-catch Mid-stream Urine Specimen

5-8 Instruct Patients in the Collection of Fecal Specimens

Procedure **5-1**

Perform Venipuncture: Syringe Draw

PURPOSE

Blood testing is a primary tool for assessing a patient's condition and assists the provider in either diagnosis or health maintenance. By using correct venipuncture techniques, medical assistants can acquire the specimen needed without undue suffering or discomfort for the patient, while also protecting themselves from exposure to blood-borne pathogens.

EQUIPMENT/SUPPLIES

- requisition slip
- PPE
- tourniquet
- syringe
- blood tubes
- alcohol wipes
- ball to squeeze

- cotton or gauze
- tape
- Band-Aids
- lab log
- pen
- sharps container

STANDARD PRECAUTIONS

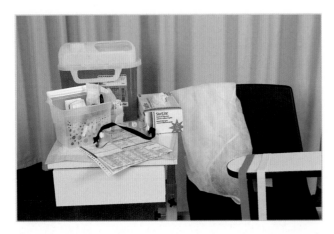

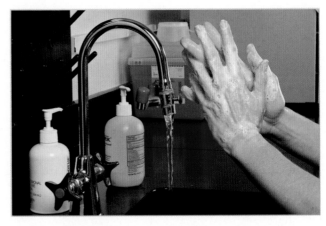

1. Gather all supplies, including the requisition slip.

ᴡʜʏ❓ *Checking the requisition slip ensures the correct specimen is collected.*

2. Wash hands.

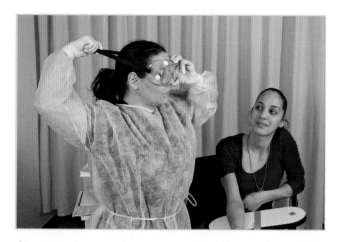

3. Apply PPE. Some offices require full PPE, some only gloves.

WHY? *Practicing Standard Precautions helps prevent the spread of infection.*

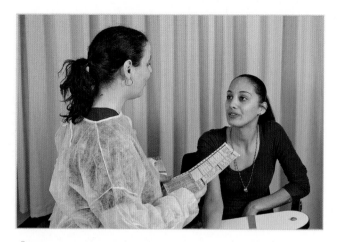

4. Identify the patient, and explain the procedure.

TIP Be sure to verify the patient's name and other identifiers, the insurance, and fasting compliance if necessary. Get a signature if the patient is a Medicare patient or for HIV testing authorization. Find out previous reactions to blood draws, and lie the patient down, if necessary.

WHY? *Proper identification avoids errors. Explaining the procedures alleviates any concerns and puts the patient at ease. Compliance with fasting ensures accurate test results; proper signatures and insurance verification ensures proper reimbursement and maintains legal guidelines.*

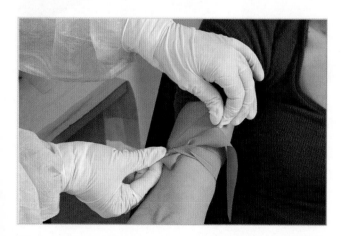

5. Apply tourniquet 3 to 4 inches above site.

:WHY? *The tourniquet causes the vein to dilate, which helps in locating the site and makes it easier to access the vein.*

TIP Ask the patient which arm is dominant or has a good vein. Many times the patient knows!

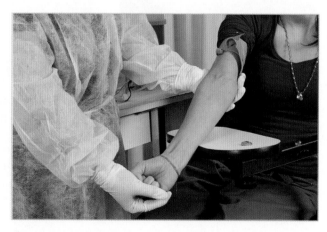

6. Instruct the patient to close the hand.

WHY? *Closing the hand makes the vein more visible.*

TIP To avoid the patient pumping the hand, give the patient a ball to hold.

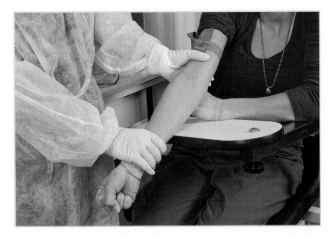

7. Place patient's arm in downward position.

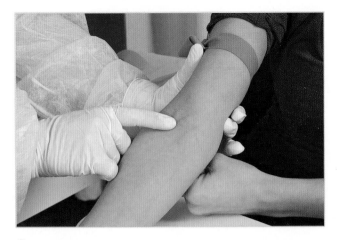

8. Palpate the vein and visualize the site.

TIP Note the direction, location, and depth of the vein.

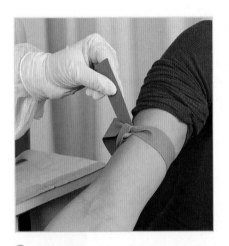

9. Release the tourniquet. (With practice this step may no longer be necessary, you can just apply the tourniquet and draw the blood.)

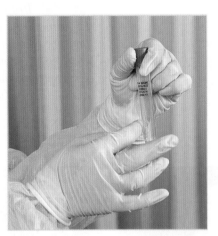

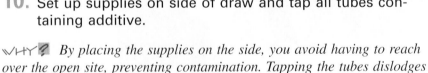

10. Set up supplies on side of draw and tap all tubes containing additive.

WHY? *By placing the supplies on the side, you avoid having to reach over the open site, preventing contamination. Tapping the tubes dislodges the additive.*

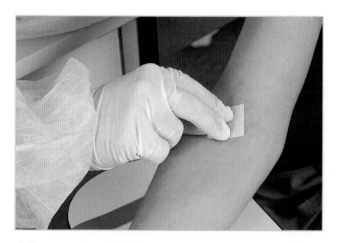

11. Clean site with alcohol.

Do not use alcohol when drawing blood for drug testing or if the patient is allergic to alcohol. Allowing the alcohol to air dry kills microorganisms more effectively than wiping the arm with clean gauze. Wipe the alcohol pad in a firm circular motion from the center of the area to be cleansed outwards.

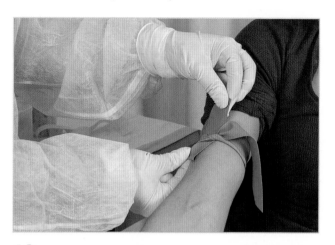

12. Reapply tourniquet, asking patient to close hand again.

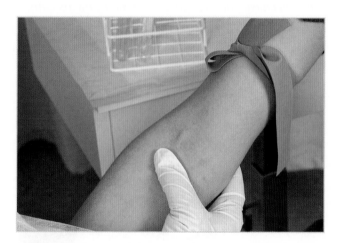

13. Anchor vein.

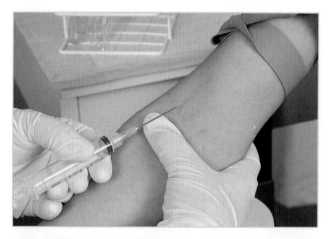

14. Position needle bevel up.

WHY? *The lumen is facing upward, which allows for smooth blood flow into the needle.*

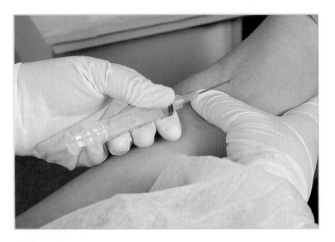

15. Insert needle quickly but gently.

w̨ʜʏ❓ *This method helps to ensure that the vein doesn't roll.*

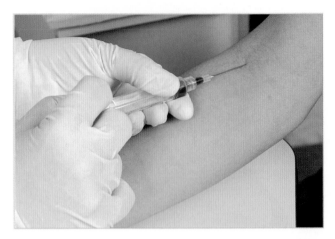

16. Anchoring the hand holding the syringe, pull back plunger slowly with the opposite hand until the syringe is full. Use an appropriate size syringe for the amount of blood needed to fill the tubes.

w̨ʜʏ❓ *Pull back on the plunger only as fast as blood flows to avoid collapsing vein. Do not switch hands because you may lose the blood flow or cause a hematoma by moving the needle and damaging the patient's vein.*

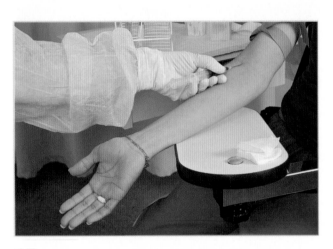

17. Ask patient to release/relax hand.

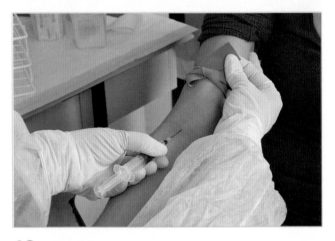

18. Release tourniquet.

w̨ʜʏ❓ *This releases pressure on the vein. Too much pressure can cause blood to leak into the nearby tissues, resulting in a hematoma.*

ⓣⓘⓟ Some phlebotomists prefer to release as soon as blood is flowing; others release when blood draw is complete, but still prior to removing needle.

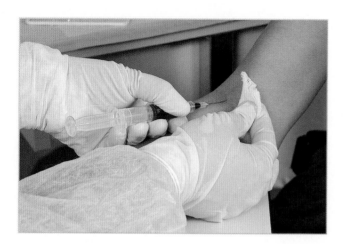

19. Lightly place gauze/cotton over site.

WHY? *This protects the puncture site.*

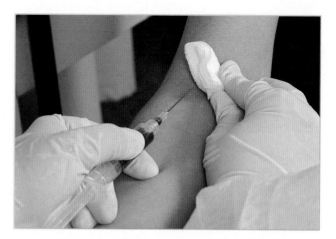

20. Remove needle from arm. Pull back on plunger slightly to avoid blood drip.

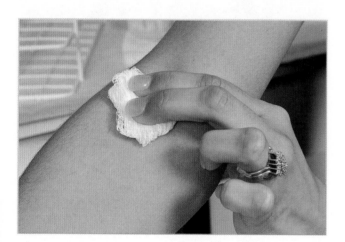

21. Apply pressure to site, or have the patient do this for you.

WHY? *Coagulation is promoted by applying pressure.*

TIP Raising the arm above the heart may help to avoid bruising.

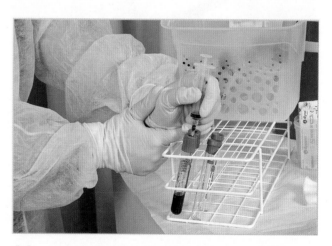

22. Aliquot blood into proper tube, using the correct order of draw. Rock the tube gently if additive is present. Do not push plunger, and do not hold tube with other hand.

WHY? *Rocking the tube mixes the blood with the additive.*

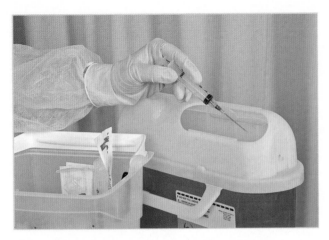

23. Put syringe directly into sharps container. If the container has a safety cover, flip it closed before placing syringe into sharps container.

ᴡʜʏ❓ *Biohazardous material must be disposed of correctly to prevent the spread of microorganisms.*

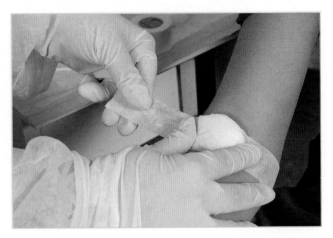

24. Place tape or bandage over patient's draw site wound. (Some phlebotomists prefer to use Band-Aids, while others prefer tape over original gauze. If new gauze is used, place old gauze into biohazard container.)

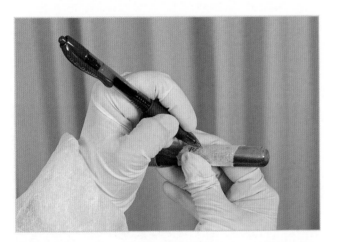

25. Label all tubes before patient leaves, either by writing on the tube or placing the numbered sticker from the requisition slip on it.

ᴡʜʏ❓ *Correctly identifying the specimens avoids errors.*

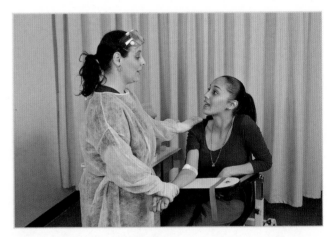

26. Ask how the patient is feeling. Ensure safety and lack of dizziness.

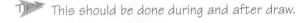
TIP▶ *This should be done during and after draw.*

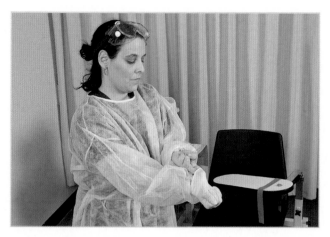

27. Remove PPE and dispose per OSHA guidelines.

 This prevents the spread of microorganisms and protects from blood-borne pathogens.

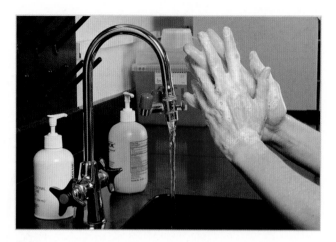

28. Wash hands.

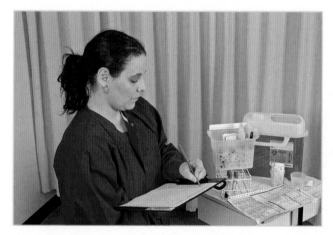

29. Document in the patient's chart if your employer requires this, or document in the lab log, and place a copy of the requisition into the patient's chart.

For all blood draws:

- To find difficult veins, use a BP cuff instead of a tourniquet, warm the site with a glove filled with warm water or with a warm washcloth, or "tap" the vein to cause it to rise.

- Be aware that you may need to spin the SST tube in a centrifuge before sending it to the lab.

- Recognize that some samples require a STAT pick up, and some need to be iced. Consult the lab book to learn which tests require special treatment and to ascertain which tests require what tubes.

- Be sure to place a copy of the requisition with each patient's samples. Consult your employer on how to correctly fill out these forms.

Charting Example

6/7/07 9:30 a.m. Venipuncture performed for CBC, pt tol. well, samples sent to lab. _____ A. Nguyen, CMA

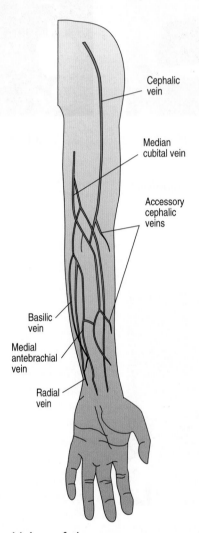

Veins of the arm.

Procedure 5-2

Perform Venipuncture: Vacutainer Draw (Evacuated Tube)

PURPOSE

Providers use blood testing to assess a patient's condition in order to ensure appropriate diagnosis and care. Performing venipuncture using the vacutainer draw method is a common way to obtain blood specimens for testing.

EQUIPMENT/SUPPLIES

- requisition slip
- PPE
- tourniquet
- vacutainer holder
- vacutainer needles

- blood tubes
- alcohol wipes
- cotton or gauze
- tape
- ball to squeeze

- Band-Aids
- lab log
- pen
- sharps container

STANDARD PRECAUTIONS

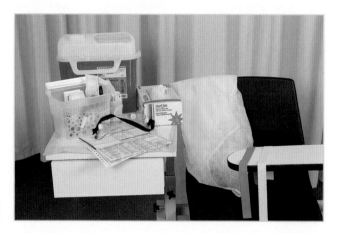

1. Gather all supplies, including the requisition slip.

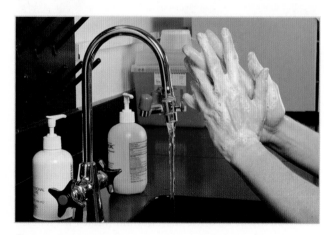

2. Wash hands.

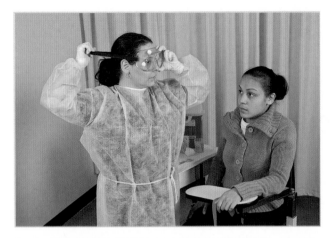

3. Apply PPE. Some offices require full PPE, some only gloves.

WHY? *Practicing Standard Precautions helps prevent the spread of infection.*

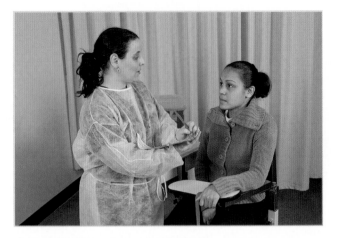

4. Identify the patient, and explain the procedure.

TIP Be sure to verify the patient's name and other identifiers, the insurance, and fasting compliance if necessary. Get a signature if the patient is a Medicare patient or for HIV testing authorization. Find out previous reactions to blood draws, and lie the patient down if necessary.

WHY? *Proper identification avoids errors. Explaining the procedure alleviates any concerns and puts the patient at ease.*

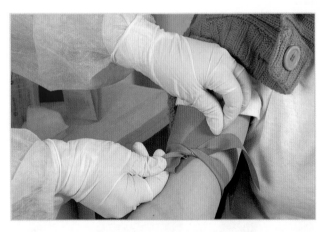

5. Apply tourniquet 3 to 4 inches above site.

WHY? *The tourniquet causes the vein to dilate, which helps in locating the site and makes it easier to access the vein.*

TIP Ask the patient which arm is dominant or has a good vein. Many times the patient knows!

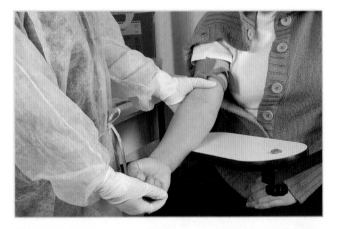

6. Instruct the patient to close the hand.

WHY? *Closing the hand makes the vein more visible.*

TIP To avoid the patient pumping the hand, give the patient a ball to hold.

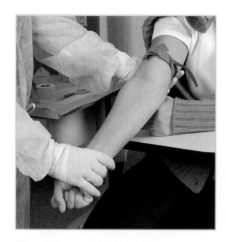

7. Place patient's arm in downward position.

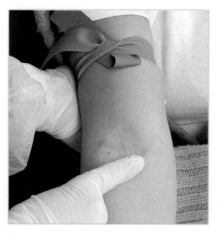

8. Palpate the vein and visualize the site.

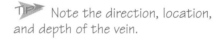 Note the direction, location, and depth of the vein.

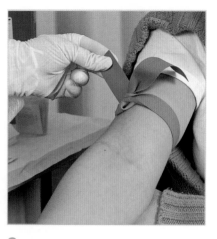

9. Release the tourniquet.

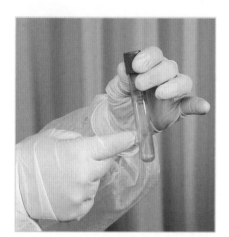

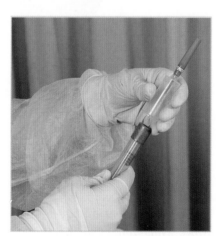

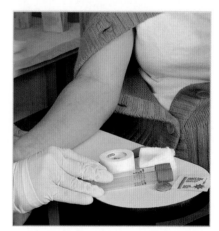

10. Set up supplies on side of draw and tap all tubes containing additive. Insert blood tube into vacutainer holder, being careful not to push all the way in or you will lose the vacuum.

WHY? *By placing the supplies on the side, you avoid having to reach over the open site, preventing contamination. Tapping the tubes dislodges the additive.*

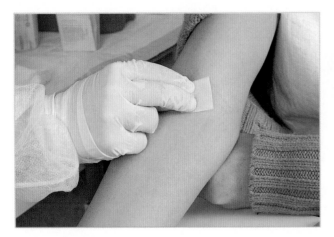

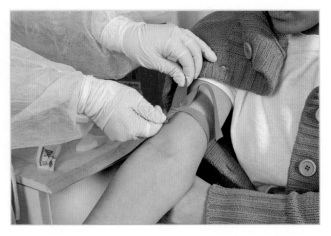

11. Clean site with alcohol.

TIP *Do not use alcohol when drawing blood for drug testing or if the patient is allergic to alcohol. Allowing the alcohol to air dry kills microorganisms more effectively than wiping the arm with clean gauze. Wipe the alcohol pad in a firm circular motion from the center of the area to be cleansed outwards.*

12. Reapply tourniquet, asking patient to close hand again.

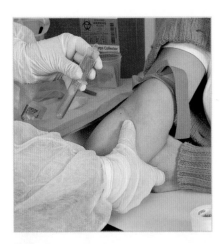

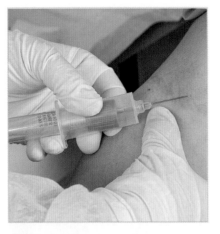

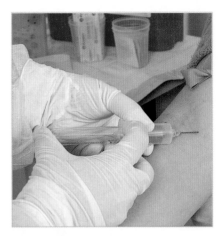

13. Anchor vein.

14. Position needle bevel up.

WHY? *The lumen is facing upward, which allows for smooth blood flow into the needle.*

15. Insert needle quickly but gently.

TIP *This method helps to ensure that the vein doesn't roll.*

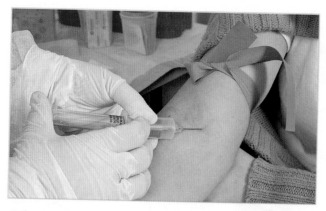

16. Push the blood tube all the way into the vacutainer holder by using the flange to allow the blood to flow. Be sure to anchor the hand holding the vacutainer holder so you do not push the needle farther into the vein. Do not switch hands.

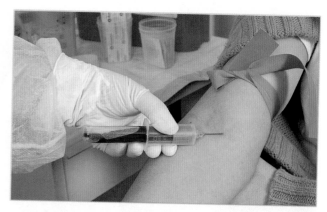

17. Fill the tube all the way. Most additives require the correct ratio of blood to additive, and the tube fills only that full due to the amount of vacuum in the tube.

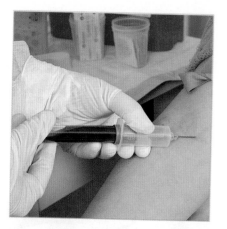
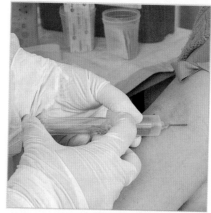
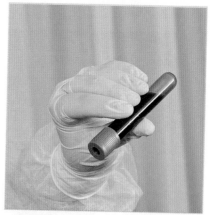

18. If more than one tube is necessary, switch tubes. (Be careful to keep your hand anchored on the patient's arm so as not to move the needle. If indicated, gently rock the tubes with additive.)

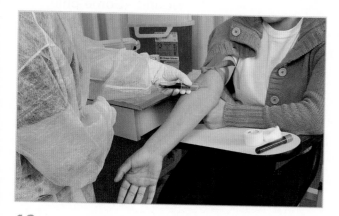

19. Ask the patient to relax hand.

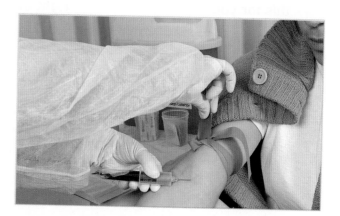

20. Release the tourniquet. (Some phlebotomists prefer to do this as the first tube is filling, others prefer to release right before withdrawing the needle from the patient's arm.)

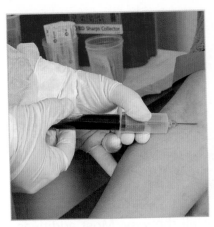

21. Pull the last tube off of the vacutainer needle.

WHY? *Doing this before withdrawing the needle prevents blood from dripping.*

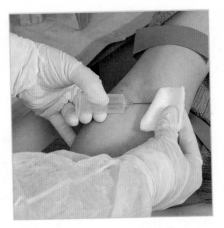

22. Lightly place gauze/cotton over site.

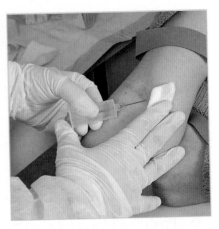

23. Remove the needle from the patient's arm.

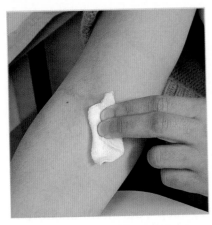

24. Apply pressure to site, or have the patient do this for you.

Raising the arm above the heart may help to avoid bruising.

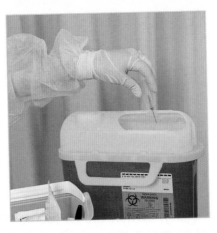

25. Discard the needle into the sharps container right away.

Some vacutainer holders have a needle guard that requires you to flip it over the needle and dispose of the whole assembly; others do not. Dispose of the entire needle assembly into the sharps container.

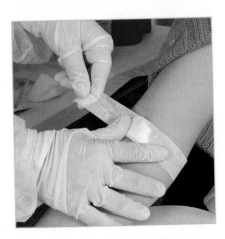

26. Place tape or bandage over patient's draw site wound. (Some phlebotomists prefer to use Band-Aids, while others prefer tape over original gauze. If new gauze is used, place old gauze into biohazard container.)

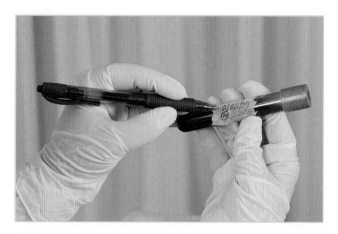

27. Label all tubes before patient leaves, either by writing on the tube or placing the numbered sticker from the requisition slip on it.

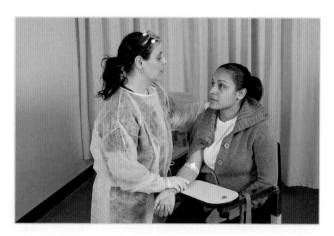

28. Ask how the patient is feeling. Ensure safety and lack of dizziness.

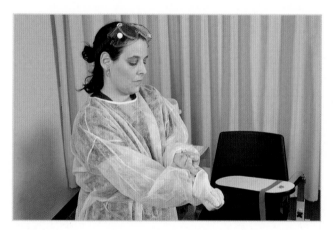

29. Remove PPE and dispose of it in the proper biohazardous container according to OSHA protocol.

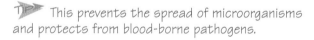 This prevents the spread of microorganisms and protects from blood-borne pathogens.

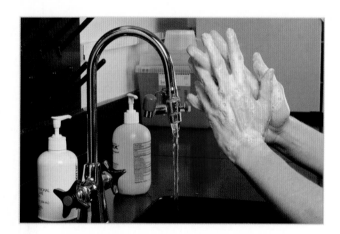

30. Wash hands.

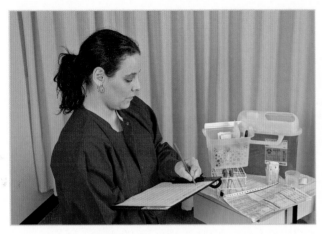

31. Document in the patient's chart if your employer requires this, or document in the lab log, and place a copy of the requisition into the patient's chart.

 Charting Example

7/2/07 9:45 a.m. Venipuncture performed for MMR titer, pt tol. well, samples sent to lab.

_____ D. Shiraz, CMA

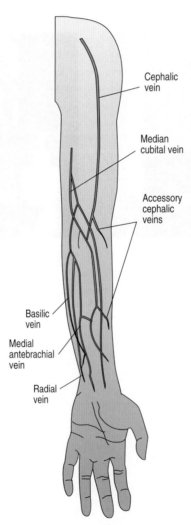

Veins of the arm.

Procedure **5-3**

Perform Venipuncture: Butterfly Draw

PURPOSE

Providers use blood testing to assess a patient's condition in order to ensure appropriate diagnosis and care. Performing venipuncture using the butterfly draw method is a common way to obtain blood specimens for testing.

EQUIPMENT/SUPPLIES

- requisition slip
- PPE
- tourniquet
- butterfly system
- vacutainer holder

- syringe
- blood tubes
- alcohol wipes
- cotton or gauze
- tape

- Band-Aids
- lab log
- pen
- sharps container

STANDARD PRECAUTIONS

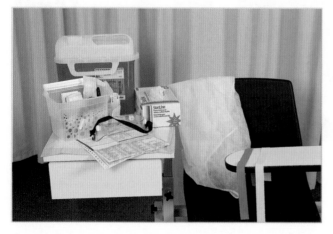

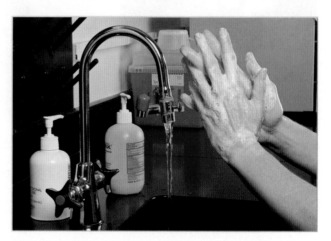

1. Gather all supplies, including the requisition slip.

2. Wash hands.

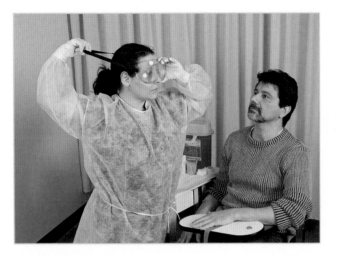

3. Apply PPE. (Some offices require full PPE, some only gloves.)

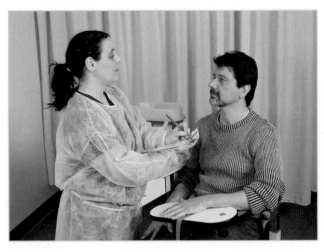

4. Identify the patient, and explain the procedure.

TIP Be sure to verify the patient's name and other identifiers, the insurance, and fasting compliance if necessary. Get a signature if the patient is a Medicare patient or for HIV testing authorization. Find out previous reactions to blood draws, and lie the patient down, if necessary.

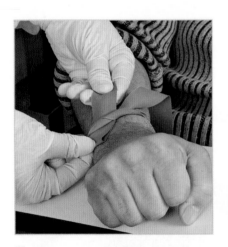

5. Apply tourniquet to wrist.

TIP A glove filled with warm water can help the veins to rise. Use this technique when a patient has difficult anticubital veins or easily collapsible veins.

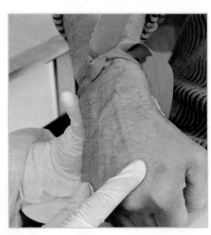

6. Palpate vein.

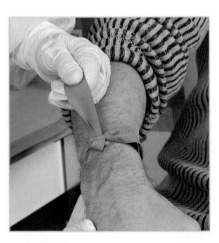

7. Release tourniquet.

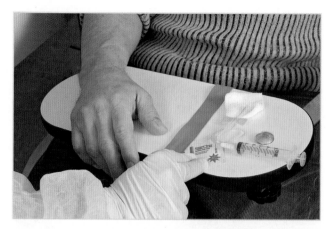

8. Set up supplies on side of draw to avoid reaching over the open site. Tap all tubes containing additive. Insert blood tube into vacutainer holder, being careful not to push all the way in or you will lose the vacuum.

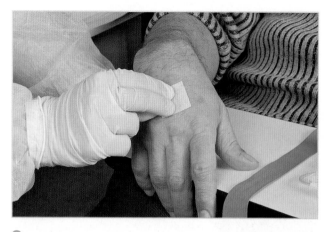

9. Clean site with alcohol.

▷ *Do not use alcohol when drawing blood for drug testing or if the patient is allergic to alcohol. Allowing the alcohol to air dry kills microorganisms more effectively than wiping the arm with clean gauze. Wipe the alcohol pad in a firm circular motion from the center of the area to be cleansed outwards.*

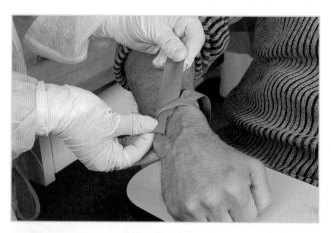

10. Reapply tourniquet.

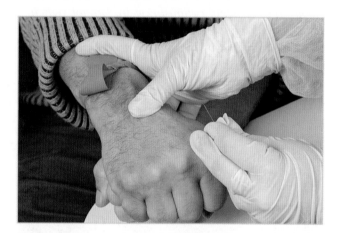

11. Anchor vein.

▷ *Hand veins have a tendency to roll, so anchor carefully.*

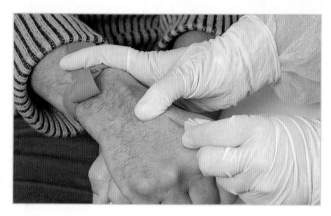

12. Position needle bevel up holding the "wings" of the butterfly needle.

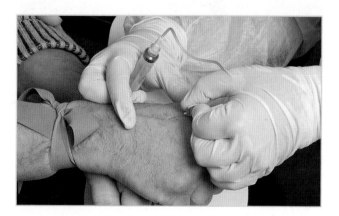

13. Insert needle quickly but gently.

If using a syringe butterfly system:

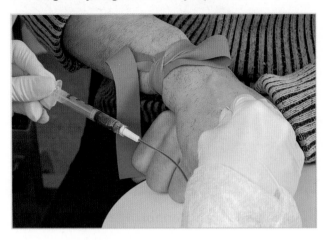

14. Using your opposite hand, pull back plunger slowly until the syringe is full. Use an appropriate size syringe for the amount of blood needed to fill the tubes.

WHY❓ *Pull back on the plunger only as fast as blood flows to avoid collapsing vein. Do not switch your hands because you may lose the blood flow or cause a hematoma by moving the needle and damaging the patient's vein.*

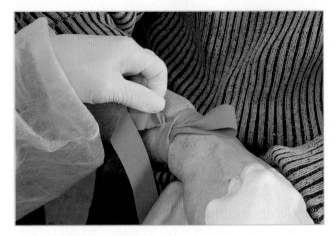

15. Release tourniquet. (Some phlebotomists prefer to release as soon as blood is flowing; others release when blood draw is complete, but prior to removing needle.)

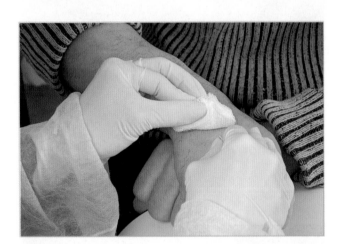

16. Lightly place gauze/cotton over site.

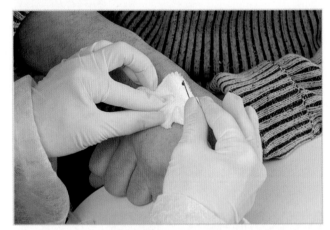

17. Remove needle from patient's hand. Pull back on plunger slightly to avoid blood drip.

If using a vacutainer butterfly system:

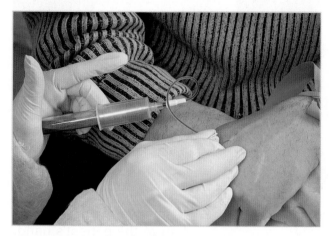

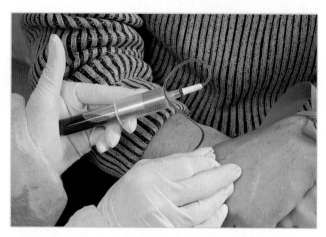

18. Push the blood tube all the way into the vacutainer holder by using the flange to allow the blood to flow. Be sure to anchor your hand holding the needle so you do not push the needle farther into the vein. Do not switch your hands.

19. Fill the tube all the way. Most additives require the correct ratio of blood to additive and the tube fills only that full due to the amount of vacuum in the tube.

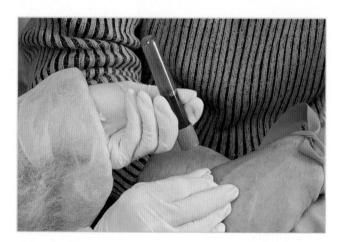

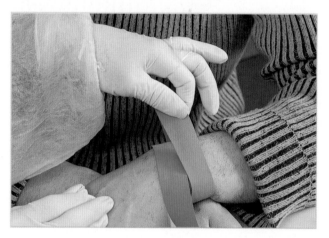

20. If more than one tube is necessary, switch tubes. (Be careful to keep your hand anchored on the patient's arm so as not to move the needle. If indicated, gently rock the tubes with additive.)

21. Release the tourniquet. (Some phlebotomists prefer to do this as the first tube is filling, others prefer to release right before withdrawing the needle from the patient's arm.)

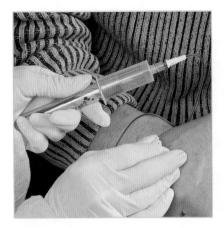

22. Pull the last tube off of the vacutainer needle.

WHY❓ *Doing this prior to withdrawing the needle prevents blood from dripping.*

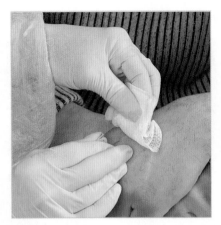

23. Lightly place gauze/ cotton over site.

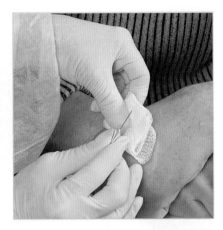

24. Remove the needle from the patient's hand.

Both types continue:

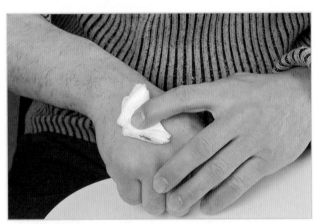

25. Apply pressure to site, or have the patient do this for you.

TIP▶ *Raising the arm above the heart may help to avoid bruising.*

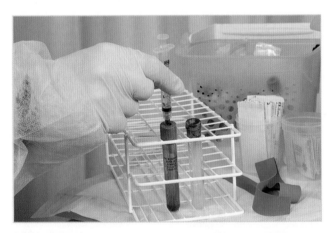

26. Aliquot blood into proper tubes. Use transfer device or new needle for safety.

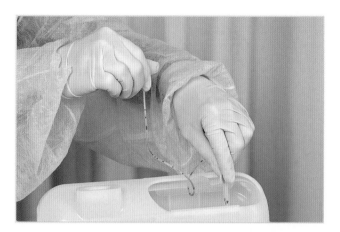

27. Discard the needle into the sharps container right away. Some vacutainer holders have a needle guard that requires you to flip it over the needle and dispose of the whole assembly; others require the removal of the needle and keeping the holder. The sharps container is designed to help you unscrew the needle without touching it.

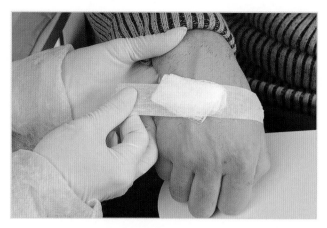

28. Place tape or bandage over patient's draw site wound. (Some phlebotomists prefer to use Band-Aids, others prefer tape over original gauze. If new gauze is used, place old gauze into biohazard container.)

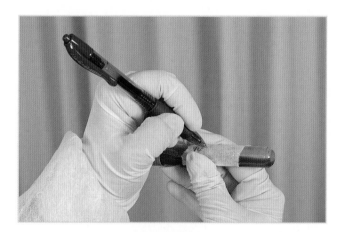

29. Label all tubes before patient leaves, either by writing on the tube or placing the numbered sticker from the requisition slip on it.

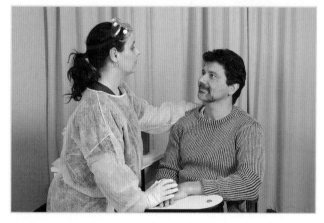

30. Ask how the patient is feeling. Ensure safety and lack of dizziness.

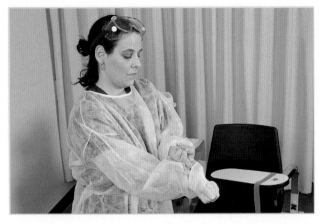

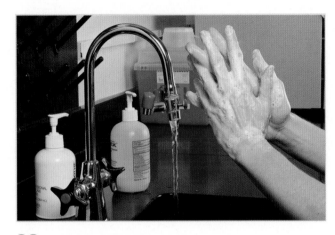

31. Remove PPE and dispose of it in the proper biohazardous container according to OSHA protocol.

ᐯᕼᒪᗩ *This prevents the spread of microorganisms and protects from blood-borne pathogens.*

32. Wash hands.

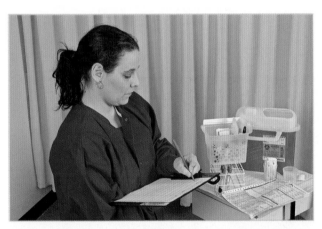

33. Document in the patient's chart if your employer requires this, or document in the lab log, and place a copy of the requisition into the patient's chart.

✎ **Charting Example**

8/7/07 10:05 a.m. Venipuncture performed for TSH, pt
tol well, samples sent to lab. _____ M. Hernandez, CMA

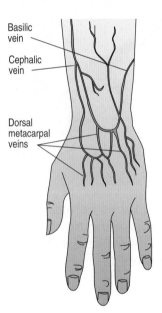

Basilic vein

Cephalic vein

Dorsal metacarpal veins

Veins of the hand.

Procedure 5-4

Perform Capillary Puncture

PURPOSE

Some patients require only a finger stick or capillary puncture to obtain a blood specimen. Performing this procedure accurately reduces trauma and pain to the patient and allow the test to be performed correctly without the need for a second stick.

EQUIPMENT/SUPPLIES

- requisition slip
- PPE
- capillary tubes (both kinds and holding tray)
- lancet
- alcohol wipes
- clay
- cotton or gauze
- lab log
- Band-Aid
- pen
- sharps container
- biohazard waste container

STANDARD PRECAUTIONS

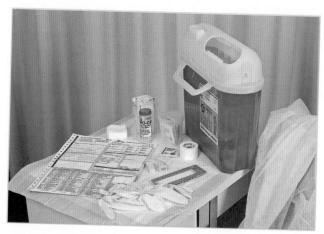

1. Gather all supplies including the requisition slip.

WHY? *Checking the requisition slip helps ensure the correct specimen is collected.*

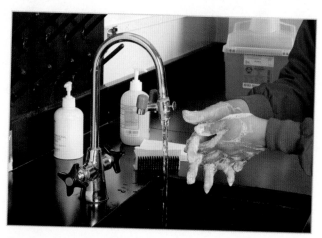

2. Wash hands.

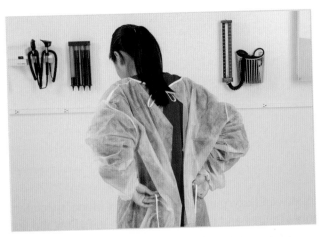

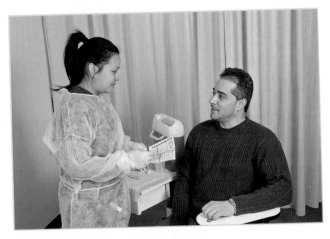

3. Apply PPE. Some offices require full PPE, some only gloves.

WHY? *Practicing Standard Precautions helps prevent the spread of infection.*

4. Identify the patient, and explain the procedure.

TIP Be sure to verify the patient's name, other identifiers, and fasting compliance if necessary.

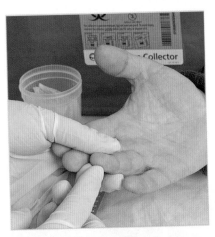

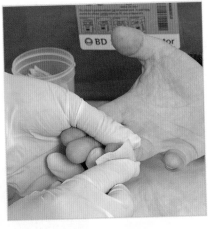

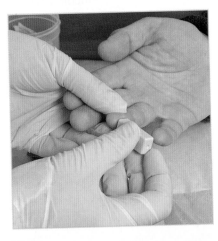

5. Select a puncture site on either the middle or ring fingers. Never use the thumb, the index, or "pinky" fingers.

WHY? *The thumb and the index and pinky fingers have many nerve sites and so are very sensitive. Going against the fingerprint grain helps obtain a large, round drop of blood.*

TIP If the patient has cold hands, fill a glove with warm water and have the patient hold it while you get ready. This improves circulation.

6. Clean the site with alcohol.

7. Puncture the finger with the lancet.

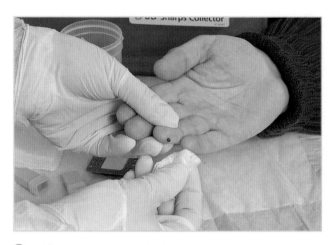

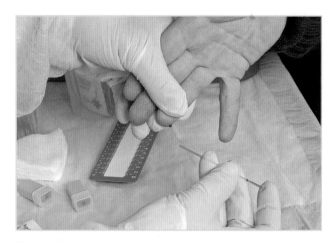

8. Wipe away the first drop.

WHY? *This allows for a clean sample without white blood cells or serum from the body's injury response.*

9. Hold the hand downward and apply gentle pressure.

WHY? *Blood flow is promoted by holding the hand downward. Be sure not to squeeze the finger as this can affect the quality of the sample.*

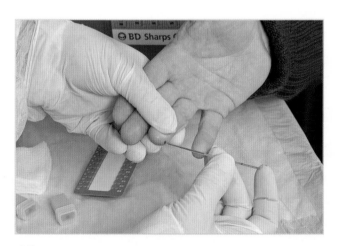

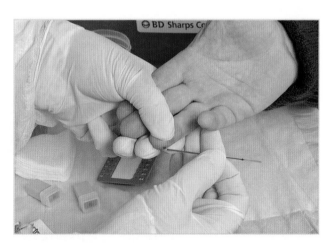

10. Fill the capillary tubes to the proper mark. Hold the tube horizontally and allow capillary pressure to fill the tube naturally; do not touch the tube to the finger.

WHY? *Touching the tube to the patient's finger may contaminate the specimen.*

TIP To avoid getting bubbles in the tube, be sure to maintain the correct position.

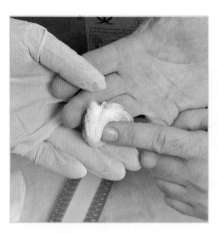

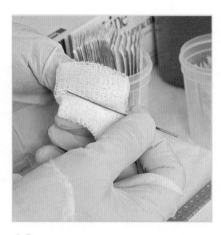

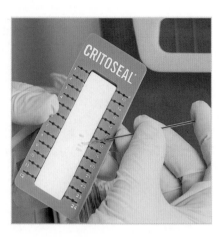

11. When all the tubes are filled to the proper amount, place gauze over the site, and ask the patient to apply pressure while holding the hand upright.

12. If using glass capillary tubes, insert the clean end into the tray of clay after wiping the sides with gauze to remove any blood.

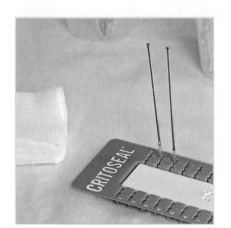

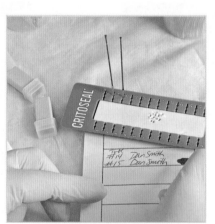

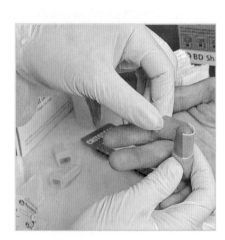

13. If using plastic sample tubes, place them in a holder to keep them upright.

14. Label all tubes appropriately before the patient leaves.

WHY? *Correctly identifying the specimens avoids errors.*

15. Apply a bandage to the patient's finger.

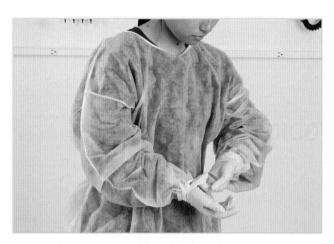

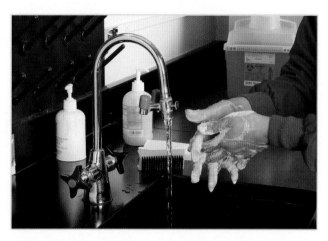

16. Remove PPE and dispose of it in the proper biohazardous container according to OSHA protocol.

WHY？ *This prevents the spread of microorganisms and protects from blood-borne pathogens.*

17. Wash hands.

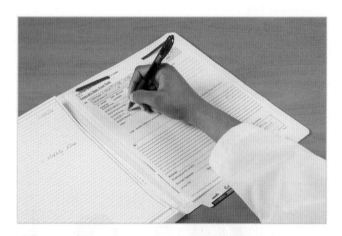

18. Document in the patient's chart if your employer requires this, or document in the lab log, and place a copy of the requisition into the patient's chart.

 Charting Example

1/17/08 11:15 a.m. Performed capillary puncture for HCT testing, left ring finger, pt tol. well, sample sent to lab for testing. _____ M. Allen, CMA

Procedure 5-5

Obtain Specimens for Microbiological Testing: Throat Culture

PURPOSE

Obtaining a throat culture for microbiological testing helps the provider ascertain if certain pathogens are present in the patient's respiratory tract. By performing this procedure accurately and quickly, the medical assistant minimizes patient discomfort and helps ensure that appropriate treatment can be initiated.

EQUIPMENT/SUPPLIES

- requisition slip or patient chart
- PPE
- sterile culture swabs
- sterile tongue depressor
- lab log

- pen
- lamp or penlight
- transport bag
- biohazard container

STANDARD PRECAUTIONS

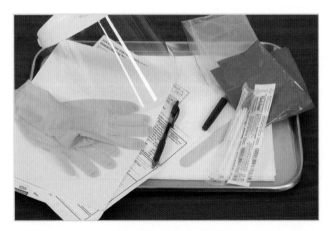

1. Gather equipment. Use a sterile tongue depressor if required by your office.

Check expiration dates on all culture tubes.

Use two swabs at once when doing a rapid strep by holding the culturette and the special rapid strep kit. Swab together, thereby avoiding a second swab.

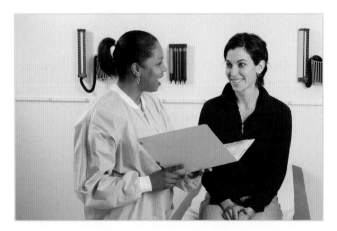

2. Explain the procedure to the patient.

Ｗ**ＨＹ** *Doing this helps alleviate any concerns and puts the patient at ease.*

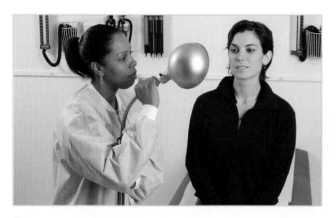

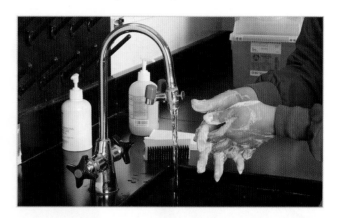

3. Position the patient and a light source if needed.

ᴠᴠʜʏ❓ *Positioning the patient and using a light source helps you better see the area of concern so a proper specimen can be obtained.*

4. Wash hands.

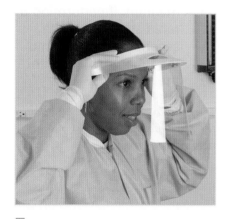

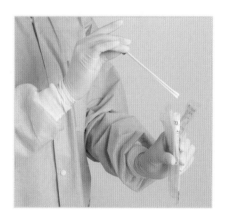

5. Apply PPE (gloves and face shield).

ᴠᴠʜʏ❓ *Practicing Standard Precautions helps prevent the spread of infection.*

6. Remove swab(s) from tube(s).

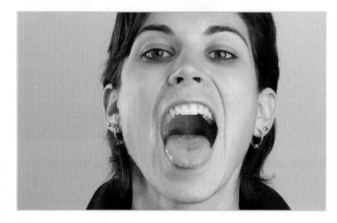

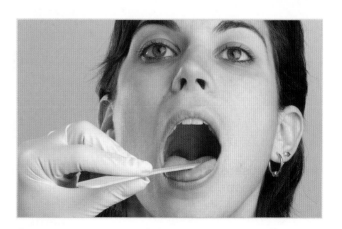

7. Ask the patient to open mouth and either say "aaaahhhhh" or pant.

ᴠᴠʜʏ❓ *Doing this helps prevent gagging.*

8. Depress the tongue with the tongue depressor.

ᴛɪᴘ ▶ Press down on the back of the tongue for the best position.

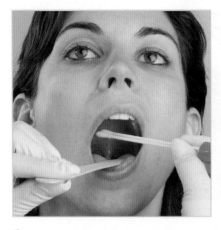

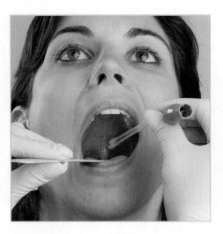

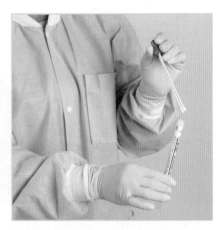

9. Swab the back of the throat, making sure to get the tonsillar area as well. You will be able to visualize the redness and possibly the areas of infection.

10. After removing the swab from the patient's mouth, place the swab into the culture tube, making sure it is in the transport medium. If performing a rapid strep, place the second strep swab into the tube provided with the strep test.

WHY? *It is important to handle the specimen properly to obtain accurate test results.*

TIP If the rapid strep is positive, it may be unnecessary to send the culture to the lab for testing; follow office policy.

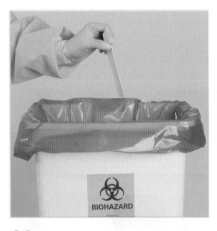

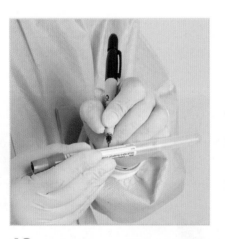

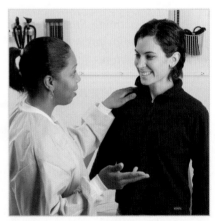

11. Dispose of the tongue depressor.

WHY? *This is biohazardous material and must be disposed of correctly.*

12. Label the culture tube, making sure to include the source, patient name, and date.

WHY? *Correctly identifying the specimen avoids errors.*

13. Thank your patient!

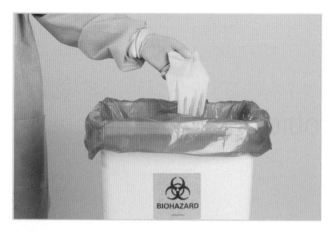

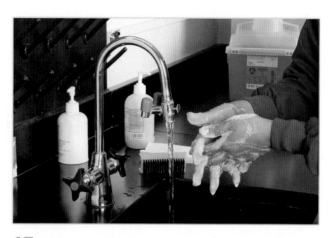

14. Remove PPE and dispose of it properly.

WHY? *Biohazardous material must be disposed of correctly to prevent the spread of microorganisms.*

15. Wash hands.

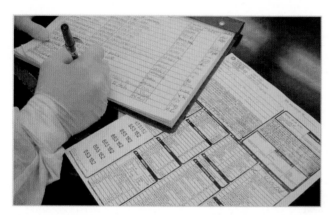

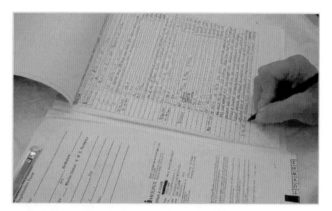

16. Document the procedure in the patient's chart if your employer requires this, or document in the lab log, and place a copy of the requisition into the patient's chart.

Charting Example

1/22/08 3:10 p.m. Performed TC for rapid strep, pat tol well, culture sent to lab to confirm neg rapid strep result in office. _____ D. Ferrar, CMA

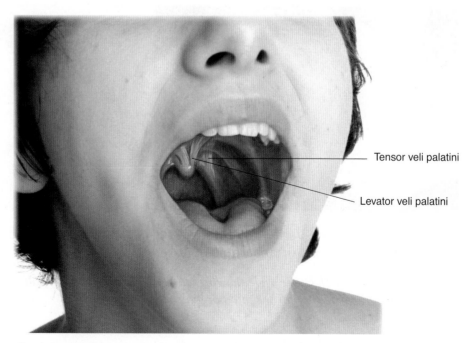

Tensor veli palatini

Levator veli palatini

Oral anatomy.

Procedure **5-6**

Obtain Specimens for Microbiological Testing: Wound Culture

PURPOSE

Obtaining a wound culture for microbiological testing helps the provider ascertain if resistant bacteria are present in a non-healing wound. By performing this procedure accurately and efficiently, the medical assistant minimizes patient discomfort and helps ensure that appropriate antibiotic treatment can be initiated.

EQUIPMENT/SUPPLIES

- requisition slip or patient chart
- PPE
- sterile culture swabs
- bandages/dressing
- lab log
- pen
- lamp or penlight
- transport bag
- biohazard container

STANDARD PRECAUTIONS

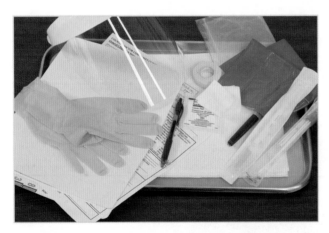

1. Gather equipment. Verify if the physician has ordered aerobic or anaerobic culture.

ᴡʜʏ❔ *Do this in order to provide the correct transport and proper testing for the microorganism the physician is looking for.*

 Check expiration dates on all culture tubes.

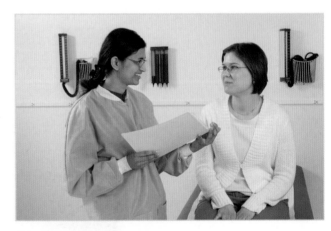

2. Explain the procedure to the patient.

ᴡʜʏ❔ *Doing this helps alleviate any concerns and puts the patient at ease.*

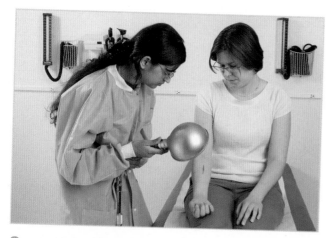

3. Position the patient and a light source if needed.

WHY? *Positioning the patient and using a light source helps you better see the area of concern so a proper specimen can be obtained.*

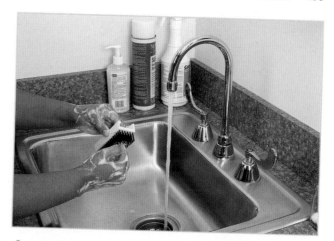

4. Wash hands.

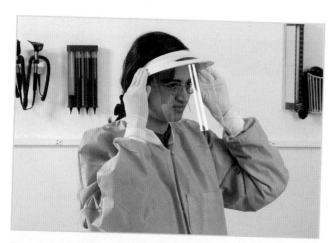

5. Apply PPE (gown, gloves, and face shield).

WHY? *Practicing Standard Precautions helps prevent the spread of infection.*

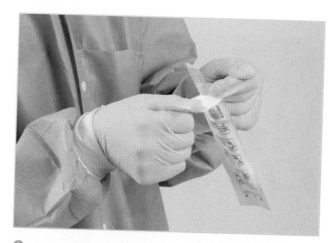

6. Remove swab(s) from tube(s).

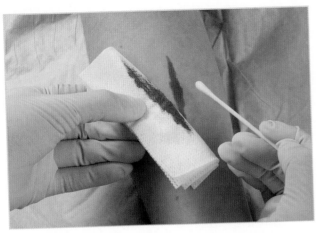

7. Swab wound, using a rolling technique, making sure to get at any areas of infection.

ᴡʜʏ❔ *Using this technique ensures that you get a variety of areas and prevents the spread of microorganisms that might cause contamination.*

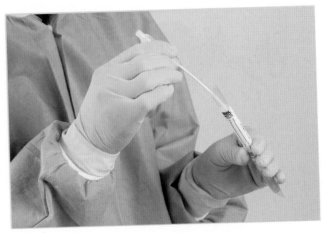

8. Place swab into culture tube, making sure it is in the transport medium.

ᴡʜʏ❔ *It is important to handle the specimen correctly to obtain accurate test results.*

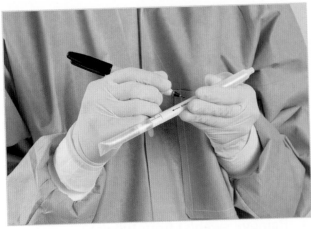

9. Label the tube, making sure to include the source, patient name, and date.

ᴡʜʏ❔ *Correctly identifying the specimen prevents errors.*

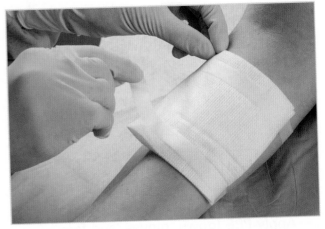

10. Bandage the wound as appropriate or as directed by provider.

TIP Assess patient vitals if necessary, and give the patient wound care instructions to take home.

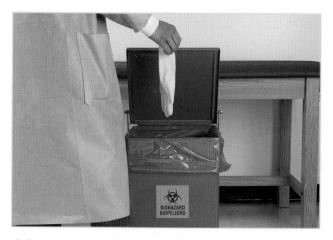

11. Remove PPE and dispose of properly.

WHY? *Biohazardous material must be disposed of correctly to prevent the spread of microorganisms.*

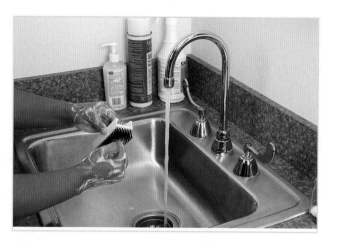

12. Wash hands.

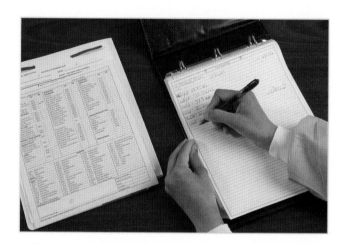

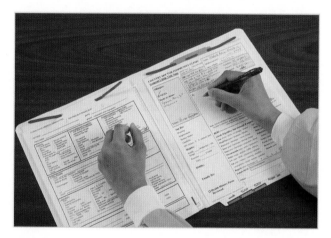

13. Document the procedure in the patient's chart if your employer requires this, or document in the lab log, and place a copy of the requisition into the patient's chart.

✎ **Charting Example**

1/16/08 9:45 a.m. Performed wound culture, right forearm laceration, pt tol. well, anaerobic culture sample sent to lab, results requested STAT. _____ J. Smythe, CMA

Procedure 5-7

Instruct Patients in the Collection of a Clean-catch Mid-stream Urine Specimen

PURPOSE

When testing urine in the ambulatory care setting for signs of a urinary tract infection, it is important to get a good, clean sample. Instructing patients on proper techniques for collecting a clean-catch mid-stream urine specimen minimizes the chance for contamination, which helps ensure accurate results.

EQUIPMENT/SUPPLIES

- requisition slip or patient chart
- PPE
- sterile urine container
- written instructions
- urinalysis strips
- urine vacutainer system
- lab log
- pen
- transport bag
- biohazard container
- internal lab slip
- antiseptic wipes

STANDARD PRECAUTIONS

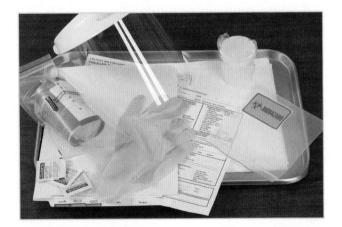

1. Gather all supplies.

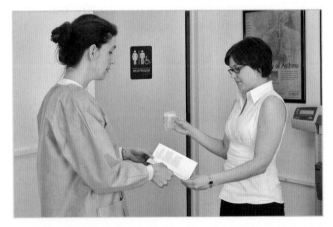

2. Show the patient to the restroom and provide a sterile urine specimen cup and antiseptic wipes.

WHY? *Only antiseptic wipes are used for the genital area because alcohol will sting and damage sensitive mucous membranes or genital tissue. Do not confuse these with alcohol wipes.*

Cleansing Steps for Women

- Wash your hands upon entering the bathroom. Remove the lid from the container and place the lid flat side down in the designated area. Be careful not to touch the inside of the lid.
- Kneel or squat over a bedpan or toilet. Spread the labia minora to expose the meatus. First, cleanse on each side of the meatus. Wipe from front to back, using a new wipe for each side. Then, using a new wipe, clean the meatus itself. Again, wipe from front to back.
- Keeping the labia separated, initially void for a second into the toilet or bedpan. It's important to do this first so the specimen will have the least contamination with the skin.
- While maintaining a stream, bring the sterile container into the stream and fill the container about three-quarters full (collect 30 to 100 mL).
- Once a sufficient amount has been collected, finish voiding into the toilet or bedpan.
- Cap the specimen container and wash your hands. Bring the container to the designated area.

Cleansing Steps for Men

- Wash your hands upon entering the bathroom. Remove the lid from the container and place the lid flat side down in the designated area. Be careful not to touch the inside of the lid.
- If uncircumcised, retract the foreskin to expose the glans penis. Clean the meatus with an antiseptic wipe. Use a new wipe for each cleaning sweep.
- Keep the foreskin retracted and void for a second into the toilet or urinal. It is important to do this first so the specimen will have the least contamination with the skin.
- While maintaining a stream, bring the sterile container into the urine stream. Fill the container about three-quarters full. Do not touch the inside of the container with the penis.
- Once a sufficient amount has been collected (30 to 100 mL), finish voiding into the toilet or urinal.
- Cap the specimen container and wash your hands. Bring the container to the designated area.

3. Instruct the patient in the proper cleansing technique (see above) and why this is necessary.

TIP If your office is crowded or noisy, you may give directions in the exam room. Be sure to tell the patient to label the container with the patient's name, or you can label it. Show the patient where to leave the specimen when completed; some offices have a small doorway into the lab from the restroom.

WHY? Using the proper cleansing technique and obtaining a sample from the middle of the urine steam helps avoid contaminating the specimen.

TIP Sometimes written instructions are on the wall of the restroom; if not, provide written instructions.

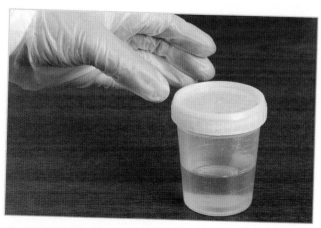

4. Wear gloves.

WHY? Gloves protect against exposure to microorganisms.

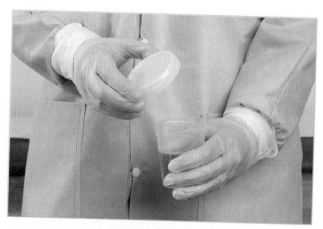

5. Process specimen (see Procedure 6-3).

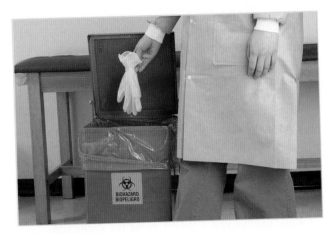

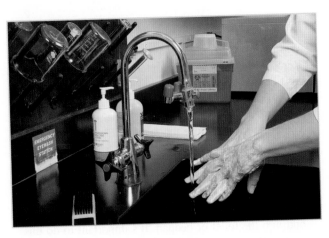

6. Dispose of PPE.

7. Wash hands.

WHY❓ *Biohazardous material must be disposed of according to OSHA protocol to prevent the spread of microorganisms.*

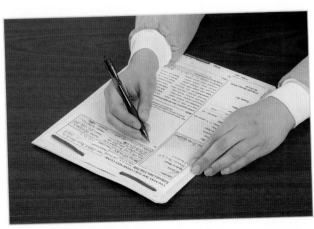

8. Document in the patient chart per office protocol.

👉 Obtaining a clean-catch mid-stream urine specimen is one of the most common procedures that medical assistants perform. It is important to practice by giving instructions to other students to overcome any discomfort felt by talking about personal bodily functions.

Box 5•1 **Chlamydia Testing Alert**

Chlamydia may now be tested with a urine specimen instead of a swab for men. This **must not** be a clean-catch specimen, as the urine will wash any of the bacteria out of the urethra. Patients must void from the start into the container without cleansing the area first.

You may need to send the urine sample to the lab for a culture and sensitivity test to find out which antibiotic is best to use.

✎ **Charting Example**

1/29/08 10:45 a.m. Patient instructed in CCMS urine sample collection. _____ A. Lubentz, CMA

Procedure 5-8

Instruct Patients in the Collection of Fecal Specimens

PURPOSE

Testing for occult blood (blood in the stool) helps with early detection of colon cancer, a leading cause of death. Accuracy in instruction is crucial to obtain a proper specimen.

EQUIPMENT/SUPPLIES

- requisition slip or patient chart
- PPE
- hemoccult cards
- developer
- "hat"

- written instructions
- internal lab slip
- pen
- transport bag
- biohazard container

STANDARD PRECAUTIONS

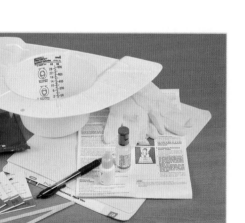

1. Gather equipment. Keep in mind that this is a three-card test. Be sure to give the patient a "hat" for collection and check the expiration dates on the cards.

WHY? *A "hat" makes collection easier for the patient. Outdated products may not give accurate results.*

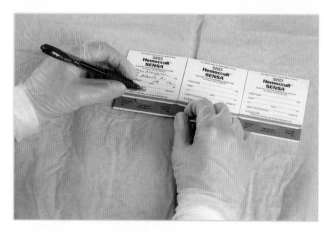

2. Label the collection cards with the patient's name and instruct the patient on how to fill in the date and time.

WHY? *Proper labeling and appropriate instructions avoid errors in specimen collection.*

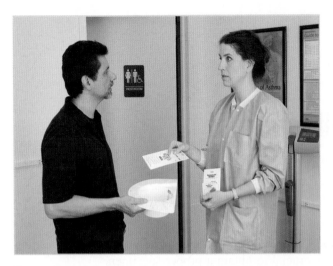

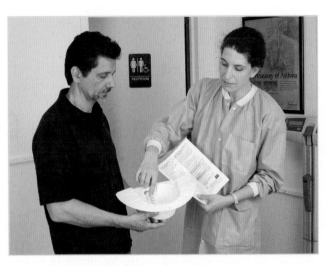

3. Explain the collection technique to the patient, emphasizing the importance of this test. Instruct the patient on proper care of the slides (e.g., keep away from light and heat and allow to dry before closing) and answer any questions.

WHY❓ *Clear instructions promote patient understanding and improve compliance.*

TIP▶ Explain foods to avoid, such as red meat, and times to avoid collection, such as during menses for women and in the presence of hemorrhoids.

4. Give the patient written instructions and show the instructions on the inner flap of the envelope.

WHY❓ *Verbal instructions should be followed up with written instructions. Always make sure the patient understands the instructions.*

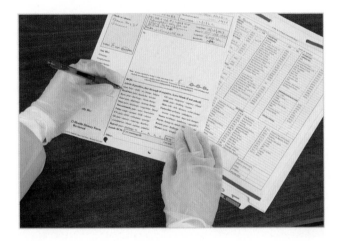

5. Document in the chart that instructions were given.

TIP▶ The provider may do this test routinely during a physical exam, and then, if positive, the medical assistant will instruct the patient on further specimen collection to be done in the home. This may require a follow-up with a gastroenterologist if the home test is positive. It is important to practice by giving instructions to other students to overcome any discomfort felt by talking about personal bodily functions.

When the slides come back:

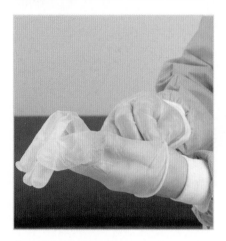

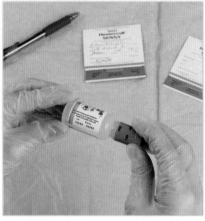

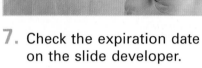

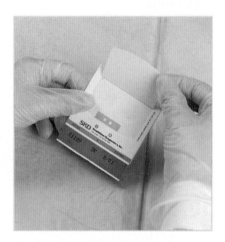

6. Wear gloves.

∨⊢Y❓ *Gloves prevent exposure to pathogens.*

7. Check the expiration date on the slide developer.

∨⊢Y❓ *Outdated products may affect test results.*

8. Open the back flaps of the slides.

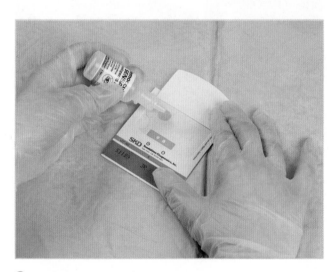

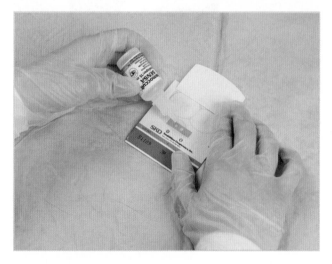

9. Apply developer to the sample and to the quality control area (two drops on each sample and one between the positive and negative control panel).

∨⊢Y❓ *Correctly applying developer ensures accurate results.*

◥▷ Be careful not to touch the tip of the developer to the slide in order to avoid contamination.

Negative

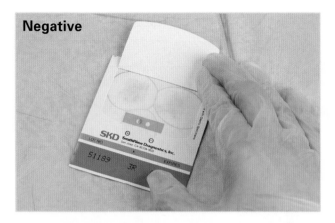

Positive

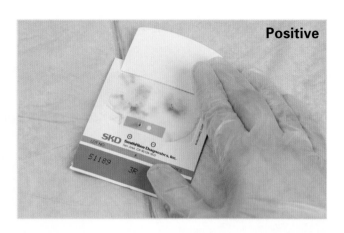

10. After 60 seconds, interpret the result.

WHY？ *Proper timing ensures testing accuracy.*

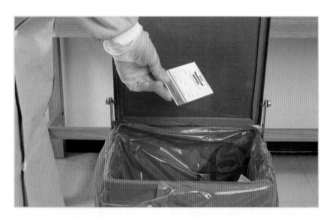

11. Dispose of PPE and finished slides properly.

WHY？ *Biohazardous material must be disposed of according to OSHA protocol to prevent the spread of microorganisms.*

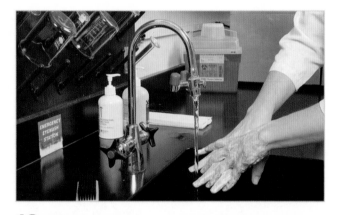

12. Wash hands.

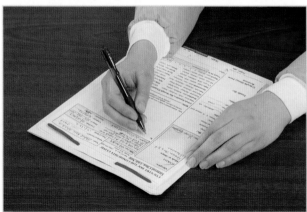

13. Document in the patient's chart and give the results to the physician.

TIP▶ Slides often are mailed back to the office in a special envelope given to the patient. It is crucial to develop slides as soon as they arrive at the office. Do not let them sit in the lab waiting for "someone else" to develop them. A good medical assistant does what needs to be done, when it needs to be done, regardless of whose patient it is!

✎ **Charting Example**

2/19/08 8:45 a.m. Patient instructed in home occult blood collection, written and verbal instructions given.
_____ C. Leschi, CMA

CHAPTER 6

Diagnostic Testing

INTRODUCTION

Diagnostic testing at the bedside using CLIA waived and other tests is a major part of a medical assistant's duties. Proper performance of testing procedures and of specimen collection is extremely important for the care and diagnosis of patient conditions. Providers count on the medical assistant to collect and/or process specimens accurately so that the patients may be treated accordingly. Accurate testing ensures that the patient is diagnosed quickly, avoiding serious health complications.

PROCEDURES

6-1 Perform Electrocardiography Using a 12-Lead, Three-Channel Electrocardiograph

6-2 Perform Respiratory Testing Using a Peak Flow Meter

6-3 Perform Urinalysis (CLIA Waived)

6-4 Perform Hematology Testing Using Sediplast Westergren ESR (CLIA Waived)

6-5 Perform Hematology Testing Using a Hemoglobin Test (CLIA Waived)

6-6 Perform Chemistry Testing of Cholesterol Using CardioChek (CLIA Waived)

6-7 Perform Immunology Testing Using a Monospot Test (CLIA Waived)

6-8 Perform Immunology Testing Using a Rapid Strep Test (CLIA Waived)

6-9 Perform Microbiology Testing: Inoculate a Culture

Procedure **6-1**

Perform Electrocardiography Using a 12-Lead, Three-Channel Electrocardiograph

PURPOSE

Electrocardiography (EKG) is a noninvasive procedure that gives the provider information needed to diagnose and treat problems with a patient's cardiac rhythm. It is crucial for the medical assistant to perform an EKG correctly and to be able to recognize artifacts (disturbances) that affect a good EKG tracing.

EQUIPMENT/SUPPLIES

- 12-lead EKG machine with the electrodes and cords
- electrolyte media
- cape or gown
- alcohol preps/antiseptic wipes
- tissue or gauze
- soap
- water
- razor
- patient chart
- pen
- gloves (if indicated by office protocol)

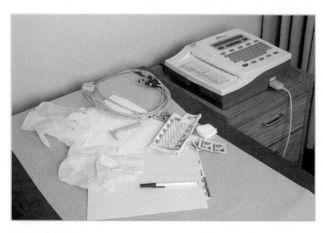

1. Gather EKG machine and equipment and supplies and wash hands.

Prepare the room and check the machine and calibration before the patient enters or before you bring a portable machine to the patient.

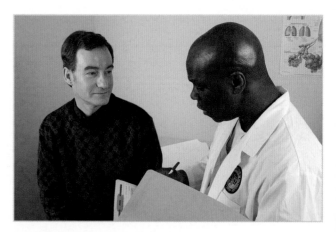

2. Identify the patient.

WHY? *This avoids errors in treatment.*

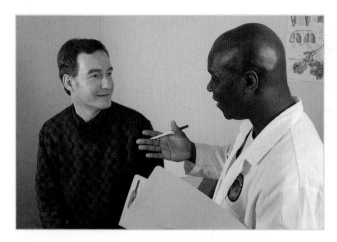

3. Explain the procedure.

ᵂᴴʸ❓ *Doing this helps alleviate any concerns and puts the patient at ease.*

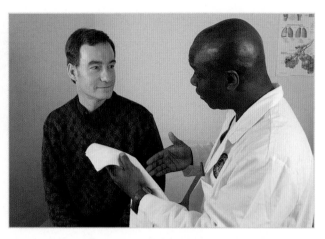

4. Provide a cape or gown and instruct patient to undress from waist up. Women must remove bra and nylons. It is also good to have the patient remove all jewelry and watches.

ᵂᴴʸ❓ *This avoids artifacts that can affect the reading.*

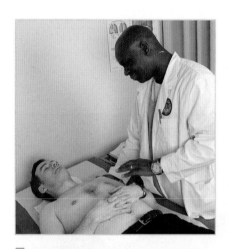

5. Position patient in the supine position.

ᵂᴴʸ❓ *If the patient is comfortable, movement is less likely, so artifacts can be avoided.*

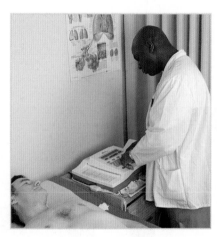

6. Turn on machine and enter all required patient information.

ᵂᴴʸ❓ *Some digital machines allow you to enter patient information on the machine; this information is then transferred directly to the recording.*

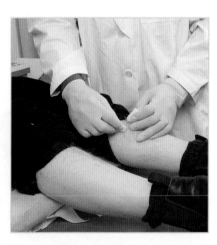

7. Prepare patient skin at sites of electrode placement by cleaning with antiseptic wipes or alcohol wipes if necessary. Shave if necessary due to too much hair.

ᵂᴴʸ❓ *Skin oil, lotion, topical medications, sun block, hair, etc. must be removed for the electrodes to have good contact with the skin.*

➤ Wear gloves per office protocol.

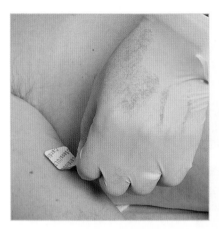

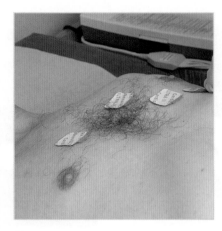

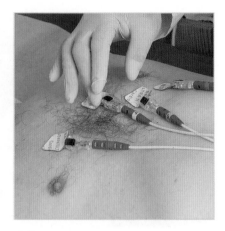

8. Apply electrodes to the arms and legs using the appropriate type and amount of conducting media (gel, lotion, pads) for the type of electrodes used with the machine.

WHY❓ *This helps ensure accurate transmission and readings.*

9. Apply chest electrodes (these may be different from those used on the limbs).

10. Connect lead wires from machine to the electrodes.

WHY❓ *Correctly placed leads ensure accurate reading and prevent having to re-test.*

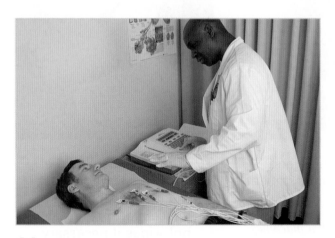

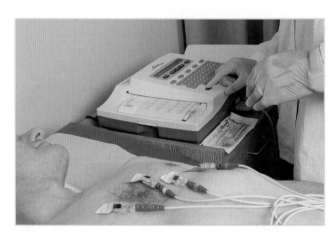

11. Instruct patient to lie still and start the EKG tracing by pressing the appropriate button (usually "automatic"). Sensitivity is usually set on 1 and speed is 25 mm/second.

WHY❓ *Having the patient lie still and not talk helps avoid artifacts.*

12. Allow tracing to complete and print.

TIP➤ If it is a single-channel EKG, it will read only one lead at a time and print a narrow continuous strip beginning with lead I and continuing through V6. This will require that the strip be cut and the best segment of each lead be mounted on a sheet to create a one-page tracing for the physician.

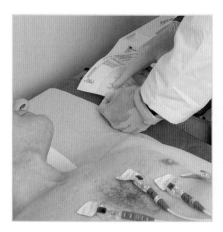

13. Verify that the standardization mark is accurate and check the tracing for artifacts.

WHY❓ *Do this to make sure the machine is operating properly.*

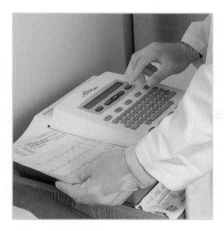

14. If any leads are inadequate, re-run those leads affected or the entire tracing until an accurate tracing is achieved.

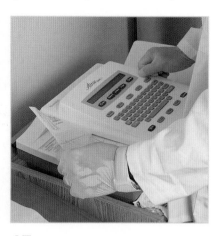

15. When a good tracing is obtained, tear off the tracing, save and clear patient data and turn off the machine.

TIP▶ If the physician is waiting, leave the patient connected and show the tracing to the physician. If not and it is a routine EKG, instruct the patient to go ahead and dress. Some providers want to see all EKGs prior to the patient leaving the clinic; follow office protocol on this.

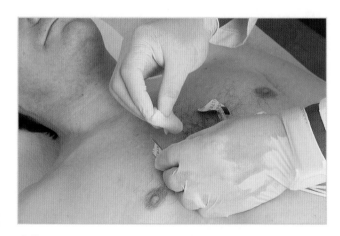

16. Clean the patient's skin of the electrolyte or provide supplies for them to do so after you leave the room.

WHY❓ *This promotes patient comfort.*

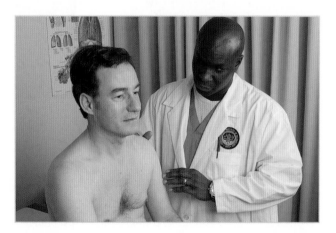

17. Assist patient in sitting up and ensure the patient is not dizzy.

WHY❓ *It is important to ensure patient safety.*

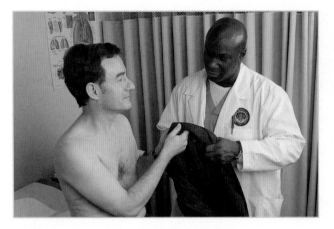

18. Instruct patient to dress.

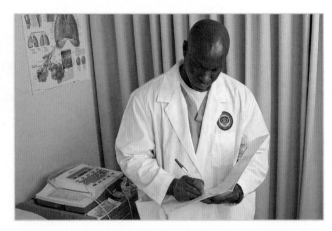

19. Document the procedure per office protocol and give the tracing with the chart to the provider.

If previous EKGs are available, mark those somehow by folding or attaching a sticky note so the provider can easily locate them.

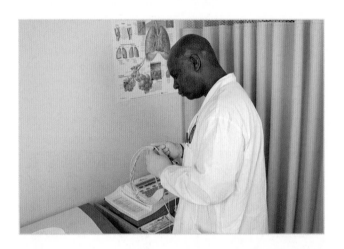

20. Clean and put away all supplies.

If the patient experiences any discomfort or problems during the EKG, discontinue and summon the physician immediately, but do not leave patient alone. Chart the situation.

Charting Examples

07/08/2007 10:00 a.m. Routine 12-lead EKG obtained, no adverse reactions. No follow-up appointment needed. _____ T. Holliker, CMA

07/08/2007 2:00 p.m. 12-lead EKG started, pt. complained of some chest discomfort, EKG discontinued and MD summoned immediately. _____ B. Lyon, CMA

Procedure 6-2

Perform Respiratory Testing Using a Peak Flow Meter

PURPOSE

Performing respiratory testing will help the provider assess pulmonary function in patients who have difficulty breathing due to asthma, bronchitis, or other diseases. Anticipating your provider by performing a peak flow measurement before the patient is seen promotes quality patient care and time management.

EQUIPMENT/SUPPLIES

- peak flow meter
- disposable mouthpiece
- normal values graph
- height bar
- patient chart
- pen

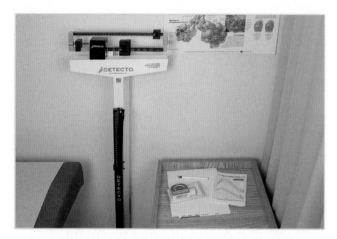

1. Gather all supplies and wash hands.

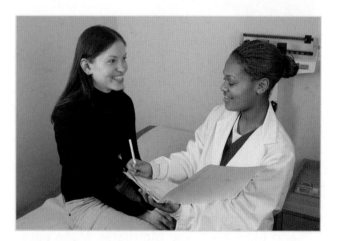

2. Identify the patient.

✓WHY？ *This avoids errors in treatment.*

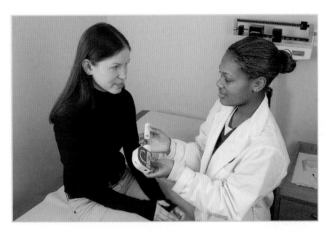

3. Explain the procedure. It is often helpful to "act" as if you are the patient and go through the motions without really blowing into the meter.

WHY? *This helps patients feel at ease when they can clearly see what they are to do.*

TIP Normal values for pulmonary function are determined by gender, age, and height, so be sure to check the chart or measure the patient's height prior to performing the test.

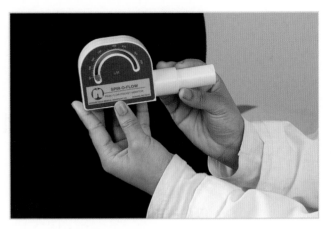

4. Assemble the peak flow meter with the disposable mouthpiece, making sure the arrow is set at 0.

WHY? *Proper assembly is essential for obtaining accurate results.*

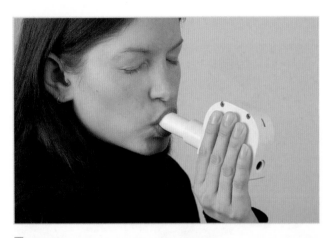

5. Instruct the patient to take a deep breath and blow hard into the meter. Make sure that their lips are sealed around the mouthpiece.

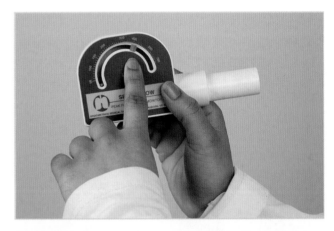

6. Read the number on the meter, reset to zero, and record the measurement.

TIP Allow the patient a minute to recover before the next breath.

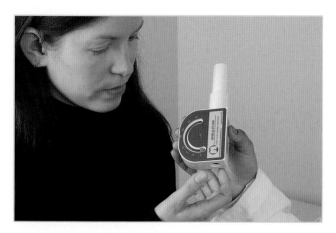

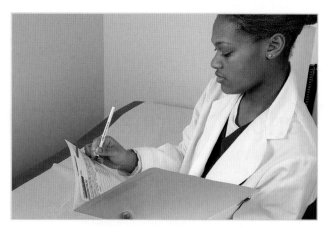

7. Repeat the procedure two more times for a total of three readings.

 If the patient is being seen for acute breathing difficulty, relay the results to the physician right away.

 It is good practice to get the O_2 saturation at this time. You may have to administer a nebulizer treatment after the provider sees the patient. Your instructor can teach you these procedures.

8. Document the procedure, being sure to note the expected or normal value for the age and gender.

 Dispose of mouthpiece per OSHA regulations.

✎ **Charting Example**

10/12/07 3:20 p.m. Age: 34, Ht. 5"6". Peak flow 450, 340, 410, Exp: 480. _____ B. Jones, CMA

Procedure **6-3**

Perform a Urinalysis (CLIA Waived)

PURPOSE

Testing urine by using a chemical strip assists the provider in diagnosing and treating urinary or metabolic disorders.

EQUIPMENT/SUPPLIES

- clean catch patient urine sample
- urine reagent test strips
- urinalysis results sheet
- PPE
- paper towel

- patient chart
- pen
- watch with second hand
- biohazard waste container

STANDARD PRECAUTIONS

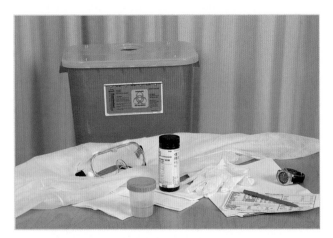

1. Gather all supplies and wash hands. Check the expiration date on the testing supplies.

   ᴡʜʏ❓ *Outdated products may not give accurate results.*

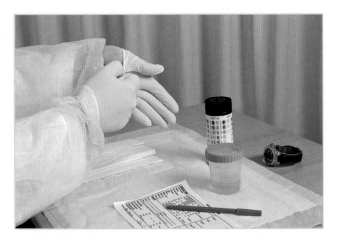

2. Apply PPE.

   ᴡʜʏ❓ *Practicing Standard Precautions helps prevent the spread of infection.*

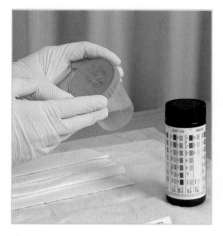

3. Identify the sample by checking the patient's name written on the container.

ᴡʜʏ❓ *Correctly identifying the specimen avoids errors.*

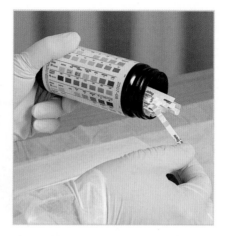

4. Remove the urine test strip by shaking the bottle and removing a strip carefully, being sure to replace the lid tightly.

ᴡʜʏ❓ *Do not contaminate other strips by touching the inside of the bottle. Strips are sensitive to moisture and light, which is why they are in a black bottle with a moisture-absorbing pack.*

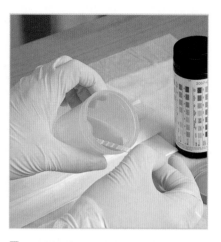

5. Open the urine container and insert the test strip.

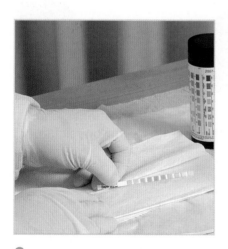

6. Tap the test strip on a paper towel to remove excess urine and set it on the towel on the counter.

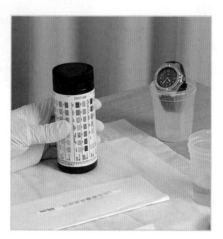

7. Observe the proper timing for each square on the test strip.

ᴡʜʏ❓ *Timing correctly is critical to obtaining proper results.*

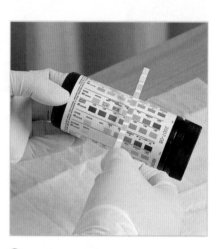

8. Hold the test strip and read the results by matching the color on the strip to the color chart on the bottle.

TIP▶ *Be careful not to touch the strip to the bottle as this will cause contamination.*

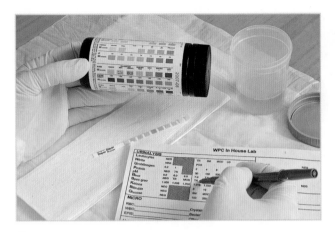

9. Document on the test results sheet.

⊳ Each office will have its own internal paperwork for logging these results. Often they match the order and type of test to the urinalysis test bottle your office uses.

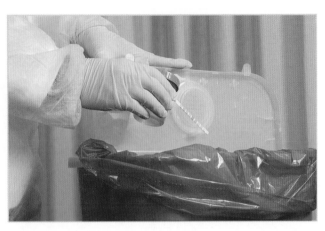

10. Dispose of all materials, put away all supplies according to OSHA regulations, and wash hands.

WHY❓ *Biohazardous material must be disposed of correctly to prevent the spread of microorganisms.*

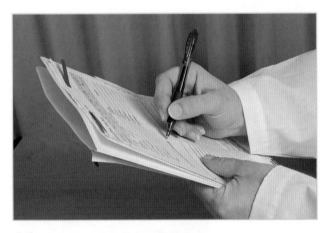

11. Document the procedure.

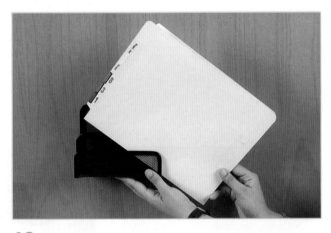

12. Place the results on the patient's chart and give the results to the physician.

⊳ It may be necessary to make sure the physician sees the results before entering the examination room to see the patient.

 Charting Example

10/24/07 11:15 a.m. Performed chemical UA, ++ protein, all others WNL, results given to physician. _____ B. Jones, CMA

Procedure 6-4

Perform Hematology Testing Using Sediplast Westergren ESR (CLIA Waived)

PURPOSE

Performing hematology testing supplies information that can help the provider diagnose and manage certain blood disorders.

EQUIPMENT/SUPPLIES

- PPE
- blood sample in EDTA tube
- Sediplast Westergren ESR kit
- gauze
- patient chart
- pen
- timer
- biohazard waste container
- requisition slip
- sedivial
- rack

STANDARD PRECAUTIONS

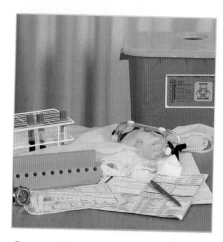

1. Gather all supplies. Check the expiration date on the testing supplies.

WHY? *Outdated products may not give accurate results.*

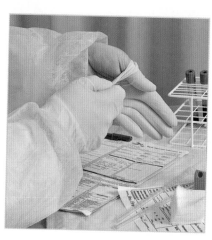

2. Wash hands and apply PPE.

WHY? *Practicing Standard Precautions helps prevent the spread of infection.*

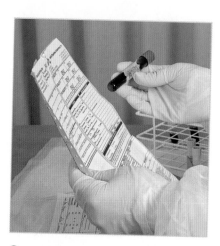

3. Identify patient sample with name and number on EDTA blood tube.

WHY? *This avoids errors in treatment.*

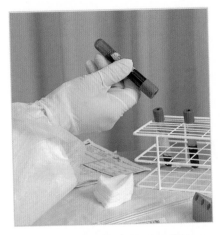

4. Gently mix blood sample from a room temperature EDTA blood tube for 2 minutes.

WHY? *Timing correctly is critical to obtaining proper results.*

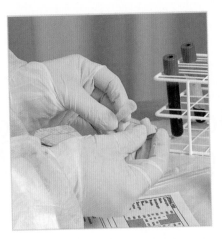

5. Remove stopper on sedivial.

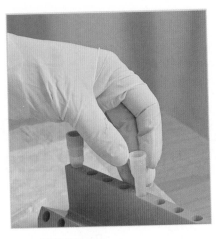

6. Place sedivial in Sediplast rack on a level surface.

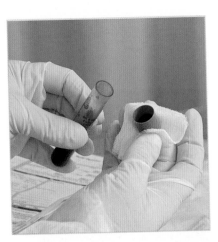

7. Carefully open the blood sample vial using gauze.

WHY? *This prevents getting blood all over gloves or spray in face.*

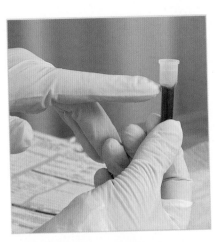

8. Fill sedivial to the indicated mark with blood sample.

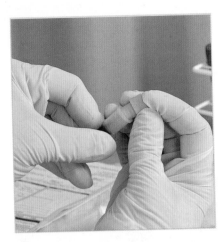

9. Replace stopper.

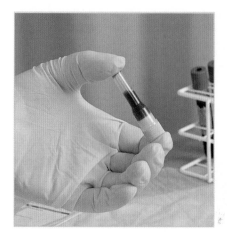

10. Invert vial several times to mix.

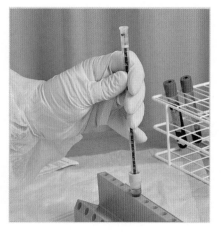

11. Replace sedivial in rack and gently insert the disposable Sediplast tube through the stopper with a twisting motion, pushing down until the tube rests on the bottom of the vial and the blood level is at 0.

ᴡʜʏ❓ *The blood level must be at 0 to ensure accurate reading.*

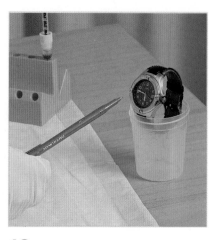

12. Set timer for 1 hour.

ᴡʜʏ❓ *Proper timing is critical for accurate results)*

▷ᴛ Testing must be performed out of the light and on a vibration-free counter to ensure accurate blood sedimentation.

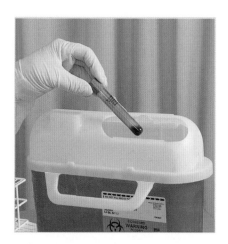

13. Dispose of blood tube per OSHA regulations or return to proper storage.

ᴡʜʏ❓ *Biohazardous material must be disposed of correctly to prevent the spread of micro-organisms.*

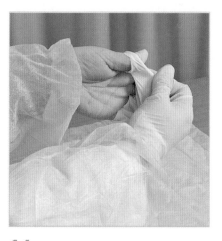

14. Remove gloves, dispose of properly per OSHA regulations, and wash hands (if not performing any other laboratory tests at this time).

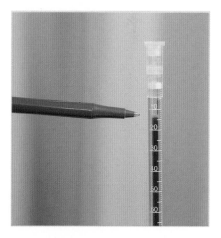

15. When 1 hour has passed, re-glove and read the results on the tube. (The scale is on the side of the tube; read from top to bottom.)

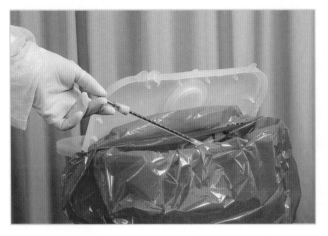

16. Dispose of all equipment, put away all supplies per OSHA regulations, and wash hands.

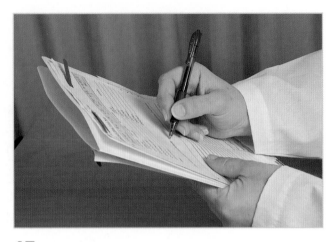

17. Document the procedure.

✎ *Charting Example*

10/30/07 1:15 p.m. Westergren ESR 12mm/hr. ___ B. Jones, CMA

Procedure 6-5

Perform Hematology Testing Using a Hemoglobin Test (CLIA Waived)

PURPOSE

Performing a hemoglobin test supplies the provider with information needed to diagnosis and treat anemia. The hemoglobin test is normally ordered for patients who have ongoing bleeding problems or chronic anemias or polycythemias.

EQUIPMENT/SUPPLIES

- PPE
- blood sample in EDTA tube or lancet
- alcohol wipes
- band aid
- hemoglobinometer
- pipette
- test strips, gauze
- patient chart
- pen
- sharps container
- biohazard waste container

STANDARD PRECAUTIONS

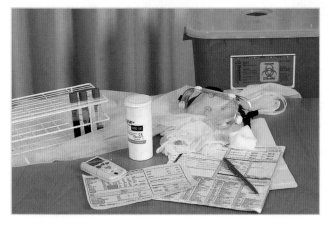

1. Gather all supplies. Check the expiration date on the testing supplies.

ᴡʜʏ❓ *Outdated products may not give accurate results.*

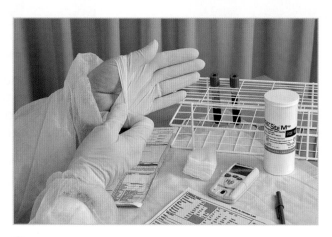

2. Wash hands and apply PPE.

ᴡʜʏ❓ *Practicing Standard Precautions helps prevent the spread of infection.*

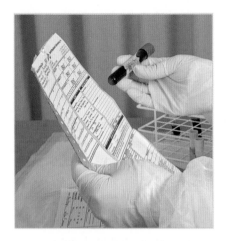

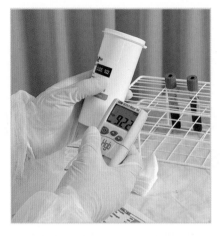

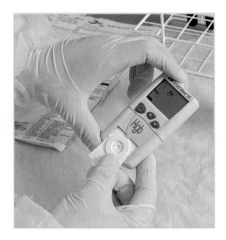

3. Identify patient, either in person or by the name on the blood tube.

ᴡʜʏ❓ *This avoids errors in treatment.*

4. Turn on hemoglobinometer, being sure to match the code on the screen with the code on the test strip vial.

ᴡʜʏ❓ *This ensures test accuracy.*

5. Insert the test strip into the machine.

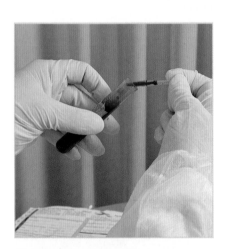

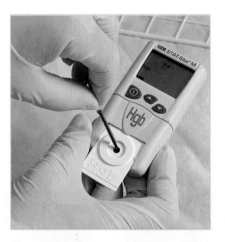

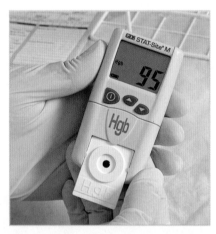

6. Obtain blood sample, either by direct finger stick or with a pipette from a room temperature EDTA blood tube that has been gently mixed for 2 minutes.

7. Apply one drop of blood onto the test strip, being sure to soak the sample area on the test strip.

ᴡʜʏ❓ *Proper sample amount ensures accurate results.*

8. Wait the appropriate time interval (the machine counts down for you and beeps).

ᴡʜʏ❓ *Proper timing ensures accurate results.*

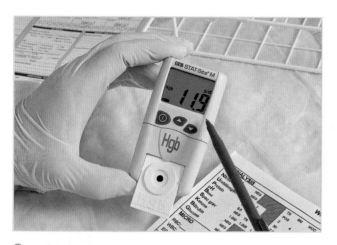

9. Read the result.

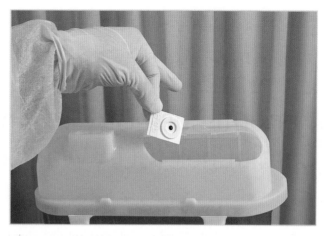

10. Dispose of all equipment and put away supplies per OSHA regulations.

WHY? *Biohazardous material must be disposed of correctly to prevent the spread of microorganisms.*

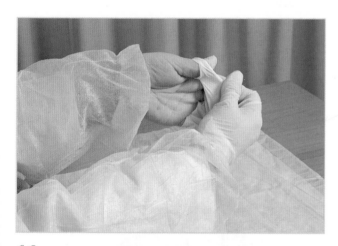

11. Remove PPE, dispose of it in the proper biohazard container according to OSHA protocol, and wash hands.

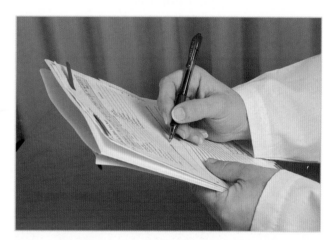

12. Document the procedure.

✎ *Charting Example*

10/12/07 9:45 a.m. Hemoglobin 11.9g/dl. _____ A. Nyguyen, CMA

Procedure **6-6**

Perform Chemistry Testing of Cholesterol Using CardioChek (CLIA Waived)

PURPOSE

Performing a cholesterol test supplies the provider with information needed to diagnosis potential high or problem cholesterol levels and avoids the patient having to return to the clinic for a blood draw.

EQUIPMENT/SUPPLIES

- PPE
- CardioChek meter
- memo chip for correct test
- test strip vial
- lancet
- calibrated capillary tube and plunger
- alcohol wipe

- gauze
- bandage
- patient chart
- pen
- sharps container
- biohazard waste container
- internal result slip

STANDARD PRECAUTIONS

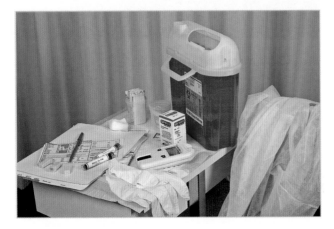

1. Gather all supplies and wash hands. Check the expiration date on the testing supplies and turn on the machine.

ᴠᴴʏ❓ *Outdated products may not give accurate results.*

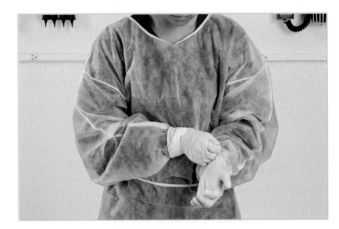

2. Apply PPE (gown and gloves).

ᴠᴴʏ❓ *Practicing Standard Precautions helps prevent the spread of infection.*

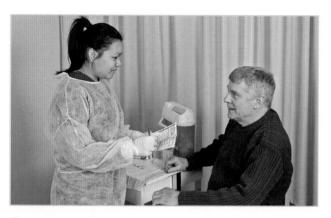

3. Identify the patient.

WHY? *This avoids errors in treatment.*

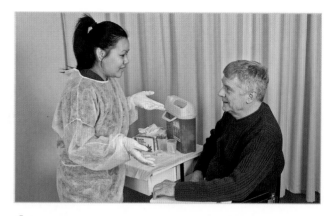

4. Explain the procedure.

WHY? *Doing this helps alleviate any concerns and puts the patient at ease.*

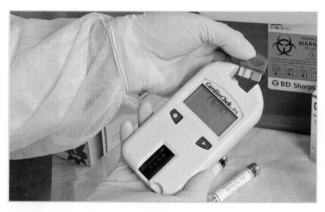

5. Insert memo chip, making sure to use the correct chip for the test you are performing.

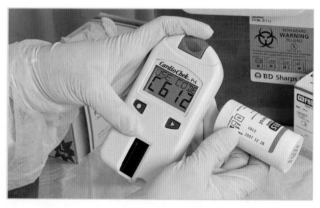

6. Check lot number on chip.

WHY? *This must match test strip vial.*

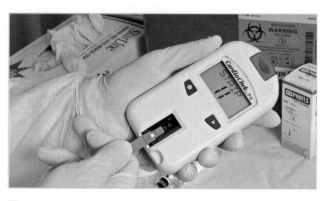

7. Insert test strip.

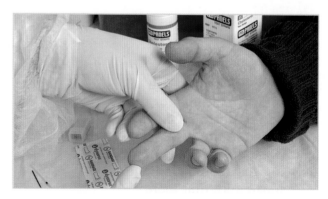

8. Select site on patient's finger. Be sure to choose 11 o'clock or 1 o'clock and go against the grain of the fingerprint.

WHY? *This is important to avoid hitting the bone or damaging nerves and to get the optimal blood drop for the collection of the specimen.*

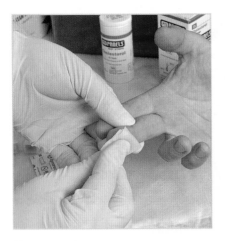

9. Clean the area with alcohol.

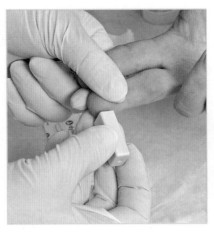

10. Stick the finger. Dispose of the lancet in the sharps container.

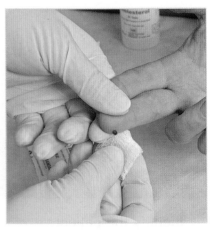

11. Wipe away first drop of blood.

WHY? *This allows for a clean sample without white blood cells or serum from the body's injury response.*

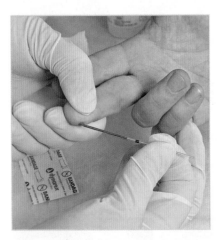

12. Collect blood drop with calibrated capillary tube. Be sure to use the correct tube for the correct test and *collect blood in the black-banded end* while holding the red-banded end. Make sure that there are no air bubbles and that the blood reaches the black band.

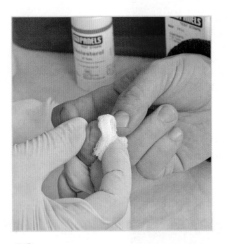

13. Give patient gauze to apply pressure on finger stick.

WHY? *Pressure promotes coagulation.*

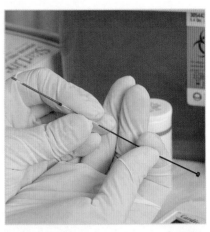

14. Insert plunger, making sure to insert the plunger in the end with the double red band.

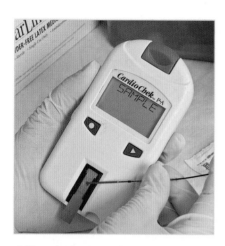

15. Dispense blood.

TIP *Wait until the meter reads "apply sample," then push on the plunger slowly and smoothly, dispensing all of the blood onto the test strip. Be careful not to get blood on the meter.*

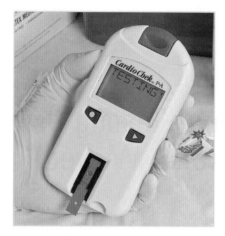

16. Wait the allotted time (the machine times for you; just wait).

WHY? *Proper timing ensures testing accuracy.*

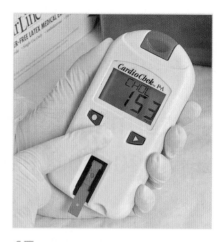

17. Read the results.

TIP *If the meter is connected to a printer, a sticker will print with the results; place this in the patient's chart.*

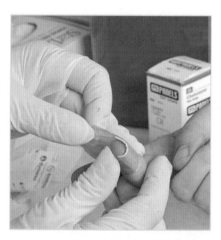

18. Bandage the patient's finger.

WHY? *This protects the puncture site.*

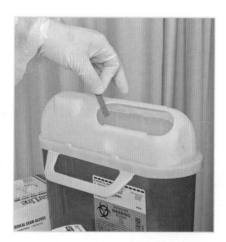

19. Clean and put away all supplies, placing spent capillary tubes and test strips into biohazard/sharps container per OSHA regulations.

WHY? *Biohazardous material must be disposed of correctly to prevent the spread of microorganisms.*

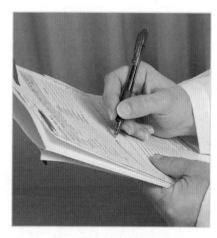

20. Document in chart.

Charting Example

10/13/07 10:45 a.m. Cholesterol 153. _____ A. Hassan, CMA

Procedure 6-7

Perform Immunology Testing Using a Monospot Test (CLIA Waived)

PURPOSE

Performing a mononucleosis test supplies the provider with information needed to diagnosis and treat mono quickly and avoids the patient having to return for a blood draw.

EQUIPMENT/SUPPLIES

- PPE
- Monospot test kit
- timer
- patient chart
- pen
- lancet
- alcohol wipe
- gauze
- bandage
- sharps container
- biohazard waste container
- internal result slip

STANDARD PRECAUTIONS

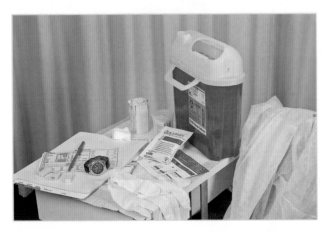

1. Gather all supplies and wash hands. Check the expiration date on the testing supplies.

ᴡʜʏ❓ *Outdated products may not give accurate results.*

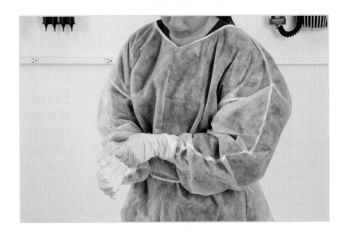

2. Apply PPE.

ᴡʜʏ❓ *Practicing Standard Precautions helps prevent the spread of infection.*

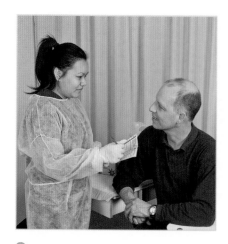

3. Identify the patient.

WHY❓ *This avoids errors in treatment.*

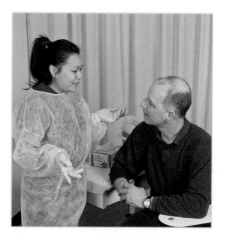

4. Explain the procedure.

WHY❓ *Doing this helps alleviate any concerns and puts the patient at ease.*

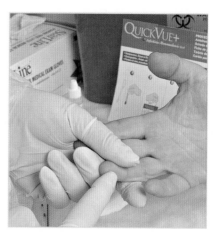

5. Select site on patient's finger. Choose 11 o'clock or 1 o'clock and go against the grain of the fingerprint.

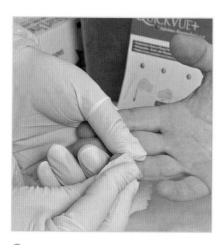

6. Clean the area with alcohol.

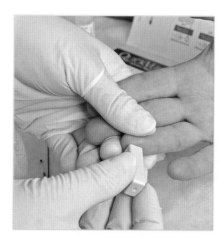

7. Stick finger. Dispose of the lancet in the sharps container per OSHA regulations.

WHY❓ *Biohazardous material must be disposed of correctly to prevent the spread of microorganisms.*

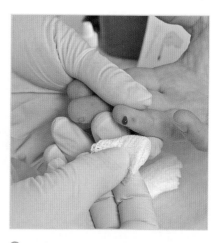

8. Wipe away first drop of blood.

WHY❓ *This allows for a clean sample without white blood cells or serum from the body's injury response*

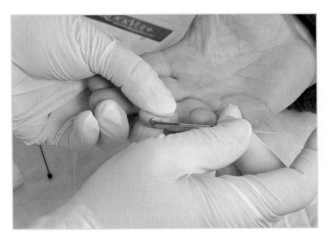

9. Collect blood drop with calibrated pipette, making sure to use the correct pipette that comes with the test.

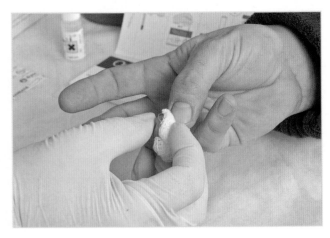

10. Apply gauze to patient's finger, having them apply pressure.

WHY? *Pressure promotes coagulation*

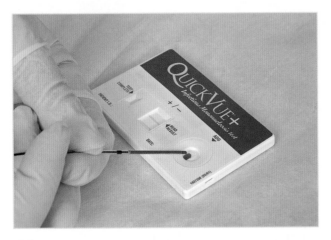

11a. Apply blood sample to test.

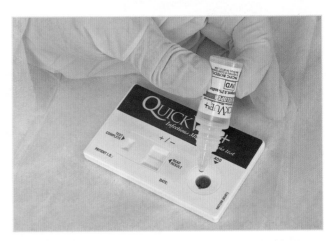

11b. Apply developer to sample.

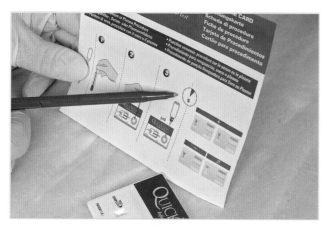

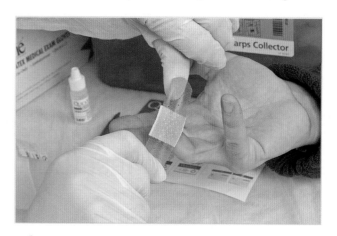

12. Wait the appropriate time interval per manufacturer's instructions.

13. Bandage the patient's finger.

WHY❓ *Proper timing ensures accurate results.*

TIP▶ Each test kit has its own instructions from the manufacturer; always be sure to follow the instructions given with any test kit.

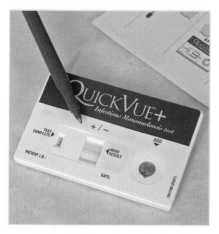

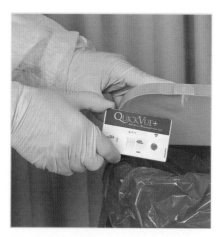

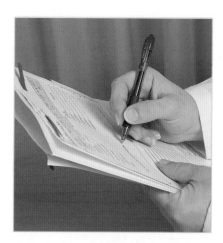

14. Read the results.

15. Clean and put away all supplies and wash hands per OSHA regulations.

16. Document the procedure.

 Charting Example

3/12/2007 9:15 a.m. Monospot negative. _____ J. Bajado, CMA

Procedure 6-8

Perform Immunology Testing Using a Rapid Strep Test (CLIA Waived)

PURPOSE

Performing a rapid strep test allows the provider to determine quickly if certain pathogens are present in the patient's throat, ensuring appropriate treatment is initiated.

EQUIPMENT/SUPPLIES

- PPE
- rapid strep test kit
- throat culture swab
- tongue depressor
- patient chart
- pen
- biohazard waste container
- internal result strip

STANDARD PRECAUTIONS

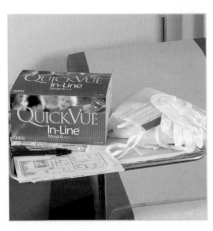

1. Assemble all equipment and wash hands. Check expiration dates on all testing supplies.

WHY? *Outdated products may not give accurate results.*

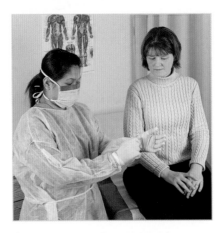

2. Apply PPE.

WHY? *Practicing Standard Precautions helps prevent the spread of infection.*

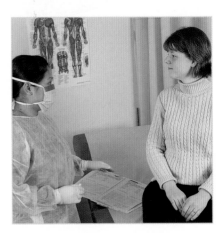

3. Identify the patient.

WHY? *This avoids errors in treatment.*

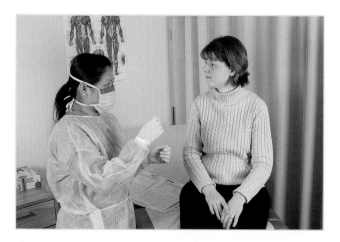

4. Explain the procedure.

WHY❓ *Doing this helps alleviate any concerns and puts the patient at ease.*

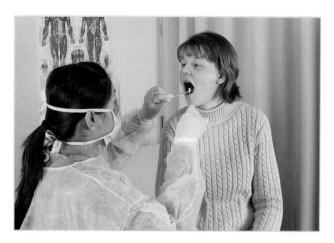

5. Obtain throat swab, using the appropriate swab that is supplied with the test kit.

WHY❓ *This ensures accurate results.*

TIP Sometimes you will use two culture swabs at once: one for the rapid test and one culture swab to send to the lab. This avoids having to swab the patient's throat twice.

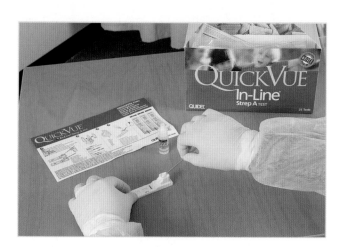

6. Insert swab into test chamber.

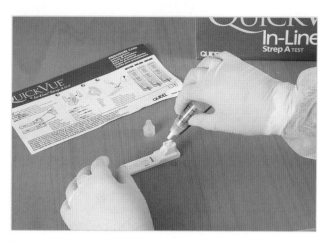

7. Apply reagents provided in the kit to the test chamber.

TIP Each test kit has its own instructions. Steps may be slightly different than those shown in this procedure. Be sure to follow all manufacturer's instructions.

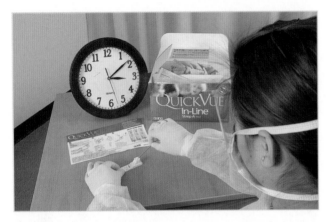

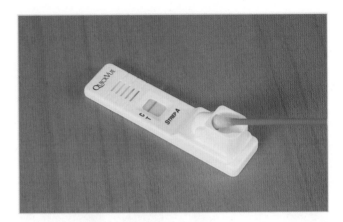

8. Wait appropriate time interval per manu-facturer instructions.

WHY? *Timing correctly is critical to obtaining proper results.*

9. Read test results.

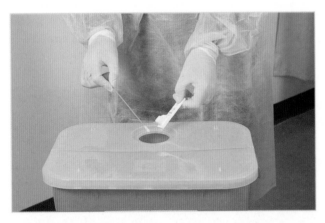

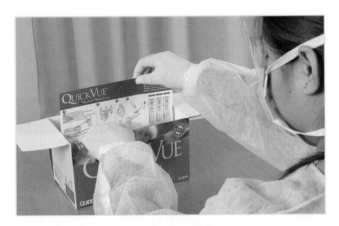

10. Dispose of used swab and test chamber per OSHA regulations.

WHY? *Biohazardous material must be disposed of correctly to prevent the spread of microorganisms.*

11. Clean and put away all supplies per OSHA guidelines and wash hands.

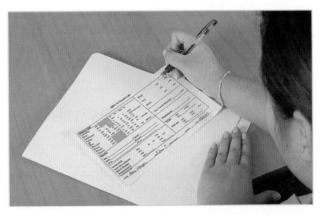

12. Document the procedure.

Charting Example

10/03/07 9:45 a.m. Rapid Strep negative, confirmatory throat culture sent to lab. _____ J. Bajado, CMA

Procedure **6-9**

Perform Microbiology Testing: Inoculate a Culture (CLIA Waived)

PURPOSE

To determine the type of bacteria causing the patient's signs and symptoms, a culture may be taken from the problem area and then applied to a culture plate that contains nutrition for the bacteria to grow. When the plate is then placed in a dark, warm incubator, the bacteria have everything needed to multiply for more extensive study.

EQUIPMENT/SUPPLIES

- patient specimen
- culture plate with medium (Petri Plate)
- disposable inoculating loop
- incubator with temperature indicator
- permanent marker

STANDARD **PRECAUTIONS**

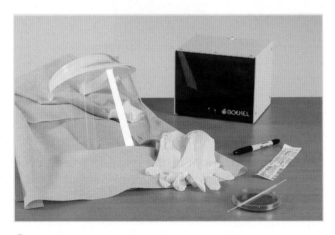

1. Gather all supplies.

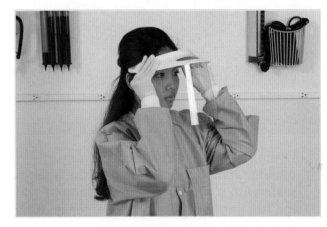

2. Wash hands and apply gloves and face shield.

WHY? *Always wear proper PPE per OSHA guidelines.*

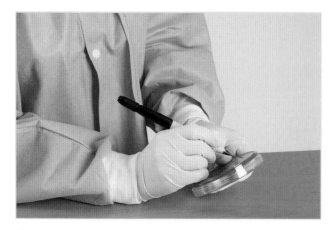

3. Label the medium side of the agar plate with the patient's name, ID number, source of specimen, time collected, time inoculated, your initials, and date.

WHY？ *Incubation may take 24 to 72 hours, so dating ensures that the plate is read at the proper time. Labeling the plate on the medium side ensures that the correct patient sample is tested and there is no confusion when replacing the lid for multiple plates.*

TIP Be sure to check the expiration date and condition of any medium.

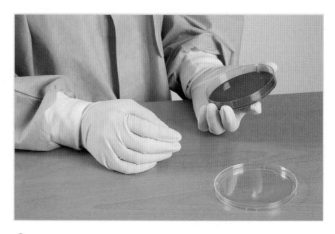

4. Remove the agar plate from the cover and place the cover opening up on the counter to avoid contamination.

TIP The plate is always stored with the cover down.

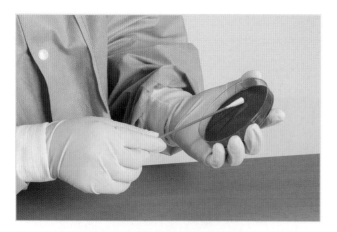

5. Using the specimen swabbed from a patient, apply the specimen to the agar plate with a rolling motion starting at the top and working to the center going almost half of the way.

WHY？ *The specimen spreads, gradually thinning across the medium to isolate colonies of bacteria.*

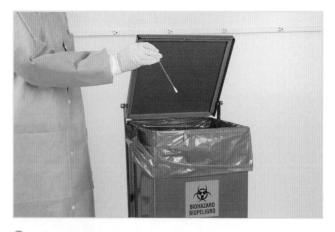

6. Dispose of the culture swab in the appropriate biohazard container.

WHY？ *Always follow OSHA guidelines for safety.*

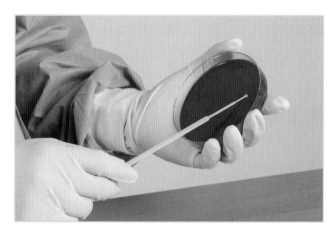

7. Rotate the plate a quarter turn and use a sterile disposable loop to spread the specimen by dragging the loop through the original inoculum and out into the agar using about one quarter of the agar area.

TIP Do not enter the originally streaked area after the first few sweeps of the loop.

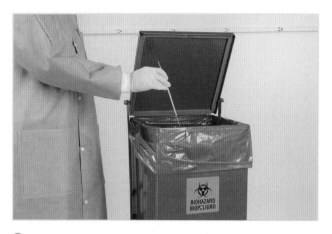

8. Dispose of this loop in the appropriate biohazard container.

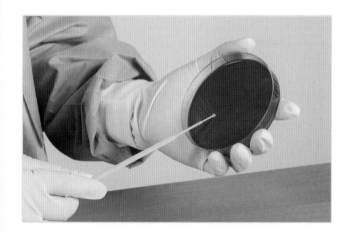

9. Rotate the plate another quarter turn so it is 180 degrees from the original smear and use a new disposable sterile loop to spread the specimen further by dragging the loop in the same manner at right angles through the most recently streaked area.

TIP Do not enter the originally streaked area after the first few sweeps of the loop.

WHY? Isolated colonies are easier to identify with this method.

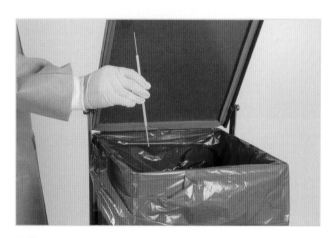

10. Dispose of this loop in the appropriate biohazard container.

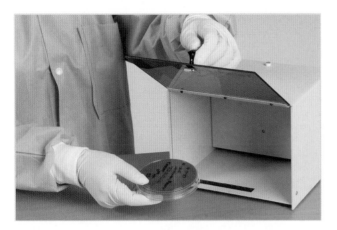

11. Replace lid on the plate and place upside down in an incubator for the appropriate time and temperature per office policy.

TIP➤ Be sure to follow office policy on any sensitivity testing required.

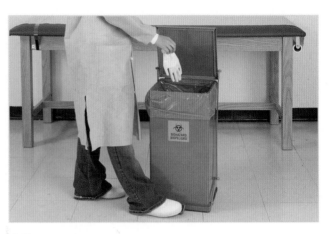

12. Remove PPE and wash hands.

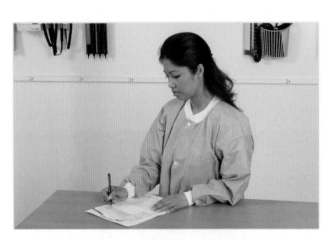

13. Document appropriately per office policy.

 Charting Example

12/13/2007 10:45 a.m. Swab of wound on right hand taken and inoculated to culture medium for incubation. To be read 12/15/2007. Sensitivity testing to be performed if indicated. Patient given both verbal and written wound care instructions. Will return to clinic in 3 days for follow-up appt. _____ A. Gregersen, CMA

CHAPTER 7

Patient Care

INTRODUCTION

Patient care is one of the medical assistant's most important jobs. Patients always come first in any medical office; they are the reason for the existence of the office and its staff. As the liaison between the provider and the patient, the medical assistant is often the first professional that patients encounter in the office. Accuracy, efficiency, and professionalism are key attributes of the medical assistant. The smooth flow of care and treatment keeps the office functioning at peak levels and enables the provider to focus on the patient. Crucial to this is a thorough knowledge of the various procedures and examinations performed, whether routine or specialty. Keeping current through continuing education and research is vital for the medical assistant to maintain quality of care and knowledge and to better assist and anticipate the patient's and the provider's needs.

PROCEDURES

Procedure 7-1

Perform Telephone Screening

PURPOSE

Telephone screening is one of the medical assistant's primary administrative duties. By carefully listening to patient concerns, asking pertinent questions, and recording the answers, the medical assistant can gather key information needed by the provider. Effective telephone screening also ensures that patients with emergencies receive immediate and appropriate care. Other aspects of telephone screening involve handling voice mail messages, returning calls, and notifying patients about lab results.

EQUIPMENT/SUPPLIES

- message pad
- patient chart
- telephone
- pen

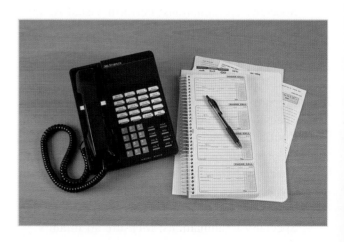

1. Gather all supplies.

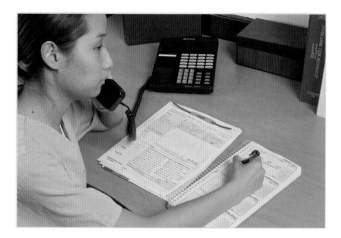

2. Identify the patient. Ask pertinent questions (location, radiation, quality, quantity, associated manifestations, aggravating factors, alleviating factors, setting, and timing).

WHY? *By gathering as much information as possible about the patient's condition or problem, the medical assistant can determine how to prioritize or handle the patient's call. If the patient's situation is life threatening, follow office protocol for emergencies.*

TIP Therapeutic communication is critical, as is maintaining the patient's confidentiality.

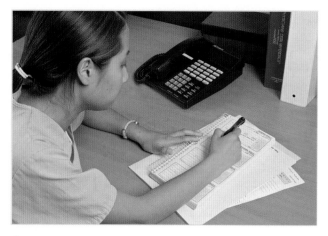

3. Document the conversation on the message pad. This will be transferred to the patient's chart after discussing the situation with the provider.

LEGAL ALERT! Always document everything concerning a patient in case of litigation. Remember: If it wasn't charted, it wasn't done.

TIP Document the date, time, patient's name, concern, and any other information given by the patient.

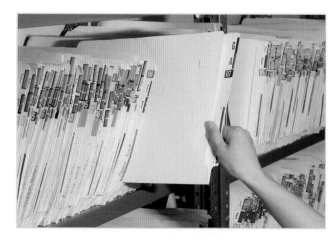

4. Pull the patient's chart.

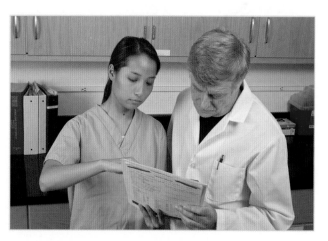

5. Discuss the patient's situation with the physician.

TIP Document any physician orders in the chart.

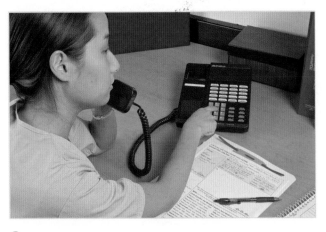

6. Call the patient back.

WHY? *By returning patient calls, the medical assistant ensures follow-up, provides for the patient's needs, and builds the patient's confidence in the practice.*

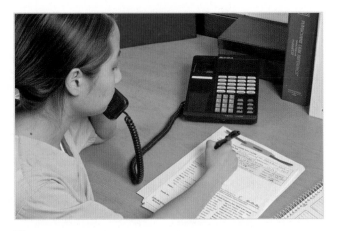

7. Get the patient an appointment, or give the physician's recommendations to the patient.

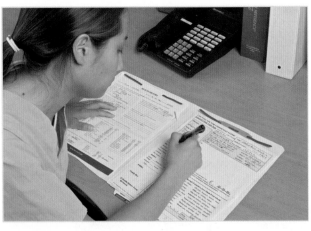

8. Document in the patient's chart (Box 7-1).

✎ *Charting Example*

6/8/07 2:25 p.m. Pt. called stating symptoms of migraine x 2d. Wants Imitrex refill. Per Dr. Jones, called in Imitrex 40mg, 1 p.o. prn, not to exceed 3xd, to Bartell's on 5th Street. _____ A. Bagdasarova, CMA

Box 7·1   **General Charting Tip**

Whenever you document in the patient's medical record, always use black ink, make corrections within legal guidelines, and only use abbreviations accepted by your office.

Procedure 7-2

Perform In-person Screening

PURPOSE

Performing in-person screening correctly is vital to maintaining smooth patient flow and providing quality care. To do this, the medical assistant must obtain all pertinent information before the physician enters the room. The medical assistant also must anticipate the physician's needs, prepare the patient for the exam, and make the patient feel at ease. Therapeutic communication is key, as is completing this task as quickly as possible.

EQUIPMENT/SUPPLIES

- confidential area
- patient chart
- any pertinent office forms
- pen
- equipment to perform vitals: scale, stethoscope, sphygmomanometer, thermometer, watch with second hand
- gown

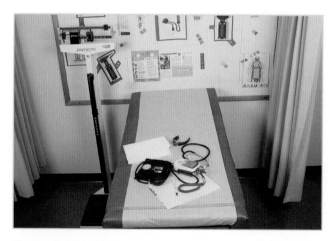

1. Gather all supplies.

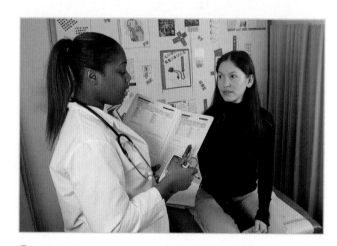

2. Identify the patient. Take the patient to the exam room and obtain vital signs.

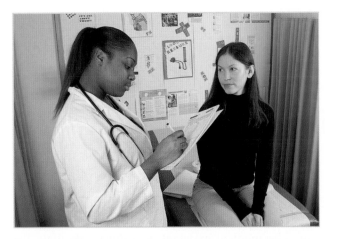

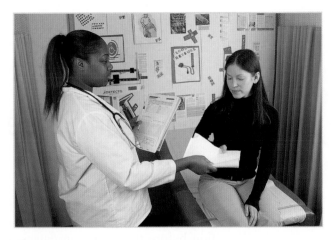

3. Determine the patient's chief complaint by asking pertinent questions (location, radiation, quality, quantity, associated manifestations, aggravating factors, alleviating factors, setting, and timing).

 Always ask about medications, allergies, and supplements at each visit. Be clear, concise and complete when taking a chief complaint.

4. Prepare the patient for the physician.

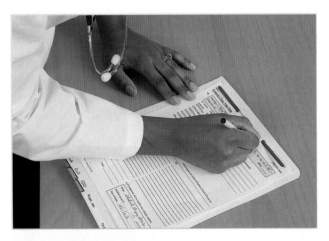

5. Document in the patient's chart.

✎ **Charting Example**

7/2/07 10:15 a.m. CC: Pt complains of backache x 1 w. Takes Advil 800mg, q 8 h with no relief. Throbbing pain radiating down left leg, pain scale 5/10, denies any injury. T 98.6 oral, P 72, R 18, BP 120/80, UA WNL, Urine preg. Neg. Takes no other meds. NKDA.

L. Forshey, CMA

Procedure 7-3

Obtain Vital Signs

PURPOSE

Vital signs, also called cardinal signs, are obtained at all patient visits. Because these measurements reflect important body functions, the medical assistant must know their normal values as well as factors that can affect them. Performing this task accurately and efficiently ensures a smooth patient flow and helps the physician provide proper care.

EQUIPMENT/SUPPLIES

- patient chart
- patient
- sphygmomanometer
- stethoscope
- scale
- height chart
- thermometer and protective sheath
- watch with a second hand
- pen
- paper towel

STANDARD **PRECAUTIONS**

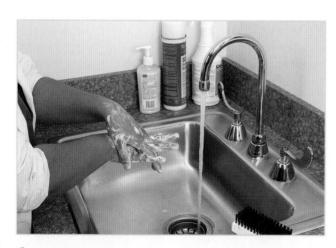

1. Wash hands.

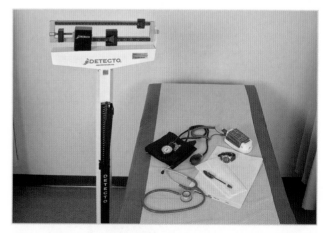

2. Gather all supplies.

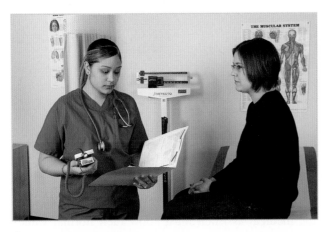

3. Identify the patient and bring the patient back to the clinical area.

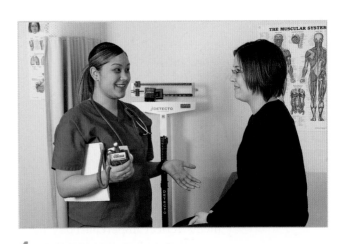

4. Explain the procedure.

WHY? *Therapeutic communication is key, as is putting the patient at ease.*

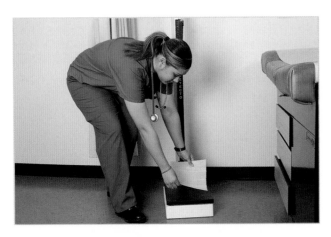

5. Place a paper towel on the scale.

WHY? *This decreases microorganism transmission.*

TIP Many offices have scales outside the exam room, and you will obtain height and weight before entering.

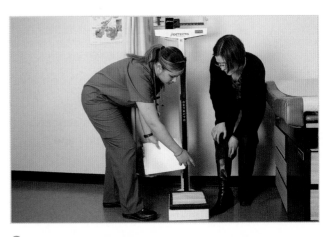

6. Instruct the patient to remove heavy items, shoes, and outerwear.

WHY? *Removing these items helps ensure an accurate measurement.*

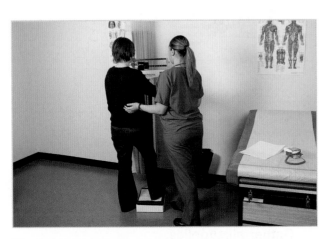

7. Assist patient onto the scale platform, positioning the patient into the center.

WHY? *This helps ensure patient safety and an accurate measurement of the real weight.*

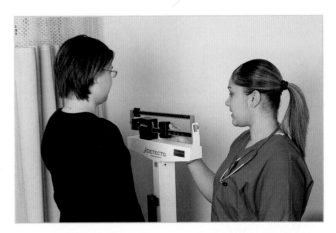

8. Move the lower weight bar to estimated number.

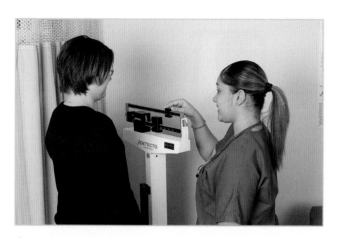

9. Slide the upper weight bar until the balance beam point is centered.

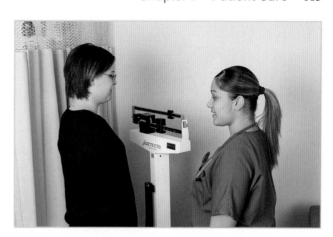

10. Read the weight accurately.

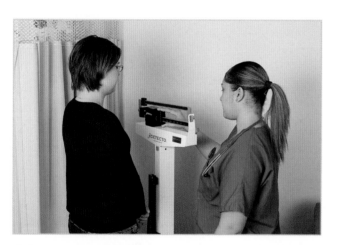

11. Return weights to 0.

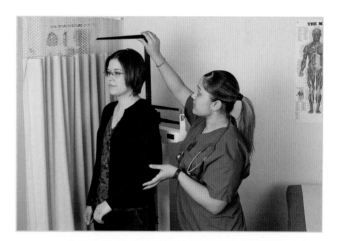

12. Assist the patient in turning on the platform so the patient's back is to the measuring bar. Assist the patient as necessary to step off first, and get back on if necessary, and to stand upright.

WHY❓ *Some patients may lose their balance when changing positions and may require assistance to avoid falling. Patients must stand erect for correct measurement of their height.*

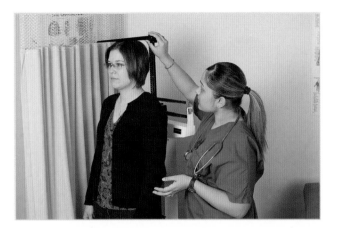

13. Lower the measuring bar until the headrest is positioned firmly atop the patient's head.

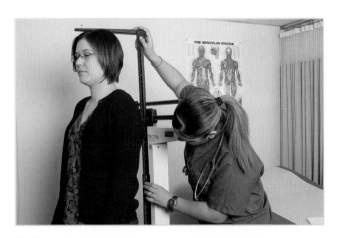

14. Read the line where the measurement falls.

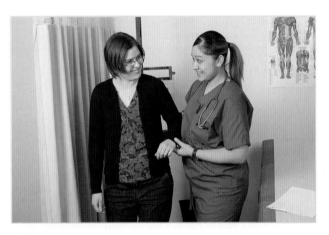

15. Assist the patient in stepping off the scale; assist with shoes, etc., as necessary.

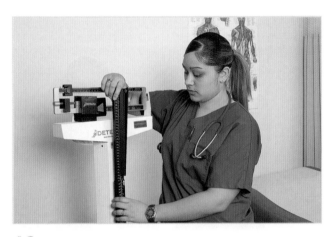

16. Lower the measuring bar to the original position.

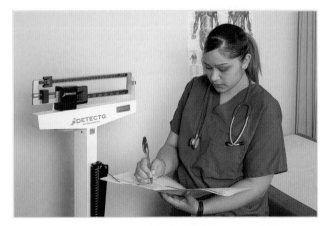

17. Record measurements in the patient chart.

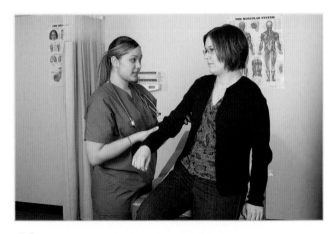

18. Take the patient to the exam room and seat the patient on the exam table.

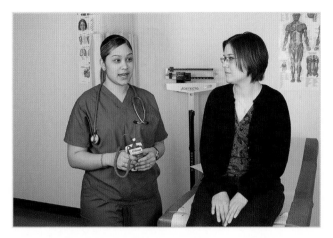

19. Determine if the patient has ingested hot or cold food or drink, or has smoked in the previous half hour.

WHY? *Eating, drinking, or smoking may alter a temperature measurement taken orally or blood pressure reading.*

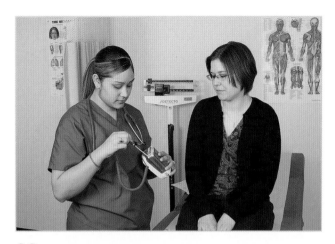

20. Select the thermometer and cover it with a probe cover.

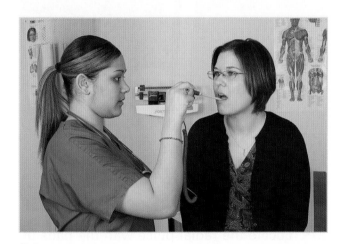

21. Insert the probe under the patient's tongue to the side of the mouth.

WHY? *This placement allows for the most accurate measurement.*

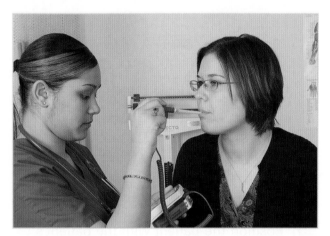

22. Instruct the patient to close the mouth around the thermometer but not to place teeth on it.

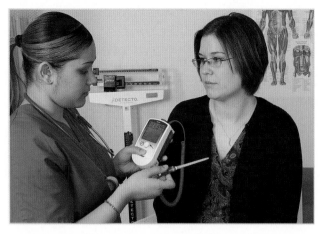

23. Leave the thermometer in place until a beeping sound is heard.

Depending on the type of thermometer used, you can measure the pulse and respiration while the thermometer is in place.

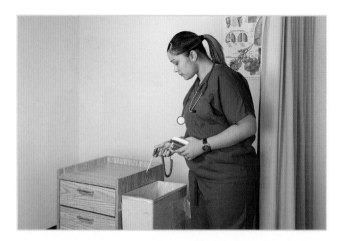

24. Discard the probe cover into the appropriate container.

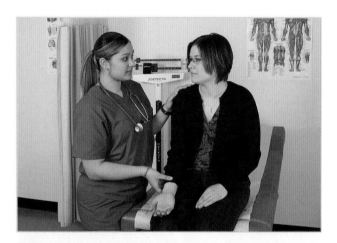

25. Position the patient with the patient's wrist resting on the lap or on the table.

WHY? *This position ensures the arm is supported and the muscles are relaxed in order to obtain an accurate measurement.*

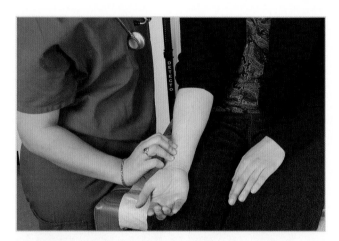

26. Locate the radial pulse with the pads of your first three fingers.

WHY? *The pulse is more easily located by using these sensitive fingertips.*

Do not use the thumb as you may feel your own heartbeat instead of the patient's.

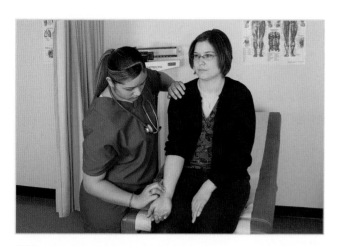

27. Gently compress the radial artery so pulsations are clearly felt.

TIP ▶ Avoid pressing too firmly, which could obliterate the pulse.

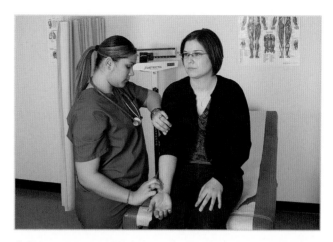

28. Using the second hand on your watch, count pulsations for one full minute (or for 30 seconds and multiply by 2).

TIP ▶ Note any irregularities in rhythm, volume, and arterial condition.

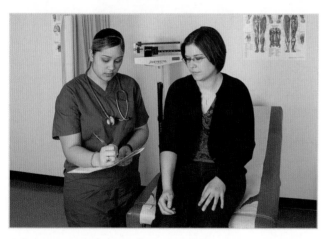

29. Note the numbers on the table paper or a notepad for now or in the patient's chart.

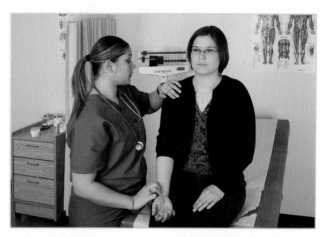

30. Continue from this position with your hand on the patient's shoulder to monitor and count the rise and fall of the patient's chest wall.

TIP ▶ Note depth of breathing, rhythm, and breath sounds while counting.

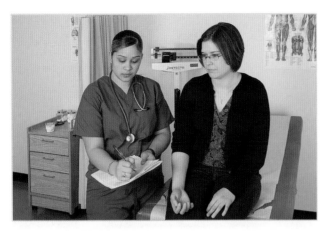

31. Accurately transfer all vital signs to the patient's chart from the notepad, if not previously charted in the chart.

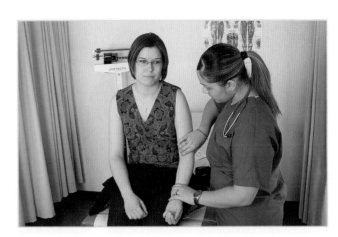

32. Palpate the patient's brachial artery.

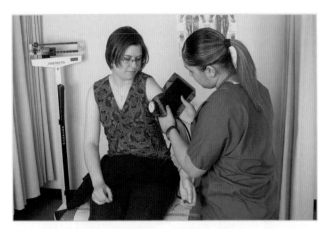

33. Apply the appropriate blood pressure cuff to the patient's arm, baring arm if necessary, and in the correct position.

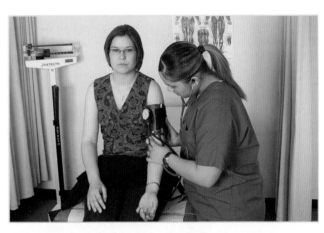

34. Position the stethoscope over the brachial artery, holding in position with fingers only.

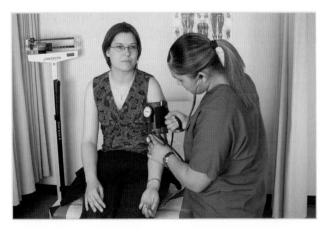

35. Inflate the blood pressure cuff, smoothly and quickly, to peak inflation level.

WHY❓ *Overinflating may cause patient discomfort; underinflating may not allow you to capture the true systolic reading.*

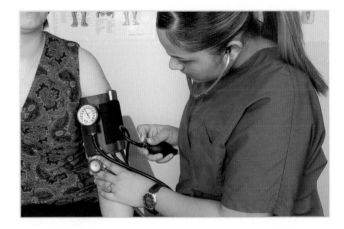

36. Deflate the cuff at 2–4 mm Hg per second.

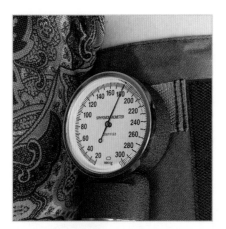

37. Listen for Korotkoff phase I, noting when it appears, while being sure not to miss the auscultory gap (Box 7-2 and Box 7-3).

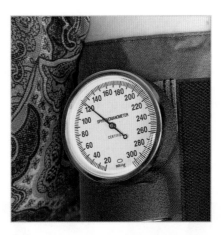

38. Continue deflation, noting each Korotkoff phase.

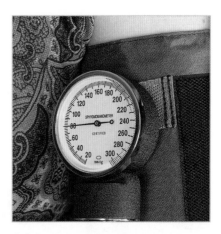

39. Note the point at which all sounds disappear, Korotkoff phase V.

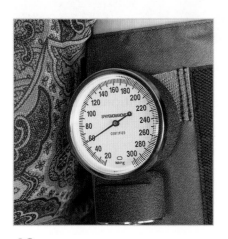

40. Continue deflating the cuff at the same rate for at least 10 mm Hg more after sounds disappear.

WHY❓ *This ensures you do not miss any trailing beats.*

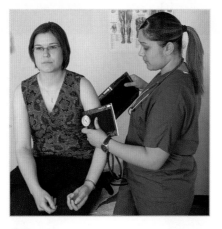

41. Deflate the cuff quickly and remove it.

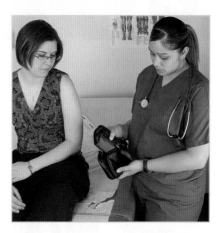

42. Replace all equipment in the appropriate place.

Box 7·2   **Korotkoff Sounds**

It is sometimes difficult to hear all the phases of the Korotkoff sounds when taking a blood pressure reading. A brief description of the various sounds may help you to identify each one:

Phase I	Faint tapping sound that is heard as the cuff is deflating (the first sound is the systolic reading)
Phase II	Light swishing sound (the auscultory gap occurs in this phase)
Phase III	Distinct tapping sound, sharp and rhythmic
Phase IV	Soft tapping sound that becomes more faint
Phase V	Very last sound heard (the diastolic reading)

Box 7·3   **Auscultory Gap**

The auscultory gap occurs in Phase II of the Korotkoff sounds. It is a period of time when the sound is no longer heard but starts again shortly. When you feel you have heard the last beat, continue to listen and deflate at least 30mm/Hg more to see if the sound resumes. If not, the diastolic reading is at the last sound you heard. If the sound starts again, continue to listen and the last sound that is heard after 30mm/Hg will be the diastolic reading.

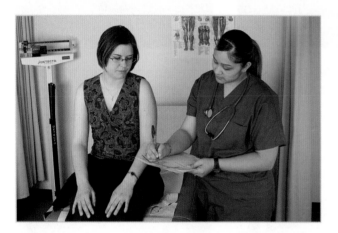

43. Document blood pressure correctly in the patient chart.

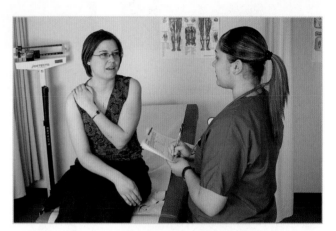

44. Take the patient's chief complaint accurately and concisely using correct abbreviations and notations.

 Make sure to list allergies and medications.

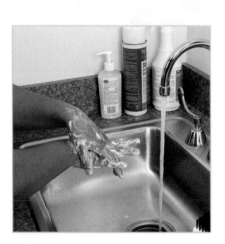

45. Wash hands.

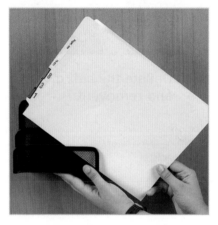

46. Place the chart in the appropriate place, flagging the physician for patient's readiness for the examination.

 Charting Example

9/12/07 9:30 a.m. CC: Pt complains of backache x 1 w. Takes Advil 800mg, q 8 h with no relief. Throbbing pain radiating down left leg, pain scale 5/10, does not remember injury.

Ht. 66", Wt. 145lbs, T 98.6 oral, P 72, R 18, BP 120/80, UA WNL, Urine preg. Neg. Takes no other meds. NKDA. _____ A. Mallen, CMA

Procedure 7-4

Obtain and Record Patient History

PURPOSE

Obtaining the patient's history is an important aspect of any first visit or for continued care of the patient. The physician uses past history as an aid in diagnosis. Family history, social history, occupational history, and past medical history are all important aspects of the patient's record.

EQUIPMENT/SUPPLIES

• patient chart
• any pertinent office forms
• pen

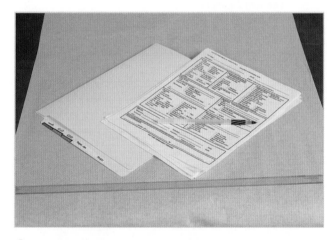

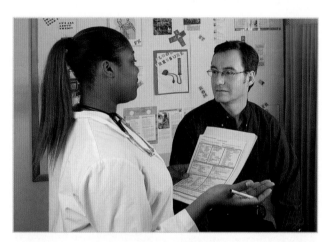

1. Gather all supplies and escort the patient to a private area or room.

WHY? *A private area ensures confidentiality for the patient.*

2. Identify the patient, introduce yourself, and explain that you are going to ask questions for the interview.

WHY? *Putting the patient at ease and maintaining confidentiality will allow the patient to feel safe to divulge pertinent information such as social habits that may affect health and/or diagnosis and treatment.*

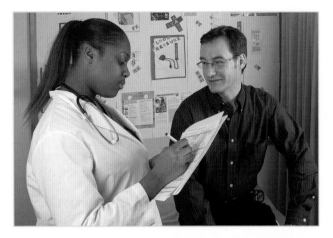

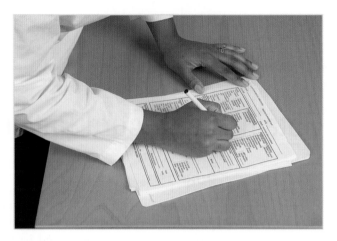

3. Interview the patient.

WHY❓ *The physician requires full and accurate information in order to provide appropriate care to the patient.*

TIP▶ Be thorough and complete using the appropriate communication skills (open-ended questions, mirroring responses, reading non-verbal clues, and covering all questions).

4. Document appropriately.

TIP▶ Always use black ink and make corrections within legal guidelines. Don't leave blank spots on pre-printed forms, noting N/A when not applicable so that the provider knows the questions have been asked.

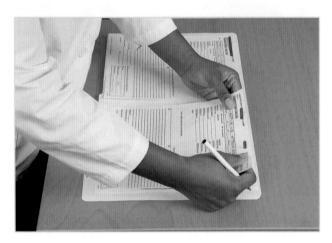

5. Place in chart.

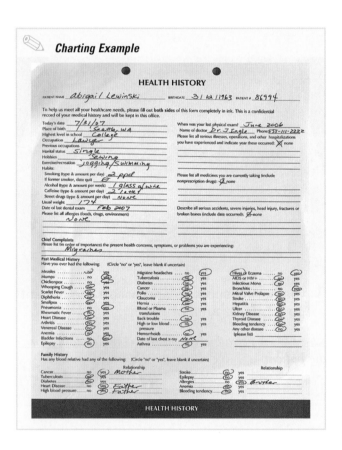

Charting Example

Procedure 7-5

Prepare and Maintain Examination and Treatment Areas

PURPOSE

Examination and treatment areas must be clean, sanitary, and safe. Keeping the rooms stocked with supplies and preventing microorganism transmission is critical both for patient treatment as well as patient and staff safety. Proper sanitization between patients must be performed routinely.

EQUIPMENT/SUPPLIES

- supplies as necessary to restock the room
- bleach and water or other disinfectant
- patient gown
- physical exam supplies (Box 7-4)

STANDARD PRECAUTIONS

Box 7·4   **Basic Physical Exam Supplies**

Patient gown and drape	Laryngeal mirror
Percussion hammer	Vaginal speculum
Tuning fork	Lubricant
Nasal speculum	Pinwheel or safety pin
Otoscope/ophthalmoscope	Urine specimen container
Examination light or gooseneck lamp	Lab requisition
Stethoscope	Tape measure
Tongue blade	Gloves
Penlight or flashlight	Gauze or cotton balls
Head light or mirror	Alcohol preps

NOTE: Not all items may be used depending on your physician and the extent of the patient's examination.

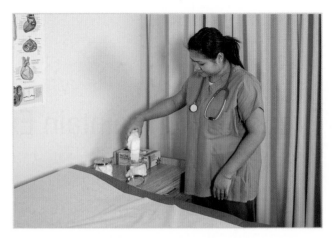

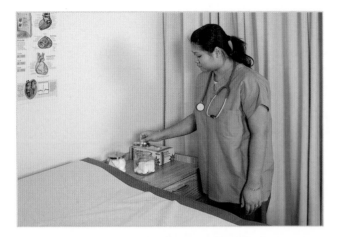

1. Inspect the examination room.

TIP Special care must be taken if small children enter the examination rooms with their parents or as patients. Sharps and other biohazardous materials must be kept safely away as must small objects.

2. Restock any supplies as necessary.

WHY? *It is best practice to keep the rooms in a state of readiness for any need that may arise; this keeps the office running smoothly.*

TIP Check all supplies such as cotton, gowns and instruments making sure room is clean and safe. Top off any soap or lotion container.

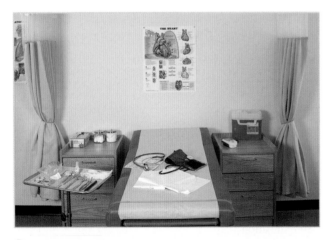

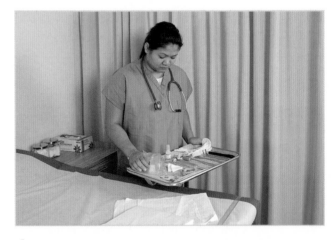

3. Gather all supplies required for the patient's examination.

4. Set up supplies for a physical exam.

TIP Many offices set up for an exam while others keep the room simple, with the provider selecting needed items from the drawers throughout the exam.

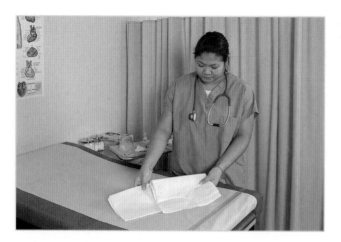

5. Select the proper gown for a male or female patient.

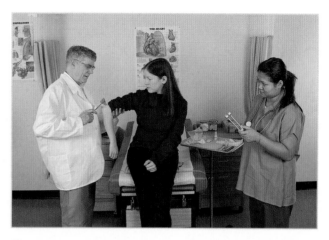

6. Assist the provider as necessary, placing the patient into the proper position, draping appropriately, and handing instruments/equipment as needed.

TIP The medical assistant may need to be present as a chaperone if the patient is female and the provider is male.

TIP Recognizing and understanding the use and function of each item will increase your efficiency in anticipating the provider's needs.

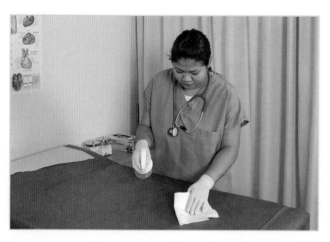

7. Properly clean and dispose of any used items.

TIP Discard any biohazardous material in the appropriate container and sterilize used equipment.

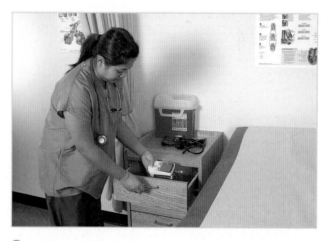

8. Return all items and unused supplies to the proper place.

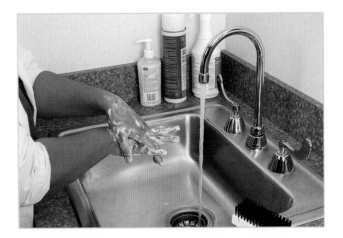

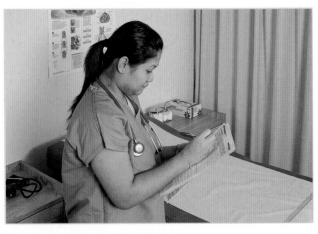

9. Wash your hands.

10. Document any tests or procedures, referrals, etc., that you complete for the provider.

➤ *Other information to be charted will include vital signs and any patient concerns or comments.*

✎ **Charting Example**

Adult Physical Exam

□ = normal

Name *Emily Weber*   Age *34*   Date *10/14/07*   Meds *Nexium, Vits.*

Vitals: Wt *153* Ht *5'8"* BP *124/78*   T *98.6* P *72* R *18*   Smoker Y Ⓝ All. *Codeine*

Present Problems: CC: *Lower back px x 10 days. No injury. ♀* LMP: *9/23/07*

BCM: *OCP*

Exam: General		Health Maintenance:	
Skin □/		DT	Pap
HEENT □/		Flu	Mammo
Neck/Thyroid □/		Pneumo	BSE/TSE
Nodes □/		Hep B	Stool Cards
Breasts □/		Dental	Sig/Colonoscopy
Heart □/		Vision	Cholesterol
Lungs □/		Exercise	Safety
Abdomen □/			

Pelvic:	Male GU:
Ext. Genitalia □/	Penis □/
Vagina □/	Scrotum □/
Cervix □/	Hernia □/
Uterus □/	Prostate □/
Adnexae □/	Rectal □/
Rectovaginal □/	Guaiac: Neg Pos
Extremities □/	Other □/
MSK □/	Laboratory None □/

Assessment   **Plan**

0) Health Maintenance

1)

2)

3)

4)

5)

Studies Pending

_____ ARNP/MD

Procedure 7-6

Prepare Patient For and Assist With Routine and Specialty Examinations: Perform Visual Acuity Test With the Snellen Chart

PURPOSE

The provider may need to assess a patient's visual acuity to provide appropriate diagnosis and treatment. Using the Snellen chart, the medical assistant tests a patient's ability to see far objects and documents the results for the provider.

EQUIPMENT/SUPPLIES

- Snellen chart
- occluder
- patient chart
- pen
- alcohol wipes

STANDARD PRECAUTIONS

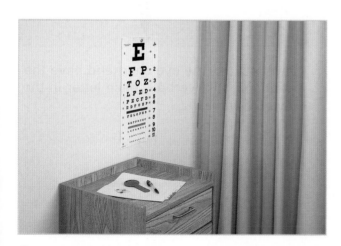

1. Gather all supplies.

▷ Wash your hands and clean the occluder with alcohol.

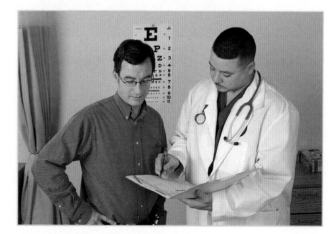

2. Identify the patient.

▷ For children, use the pediatric Snellen chart with shapes instead of letters. If they wear corrective lenses, have them keep them on and note this in the chart.

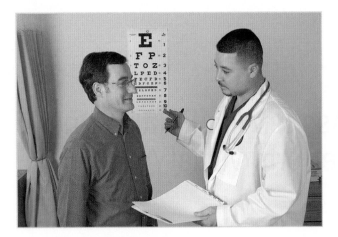

3. Explain the procedure.

TIP▶ *Being able to explain the procedure to the patient and help the patient remain at ease is the MA's duty, as is observing the patient for any adverse reactions.*

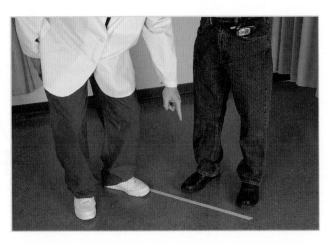

4. Instruct the patient to stand behind the 20-foot mark.

WHY❓ *The patient must stand 20 feet from the chart because that is the standard of comparing normal visual acuity to the patient's visual acuity.*

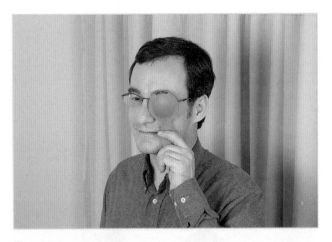

5. Have the patient cover the left eye with the occluder.

WHY❓ *Make sure the patient keeps the left eye open and does not apply pressure, because pressing the occluder against the eye will cause blurred vision and affect the test results when the left eye is tested.*

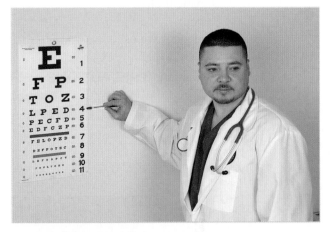

6. Stand next to the eye chart and have the patient identify verbally each letter in the row you point to.

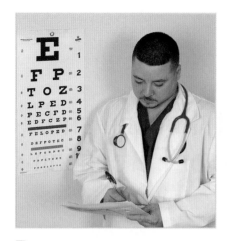

7. Record the results of the smallest line the patient is able to read with two or fewer errors.

Record the patient's reactions such as squinting, leaning, or tearing.

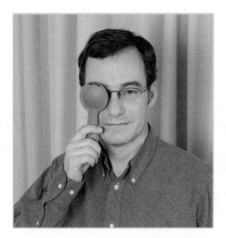

8. Repeat the process with the patient covering the right eye with the occluder.

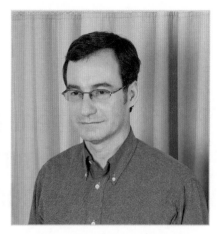

9. Repeat the process with the patient using both eyes (uncovered).

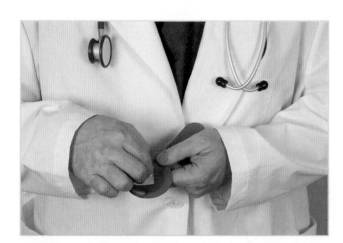

10. Clean the occluder with alcohol.

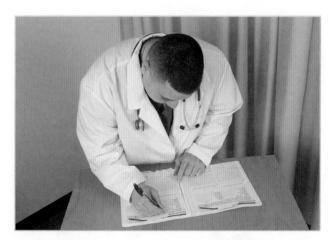

11. Document the procedure.

If the patient is wearing corrective lenses, document that.

 Charting Example

6/21/07 10:15 a.m. Performed Visual Acuity with Snellen, right eye 20/30, left eye 30/20, both eyes 20/20 with corrective lenses. _____ Liz Foster, CMA

Procedure 7-7

Prepare Patient For and Assist With Routine and Specialty Examinations: Perform Color Perception Test With Ishihara Plates

PURPOSE

Ishihara Plates are used to assess color perception and determine if the patient has any deficits.

EQUIPMENT/SUPPLIES

- Ishihara plates
- daylight room
- patient chart
- pen
- chair

STANDARD PRECAUTIONS

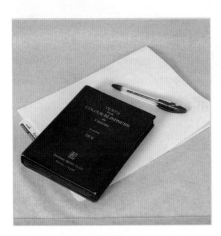

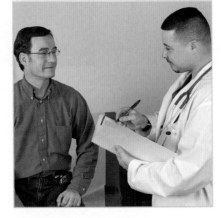

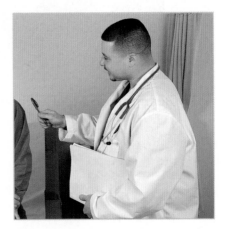

1. Gather all supplies.

2. Identify the patient.

3. Explain the procedure.

 Wash your hands.

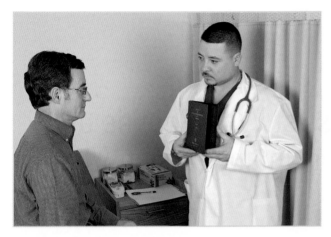

4. In a well-lit room, preferably lighted with daylight, seat the patient in a chair and hold the plates 30 inches from the patient.

WHY? *Daylight ensures that electric lighting does not alter the appearance of the plates.*

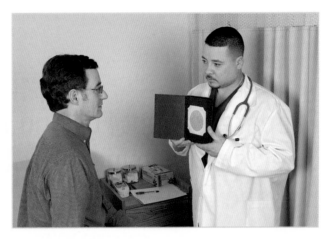

5. Show the patient plate number twelve as an example.

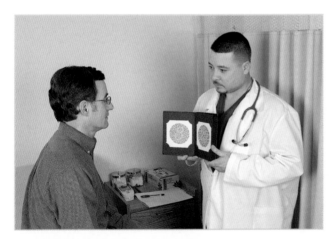

6. Show the patient each plate and record the patient's response.

WHY? *Because differences in red-green deficiencies will make the patient see other numbers, record each response and compare to the score sheet included with the book.*

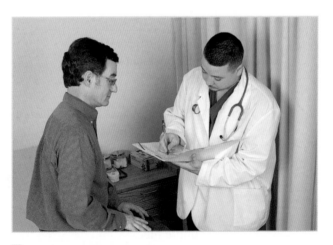

7. Assess the patient's responses and document in the chart.

TIP Keep the Ishihara Plate book covered when not in use to maintain the integrity of the plates.

 Charting Example

12/5/07 10:30 a.m. Performed color perception with Ishihara, pt. scored 10/10, color vision WNL. _____ J. Fuentes, CMA

Procedure **7-8**

Prepare Patient For and Assist With Routine and Specialty Examinations: Set Up and Assist With Routine Prenatal Visit

PURPOSE

Prenatal patients need to have certain tests or procedures at specific points in their pregnancy. The medical assistant must be aware of office policy regarding these tests and procedures in order to ensure that equipment needed by the provider is available and that the patient is prepared appropriately.

EQUIPMENT/SUPPLIES

- scale
- urine specimen cup
- urine dip sticks
- sphygmomanometer
- stethoscope
- Doppler
- pregnancy Wheel for due date calculation
- sterile and non-sterile gloves
- sterile speculum
- patient gown
- possibly gynecological supplies (Box 7-5)
- measuring tape
- lab slip
- culture tubes
- patient chart
- pen

STANDARD PRECAUTIONS

Box 7·5 **Gynecological Supplies for a Routine Exam**

Gown and drape	Cotton-tipped applicators
Vaginal speculum	Various STD cultures and appropriate lab requisitions
Lubricant (water soluble)	Pap kit (or cervical spatula or cytology brush, slide,
Gloves	fixative, lab requisition)
Examination light or gooseneck lamp	Tissues

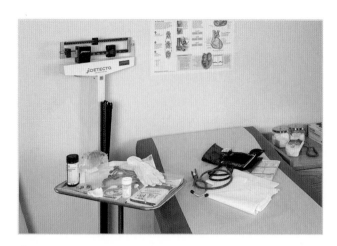

1. Gather all supplies.

TIP Some offices have an "OB Tray" that includes a measuring tape, Doppler, doppler conductivity gel, birth date calculator or wheel, litmus paper for amniotic fluid testing, a sterile speculum, and sterile gloves.

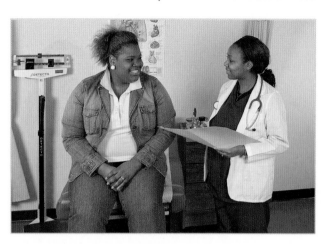

2. Identify the patient.

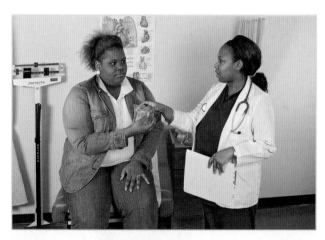

3. Have the patient leave a urine sample.

WHY? *This is done for each visit so that the patient's urine protein and glucose levels can be assessed.*

TIP If it is an initial visit, you may also perform a UA and HCG test as well as send a urine sample to the lab.

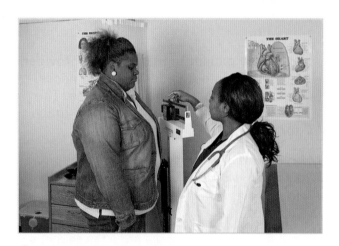

4. Obtain the patient's weight.

WHY? *This is done each visit to determine weight gain during pregnancy.*

TIP Some patients do not want to know their weight; be discreet and empathetic to their feelings.

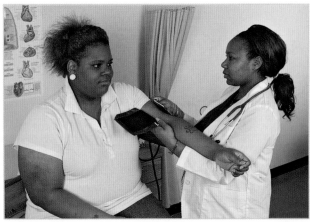

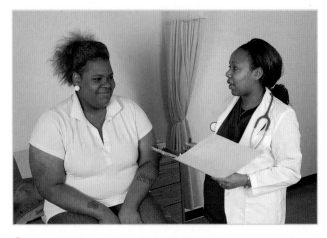

5. Obtain vital signs.

WHY? *Blood pressure is obtained for every exam and is critical to watch because high blood pressure can be an indicator of complications such as pre-eclampsia.*

TIP Some offices may want all vital signs obtained, while others only want BP; know your office's policy.

6. Ask the patient if she has any questions or concerns and note this in the chart.

TIP Some offices may only want the provider to do this, some may expect the medical assistant to ask. Tailor your questions to the patient's gestational weeks, i.e., if the patient is in the first trimester, you may ask about nausea; if in the last, you may ask about heartburn or edema and fetal movement.

7. Have the patient prepare for the provider by getting into a patient gown if necessary and sitting on the exam table. The nmedical assistant may provide a drape for privacy.

WHY? *Having the patient ready for the provider avoids delays and ensure smooth operation of the medical office.*

TIP If this is the first exam, the patient may undress and have a pelvic exam and a Pap smear as if it were a routine gynecological exam. Patients in the second trimester may only be examined for fetal growth and may not need to undress. Patients in their last weeks prior to delivery may need to undress from the waist down and have a pelvic exam to determine cervical effacement.

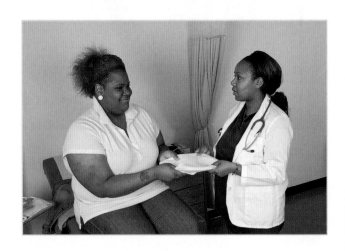

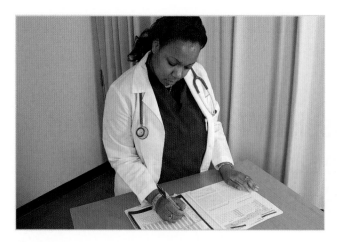

8. Document in the patient's chart.

Many offices use special forms for pregnancy; be aware of what your office uses.

Certain prenatal tests or procedures occur at specific intervals. At the initial prenatal visit, for example, blood tests and cultures are required. At 16 weeks, a hematocrit and genetic testing or an ultrasound may be performed. Some patients may need a glucose tolerance test; others may need Rhogam if it is their second pregnancy and they are Rh-. In the last trimester, a fetal stress test may be done.

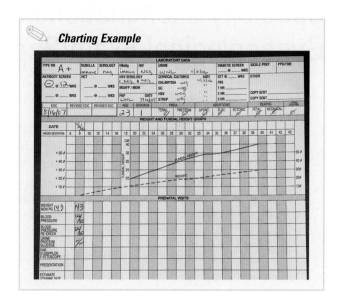

Procedure **7-9**

Prepare Patient For and Assist With Routine and Specialty Examinations: Set Up and Assist With Gynecological Exam/Pap Smear

PURPOSE

A yearly pelvic exam and Pap smear are critical for early detection of cervical cancer and other conditions and diseases. Many women use their annual exam with a gynecologist as a yearly physical. Be aware of routine tests that may occur with this exam, such as STD testing, EKG, blood work, and so on. Many patients also obtain medication refills, especially birth control, during this exam. Know your office's policy surrounding these issues in order to ensure that equipment needed by the provider is available and that the patient is prepared appropriately.

EQUIPMENT/SUPPLIES

- scale
- urine specimen cup
- urine dip sticks
- sphygmomanometer
- stethoscope
- patient gown
- speculum
- Pap kit
- lubrication gel
- swabs
- lab slip
- culture tubes
- patient chart
- pen
- cape and drape as appropriate
- non-sterile gloves
- 10% bleach and water solution
- paper towels

STANDARD PRECAUTIONS

1. Gather all supplies.

ᴡʜʏ❓ *Gathering supplies and equipment before the patient is brought into the room will make the exam run more efficiently and avoid alarming the patient by seeing the items to be used.*

TIP Many offices set up for an exam while others keep the room simple, with the provider selecting needed items throughout the exam from the drawers. In offices where gynecological exams are routinely done, the supplies and equipment are often in the drawers at the end of the table where they are convenient for the provider to access during the exam. Other offices will require a tray to be set up and all of the items gathered.

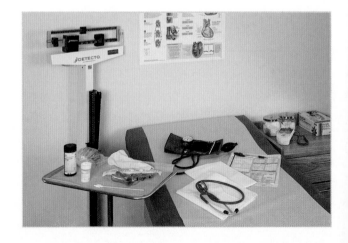

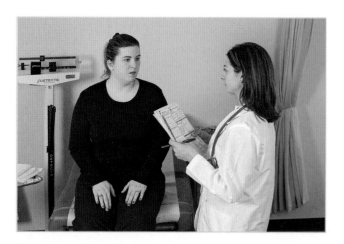

2. Identify the patient.

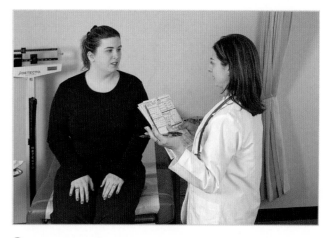

3. Explain the procedure.

WHY? *A patient will usually cooperate better and feel more at ease when she knows what to expect.*

TIP Some offices require patients to leave a urine sample so you may need to give instructions on collecting the urine.

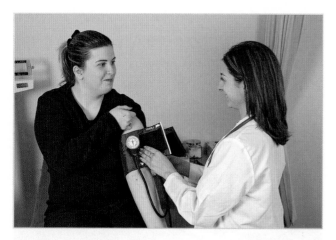

4. Obtain vital signs.

WHY? *This is critical at most exams (of any kind) to provide the physician with the basic indications of the patient's overall condition. For example, in gynecological patients, elevated blood pressure may affect the provider prescribing birth control medication; in obstetric patients, it may indicate pre-eclampsia.*

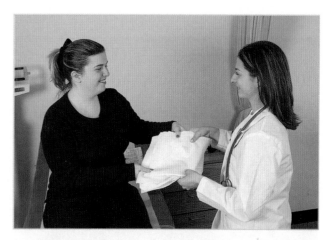

5. Select the proper gown and drape and have the patient undress.

TIP The gown needs to be open in the front for the breast exam; the patient must remove her bra and underwear and the drape is placed lengthwise across the patient's lap as she sits on the end of the exam table.

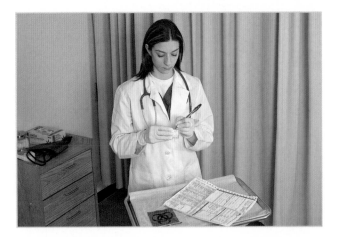

6. Assist with the exam as needed by your provider, handing instruments and supplies, labeling specimens, and reassuring the patient during the exam.

Anticipate the items and supplies needed and hand them to provider before being asked, assist patient into appropriate positions, and maintain draping for privacy.

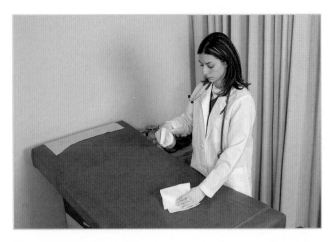

7. Properly clean or dispose of used equipment. Prepare any specimens and route them to the lab.

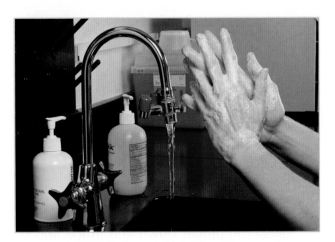

8. Wash hands.

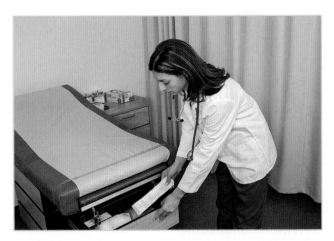

9. Return all items and unused supplies to the proper place.

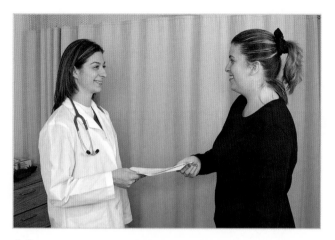

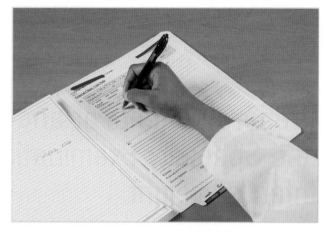

10. Ensure that the patient receives any referrals, information about required tests, or medication refills as ordered by the provider.

11. Document what you did yourself, such as obtaining vital signs, measuring weight, or patient teaching of the breast self-exam, as a few examples.

The procedure or exam itself is documented by the provider.

Charting Example

10/30/07 10:45 a.m. Annual GYN exam, see GYN worksheet. _____ D. Bedford, CMA

Procedure 7-10

Prepare Patient For and Assist With Routine and Specialty Examinations: Measuring an Infant's Weight

PURPOSE

Weight is an important parameter for assessing health. Measuring an infant's weight and documenting the results helps the provider to determine if growth is within normal limits.

EQUIPMENT/SUPPLIES

- scale
- protective cover
- pediatric growth chart
- patient chart
- pen
- gloves
- water-resistant drape or towel
- 10% bleach and water solution
- paper towels

STANDARD PRECAUTIONS

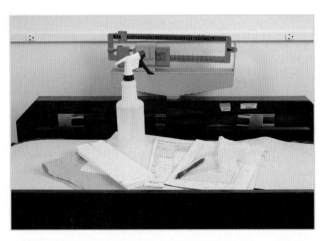

1. Gather all supplies.

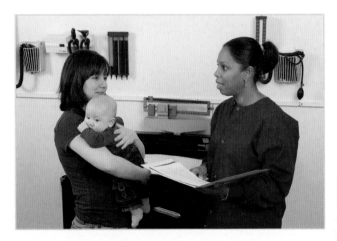

2. Identify the patient.

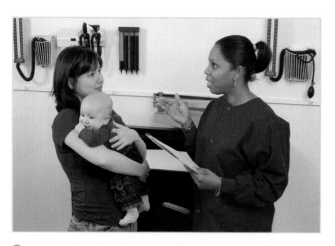

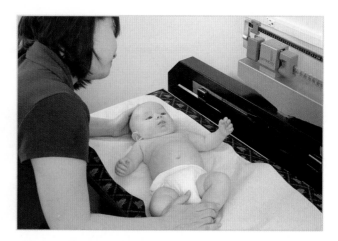

3. Explain the procedure to the parent.

ᴡʜʏ❓ *It is vital to obtain the parent's understanding and assistance, as many babies are frightened by this exam.*

4. Have the parent remove all of the infant's clothing.

ᴡʜʏ❓ *Diapers have weight and it is critical to get the infant's exact weight to the ounce so as to assess proper growth and development.*

TIP➤ If you will be removing the clothing and anticipate contact with urine or feces in the diaper, your employer may require you to wear non-sterile gloves or may not. Always follow your employer's directives.

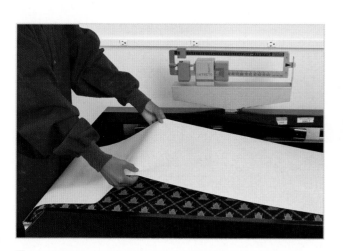

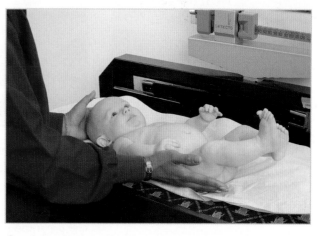

5. Place a protective covering on the scale, then turn on the scale (if electronic) or balance it (if manual) to ensure you are not weighing the covering as well.

ᴡʜʏ❓ *The covering provides warmth and helps to prevent transfer of microorganisms.*

TIP➤ Scales may be digital or manual; know how to use both types.

6. Place the infant on the infant's back on the scale.

TIP➤ Male infants may urinate at this time so it is prudent to hold a diaper or a fluid-resistent drape/towel hovering above the infant but not on the infant (to avoid extra weight). This will also keep your hand near-by to ensure the infant doesn't roll or fall off of the scale.

TIP➤ Babies are wiggly, or they may not like this, as it can be cold and scary. Talk to them and make them smile so as to get better results. Have the parent assist if necessary.

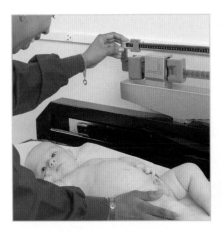

7. Weigh the infant.

If using a manual scale, move the weight down the weight bar and balance; a digital scale weighs the infant for you.

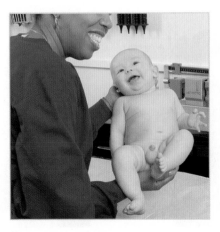

8. Remove the infant and diaper the baby (parent can assist).

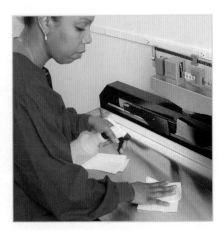

9. Sanitize the scale.

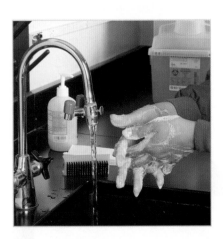

10. Wash hands.

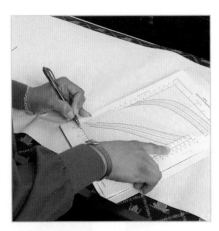

11. Document in the patient's chart.

This may be done on the pediatric growth chart as well as the progress note. There may be variations of charting forms and requirements depending on the type of pediatric visit the patient is in for—a well child visit or a sick child visit.

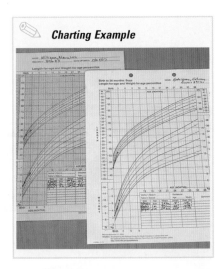

Charting Example

Procedure 7-11

Prepare Patient For and Assist With Routine and Specialty Examinations: Measuring an Infant's Length

PURPOSE

An infant's length can indicate health status. The medical assistant obtains this measurement to help the provider assess the infant's growth and development patterns.

EQUIPMENT/SUPPLIES

- measuring board or exam table
- measuring tape
- pediatric growth chart
- patient chart
- pen

STANDARD **PRECAUTIONS**

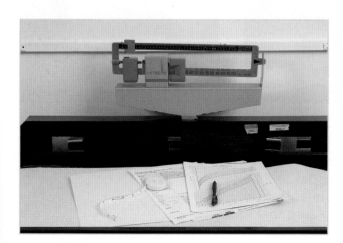

1. Gather all supplies.

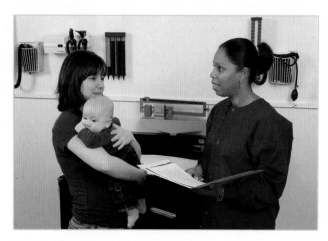

2. Identify the patient.

Note that measuring an infant's weight, length, and head circumference are all done together.

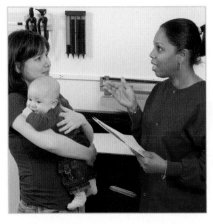

3. Explain the procedure to the parent.

WHY❓ It is vital to obtain the parent's understanding and assistance, as many babies are frightened by this exam.

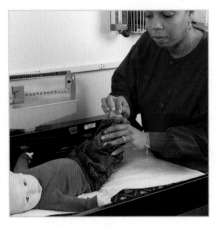

4. Remove infant's shoes if wearing any.

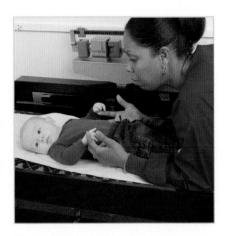

5. Lay the infant on the infant's back on the exam table.

WHY❓ All infants up to two years must be measured laying down for accuracy.

TIP❯ Some offices have special measuring boards or attached measuring units on the exam table for infants, while others just use the method described here.

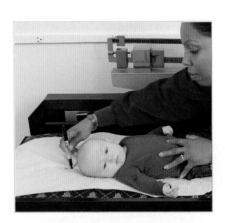

6. While gently holding the infant's head, place a mark on the table paper at the top of the head.

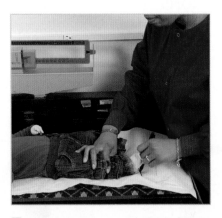

7. While gently holding the infant at the knee, stretch the leg and make a mark on the table paper at the point that the infant's heel reaches, being sure that the head position does not move and the leg is as straight as possible.

WHY❓ The infant's legs must be extended to obtain an accurate measurement at the heel.

TIP❯ Ask the parent to assist if necessary.

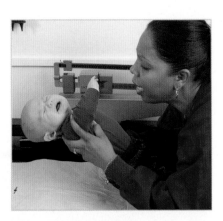

8. Lift up the infant and give to the parent to comfort.

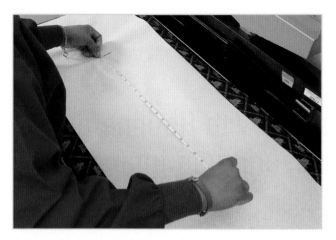

9. Using a measuring tape, measure the marks on the table paper or use the measuring board to determine length.

▷ *Some parents may want to keep the table paper with measurements on it for their scrapbook. Give it to them at the end of the exam.*

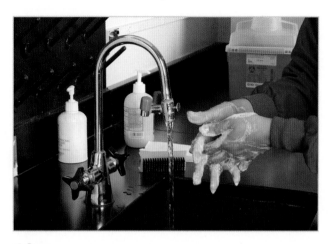

10. Wash hands.

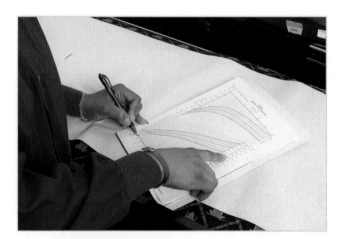

11. Document in chart.

▷ *There may be variations of charting forms and requirements depending on the type of pediatric visit —a well child visit or a sick child visit.*

▷ *Give attention to infants as well as the parents, and attempt to make the infants smile to gain their trust and cooperation.*

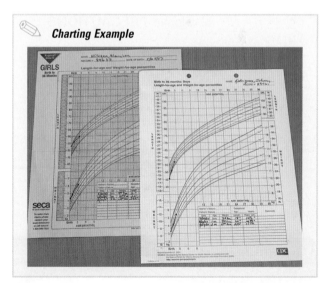

Charting Example

Procedure 7-12

Prepare Patient For and Assist With Routine and Specialty Examinations: Measuring an Infant's Head Circumference

PURPOSE

Along with weight and length, an infant's head circumference is a key indicator of appropriate growth and development. It is important for the medical assistant to obtain this measurement at well child visits.

EQUIPMENT/SUPPLIES

- exam table
- measuring tape
- pediatric growth chart
- patient chart
- pen

STANDARD **PRECAUTIONS**

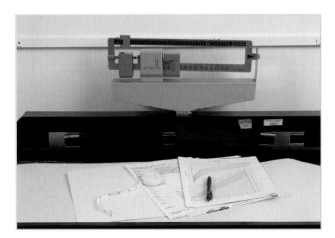

1. Gather all supplies.

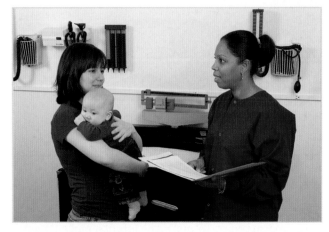

2. Identify the patient.

TIP   Note that measuring an infant's weight, length, and head circumference are all done together.

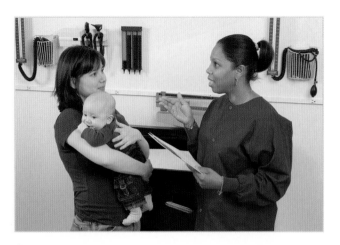

3. Explain the procedure to the parent.

WHY? *It is vital to obtain the parent's understanding and assistance, as many babies are frightened by this exam.*

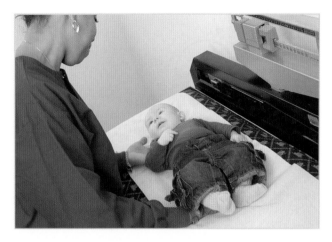

4. Lay the infant on the exam table (if the infant can sit, sit the infant on the table) or allow the parent to hold the infant.

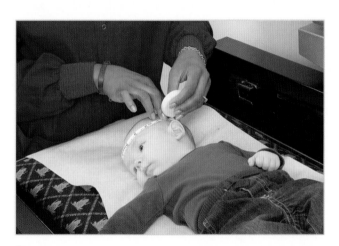

5. Place a measuring tape snuggly around the infant's head from the occipital protuberance to the supraorbital protuberance.

TIP Use a flexible measuring tape or a special pediatric head circumference measuring device, available in some offices.

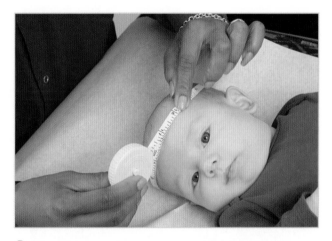

6. Read the measurement to the exact quarter of an inch or centimeter.

WHY? *Since infants are very small, the smallest measurement increment must be used to record the true growth of the child. An error of an inch, for example, would be very significant in an infant compared to an adult.*

TIP If the infant has been lying on the table, you can pick the infant up and hand to the parent to hold and/or comfort prior to the next part of the exam.

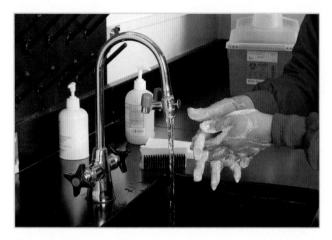

7. Wash hands.

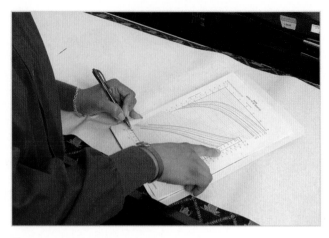

8. Document in chart.

There may be variations of charting forms and requirements depending on the type of pediatric visit —a well child visit or a sick child visit.

Give attention to infants as well as the parents, and attempt to make the infants smile to gain their trust and cooperation.

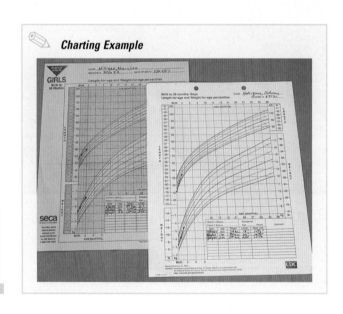

Charting Example

Procedure **7-13**

Prepare Patient For and Assist With Routine and Specialty Examinations: Recording Infant Measurements on a Growth Chart

PURPOSE

A pediatric growth chart displays in graphic format a child's growth patterns, which can be compared with same-age children. The provider uses this information to assess a child's development and spot potential health concerns.

EQUIPMENT/SUPPLIES

- pediatric growth chart
- patient chart
- pen

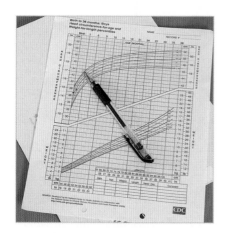

1. Gather all supplies.

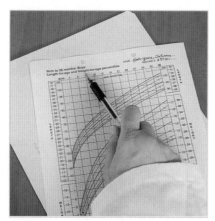

2. Choose the correct growth chart for boys or girls and age.

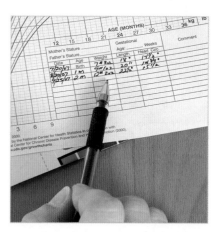

3. Fill out the date, age, and measurements in the space at the bottom or top of the chart.

TIP If this is a new baby, ask the parents the birth weight and length. Complete the demographic data for the infant on the graph, and place in child's chart to become part of the permanent record.

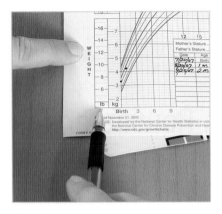

4. Locate the weight value in the vertical column of the physical growth percentile chart.

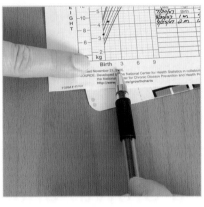

5. Find the child's age in months in the horizontal rows.

> TIP▶ Remember that an infant growth chart is from birth to 36 months; the appropriate growth chart for older children spans 36 months through the teens.

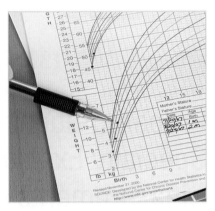

6. Locate the area where the growth value lines intersect on the graph and plot the weight by marking with a dot.

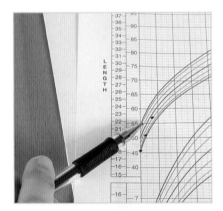

7. Repeat the steps for length or height.

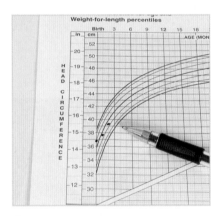

8. Repeat the steps for head circumference.

> TIP▶ Head circumference is measured up until age 5.

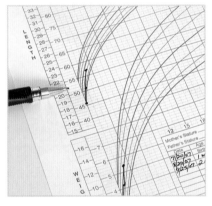

9. Connect the dots from the previous measurements so that a line is formed in each area of the graph.

> WHY？ *This shows the provider the child's growth pattern and percentile according to the average child of that age.*

> TIP▶ Many children are "off the charts" and don't follow the average. As long as they are following the curve and not trending downward or failing to move up, this is normal. Many parents are concerned that their child is not at the top of the child's percentile. Use therapeutic communication to reassure parents that it is not necessary to always be in the 90th + percentile.

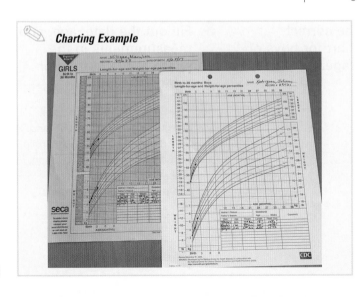

Charting Example

Procedure **7-14**

Prepare Patient For and Assist With Procedures, Treatments and Minor Office Surgeries: Perform Ear Lavage

PURPOSE

Ear lavage is commonly performed in order to remove impacted cerumen from the patient's ears. Other reasons for ear irrigation may include pain relief or removal of a foreign object.

EQUIPMENT/SUPPLIES

- irrigation syringe
- towel
- irrigation solution
- ear basin
- otoscope with disposable speculum
- bowl
- cotton/gauze
- wax softener
- patient chart
- pen
- gloves

STANDARD PRECAUTIONS

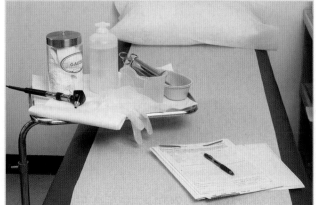

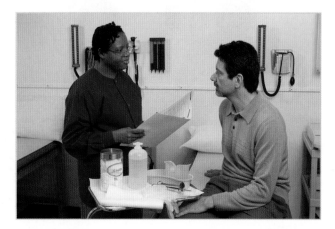

1. Gather all supplies

WHY? *The ability to anticipate your provider's needs as well as the patient's needs is critical.*

TIP Some offices use special solutions, others use sterile water, and still others use a mixture of 50/50 hydrogen peroxide and water. Many providers instill wax softening solution prior to the irrigation. Follow office protocol.

2. Identify the patient.

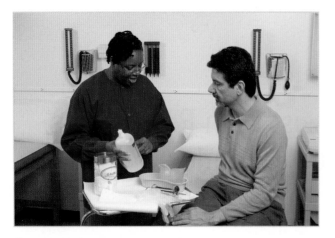

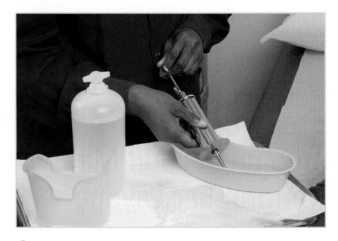

3. Explain the procedure.

WHY❓ Helping to maintain the comfort of the patient as well as enlisting cooperation ensures a smooth flow in the treatment process as well as the patient flow of that day. Knowledge of procedural steps and processes helps you to keep interruptions at a minimum as well as helping to keep the examination running smoothly.

Inform the patient that some dizziness or discomfort may occur due to fluid coming in contact with the tympanic membrane. If the patient feels pain, stop and consult the provider. Always be patient and gentle, and always monitor your patient's reaction to this procedure.

4. Prepare the solution and draw up in a large syringe.

The solution should feel warm to the touch, like a baby's bath water. Cold water makes patients dizzy; hot water burns. Some offices use a 50cc syringe, others have special metal syringes for ear lavage, while specialists may have a device for this attached to the wall with a water source, somewhat like a water pic.

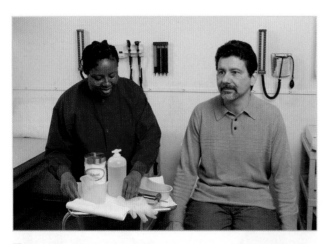

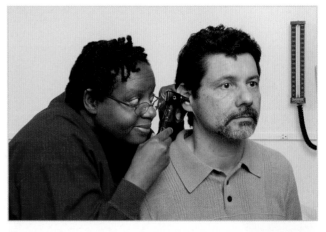

5. Have the patient sit on the examination table.

6. Visualize the patient's ear canal with the otoscope.

WHY❓ You must visualize the area to be irrigated before beginning the procedure to assess the cerumen that needs to be removed.

Pull back on the pinna, hold the otoscope sideways, and always keep a finger or two in contact with the side of the patient's head.

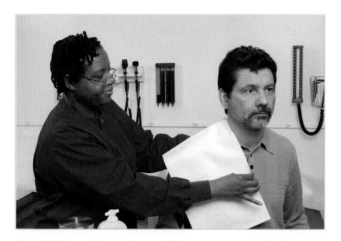

7. Place a towel on the patient's shoulder.

WHY? *This avoids getting the patient's clothing wet with the solution.*

TIP It is best to put a liquid-resistant drape such as a plastic-lined tray cover or a Chux beneath the towel to further avoid the patient getting wet.

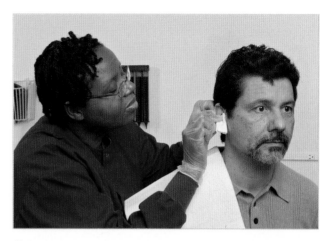

8. Apply gloves and cleanse the outer ear with a cotton ball dipped in cleaning solution.

WHY? *It is important to remove any visible particles in the outer ear before beginning the procedure to avoid washing debris back into the ear canal.*

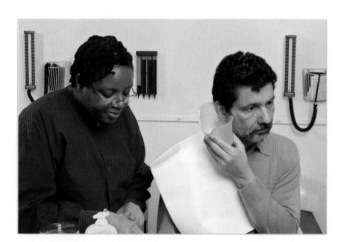

9. Have the patient hold the ear basin in close contact with the head, under the ear, leaning the head slightly towards you.

WHY? *Leaning the head helps the solution flow out of the ear.*

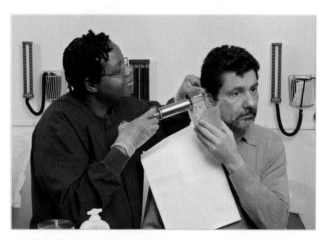

10. Pull back gently on the pinna to straighten the ear canal.

WHY? *The ear canal must be straight to allow proper treatment.*

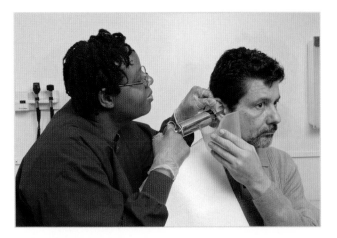

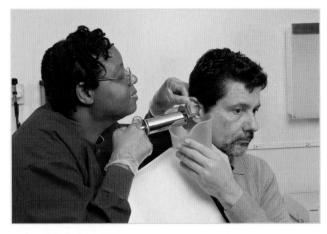

11. After expelling any air from the syringe, insert the tip into the ear canal and gently apply pressure to the plunger, directing the flow of fluid to the top of the ear canal and not directly at the tympanic membrane. Do not block the draining of fluid at the bottom of the outer ear.

TIP Many offices attach the tip from a butterfly needle, with the needle cut off, to the syringe for use in the lavage process.

12. Repeat the process until the impacted cerumen is cleared.

TIP Some offices may want you to record the amount of fluid in and out, while others just want you to continue irrigation until the cerumen is ejected. Describe the color, size, and texture of any cerumen particles removed.

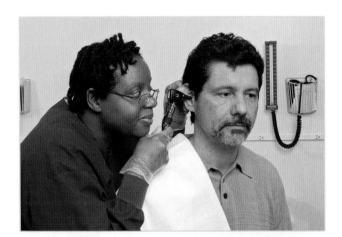

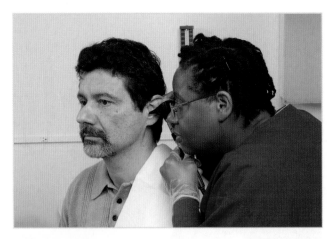

13. View the ear canal as needed with the otoscope to see if the tympanic membrane is visible yet or to visualize any change in the cerumen that you are trying to remove.

TIP If the cerumen cannot be removed sufficiently before the patient has too much discomfort to continue, the physician may use an ear curette to manually remove it or may order medication that softens cerumen be instilled into the ear.

14. Repeat the process with the other ear if necessary.

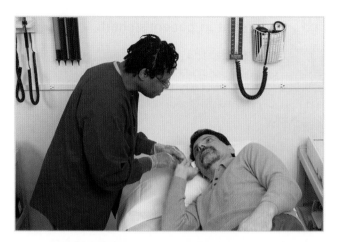

15. When the irrigation is complete and all cerumen is cleared or the patient cannot go on due to discomfort, remove the basin and towel and have the patient lie on the side with a tissue or cotton ball on the ear to facilitate drainage and to alleviate any dizziness.

WHY? *It is important to allow the solution to completely drain out of the ear to prevent patient discomfort.*

TIP Never let the patient just get up and leave. Many patients do not tolerate this procedure well; always monitor for dizziness and discomfort.

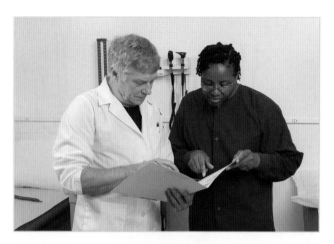

16. Inform the provider that the irrigation is complete.

WHY? *The provider must complete the examination of the ear and tympanic membrane now.*

TIP If the provider has completed the exam and you are simply removing cerumen for cleaning, the provider would not have to be informed at this point.

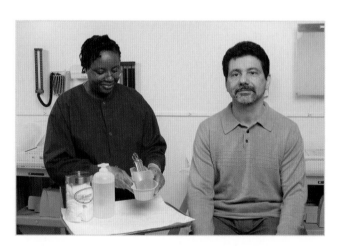

17. Clean up all supplies.

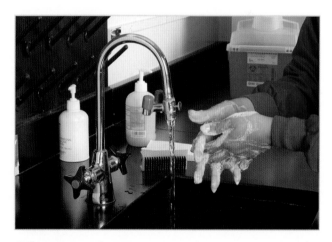

18. Wash hands.

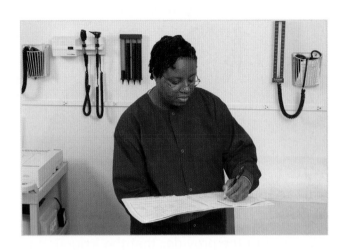

19. Document in patient's chart.

 Be sure that the amount, name, and strength of the fluid used to irrigate is recorded (if the provider has required you to keep track of the amount used) and to describe the cerumen per office protocol.

 Because this procedure is time consuming, have another medical assistant prepare your other patients and inform your co-workers that you are doing an ear lavage. Also ask your colleague to check if your provider needs something for another patient. It is important to keep a smooth flow of clinic patients for your physician even when you are doing a lengthy procedure.

✎ **Charting Example**

9/30/07 11:15 a.m. Performed ear lavage, AU, 100cc's in/100cc's out 50/50 hydrogen peroxide/water, removed 6 large cerumen particles AD, 5 large particles AS, pt. tol. well, no adverse reactions, remained in office 20 minutes post procedure, no dizziness noted. Pt. left fine. _____ A. Christopher, CMA

Procedure **7-15**

Prepare Patient For and Assist With Procedures, Treatments and Minor Office Surgeries: Apply Sterile Gloves

PURPOSE

Sterile gloving is required in order to maintain sterile technique and ensure safety when assisting with invasive procedures.

EQUIPMENT/SUPPLIES

- sink
- soap
- sterile towels
- sterile glove package

STANDARD PRECAUTIONS

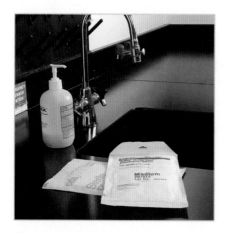

1. Gather all supplies.

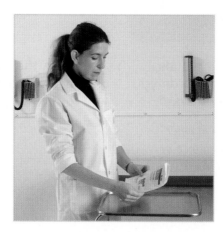

2. Inspect the package of sterile gloves for any tears or signs of disrepair.

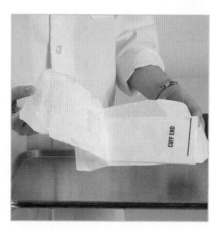

3. Open the outer package on a clean counter, being careful not to touch the inner wrap.

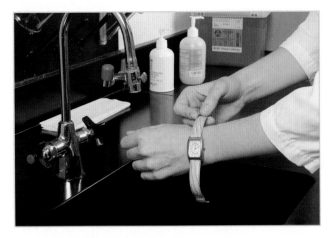

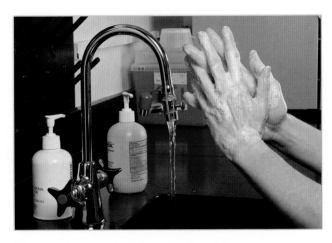

4. Remove all jewelry.

WHY? *Jewelry can harbor microorganisms and can tear the gloves. If tearing occurs, the procedure will be contaminated.*

5. Perform a surgically aseptic hand wash.

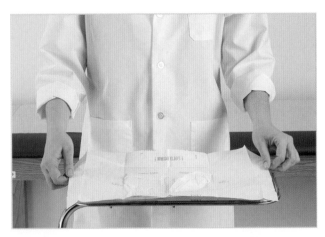

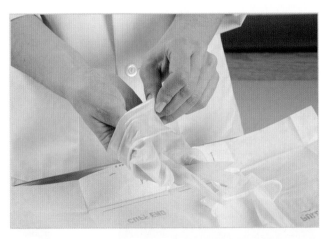

6. Open the inner package of the gloves, being sure that the cuffs are towards you and the thumbs are pointing outward.

WHY? *Positioning the gloves in this manner allows for easier application and less chance of contaminating gloves while putting them on.*

TIP If the gloves are not positioned properly, turn the package around, being careful not to reach over the sterile area or touch the inner surface of the gloves.

7. With the index finger and thumb of one hand, grasp the *inner*, cuffed edge of the opposite glove.

TIP The glove should be picked straight up off the package surface without dragging or dangling the fingers over any non-sterile area.

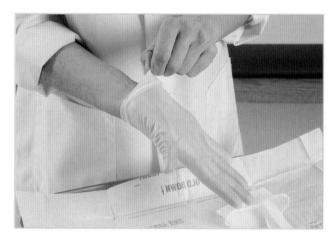

8. With the palm up of the hand you are placing in the glove, fully slide the hand into the glove.

▶ Always keep hands above waist level so as not to breach sterility.

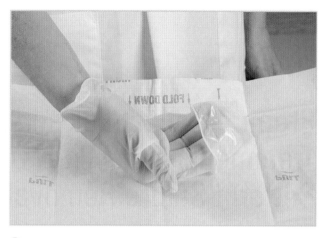

9. With the gloved hand, pick up the glove for the non-gloved hand by slipping four fingers under the *outside* of the cuff.

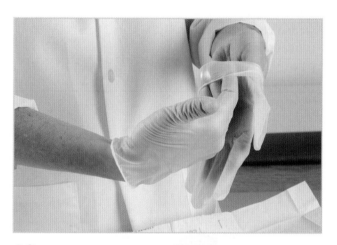

10. Lift the second glove up, keeping it above waist level, and slide the non-gloved hand into it palm up.

Do not allow the glove to drag or touch any non-sterile surface.

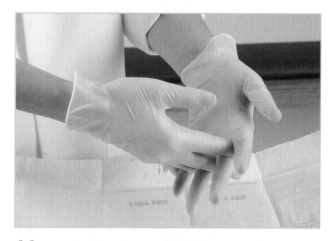

11. Adjust the gloves as needed, only touching the sterile parts of the gloves, not the arm or wrist.

WHY❓ *This avoids contaminating the gloves.*

▶ Keep gloved hands above waist level so as not to breach sterility. Do not touch non-sterile surfaces with gloved hands.

Procedure 7-16

Prepare Patient For and Assist With Procedures, Treatments and Minor Office Surgeries: Perform Suture Removal

PURPOSE

When non-absorbable sutures are used to close a wound, they will need to be removed after healing has occurred.

EQUIPMENT/SUPPLIES

- sterile suture removal scissors
- sterile thumb forceps
- sterile gauze
- bandaging
- antibacterial ointment
- gloves
- sterile water
- wound care instructions
- patient chart
- pen

STANDARD PRECAUTIONS

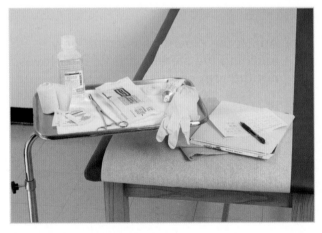

1. Gather all supplies.

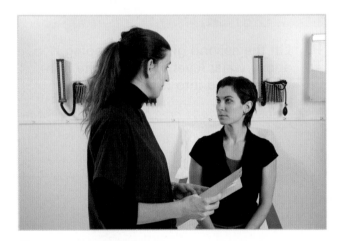

2. Identify patient.

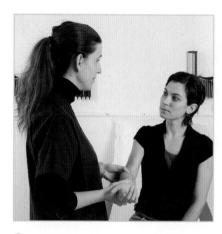

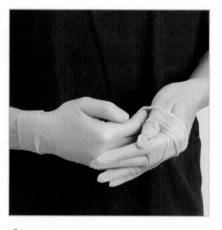

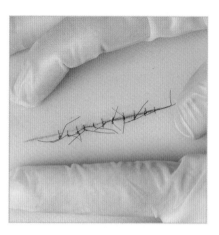

3. Explain the procedure.

4. Apply gloves.

▷ Use either sterile or regular gloves per office protocol. If you are using sterile, use regular gloves to inspect the wound and apply sterile gloves after preparation.

5. Examine the wound for any signs of infection and readiness for the sutures to be removed.

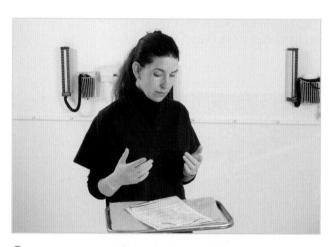

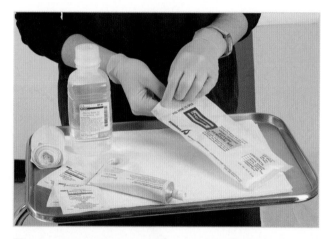

6. Check the chart for how many sutures were placed.

▷ If this was done elsewhere, you should have chart notes from that facility. If there seem to be fewer sutures, ask the patient if any fell out, if they took them out, or if any are impacted into the wound. If impacted, consult the provider.

7. Prepare your sterile instruments.

WHY❓ *It is important to touch the sutures with only sterile instruments.*

▷ Some offices many have you set up a sterile field and use sterile gloves to remove sutures, others may have you use regular gloves and use a sterile package of suture removal instruments. Always use sterile instruments to remove sutures. Some offices use pre-packaged suture removal kits, while others sterilize their own kits. Follow office protocol regarding this procedure.

▷ Assess the wound and sutures for signs of infection, non-healing, and cleanliness. If it appears infected or non-healing, inform the provider first. If the wound is not clean, cleanse prior to removing sutures.

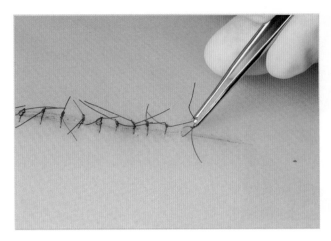

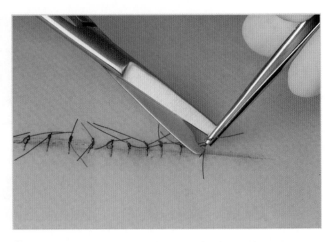

8. Using the thumb forceps, gently pick up one knot of a suture while gently pulling upward toward the suture line.

9. Using suture removal scissors, cut one side of the suture as close to the skin as possible so as not to drag any of the sutures through the wound.

WHY❓ *This helps to protect against infection.*

TIP▶ If sutures are stuck, you may use sterile water or a mixture of 50/50 hydrogen peroxide on sterile gauze to soak and loosen them as per office protocol and provider approval.

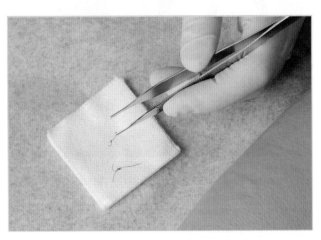

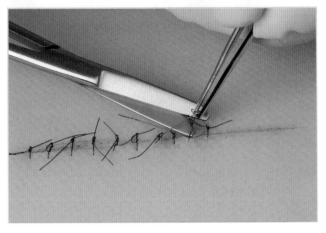

10. Pull out the suture, placing it on a piece of gauze so as to keep track of suture count.

WHY❓ *A correct count of sutures removed compared to number of sutures inserted will ensure that no suture is left in the tissue.*

TIP▶ As with any procedure, constantly assess the patient by checking skin color and reactions and asking how he or she feels. Stop any procedure if the patient has an adverse reaction and notify the provider.

11. Repeat the process with the remaining sutures.

TIP▶ If the wound is long and there are many sutures, it is best to remove one or two sutures at one end of the site, then one or two sutures at the other end of the site. This avoids too much pulling on the wound at one end, which can cause it to open.

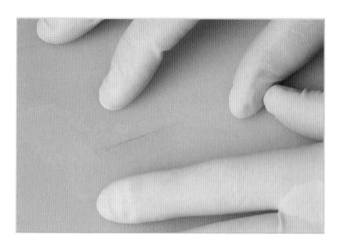

12. Examine the wound for any sign of bleeding and to ensure that all sutures have been removed.

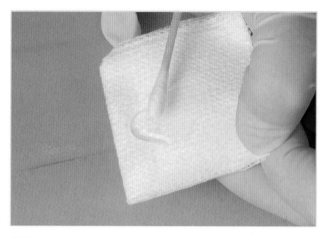

13. Apply medication as per provider order.

TIP This may not be necessary, or you may apply anti-bacterial ointment or Betadine as per office policy.

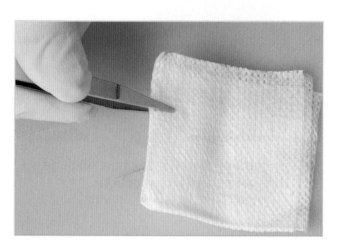

14. Apply bandage or sterile dressing as per provider order.

TIP Most times this will not be necessary, as when sutures come out, healing has already occurred, and air needs to circulate around the suture site to promote healing.

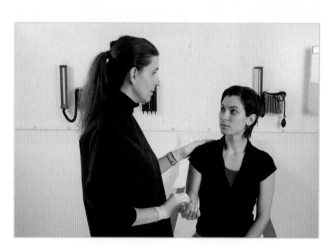

15. Examine patient for any adverse reactions, taking vitals if necessary.

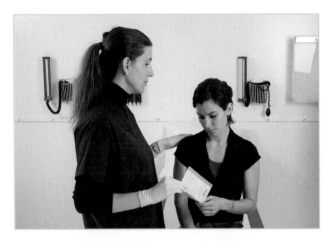

16. Provide both oral and written wound care instructions.

WHY? *Providing instructions orally and in writing helps promote patient understanding.*

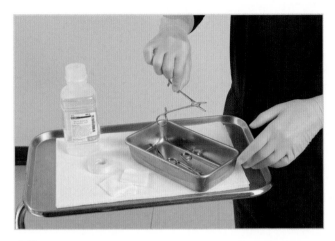

17. Clean up and dispose of items as per OSHA guidelines.

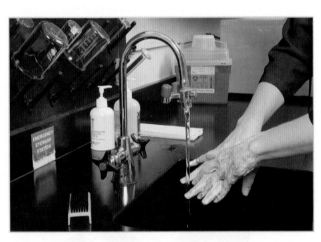

18. Wash hands.

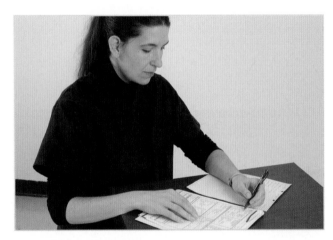

19. Document in patient's chart (include suture count and any reaction).

✎ *Charting Example*

3/21/07 1:00 p.m. Performed suture removal, left wrist. (6 sutures placed, 10/03/05), removed 6 sutures 10/15/05, suture count OK. Wound healing well, no signs of infection. Pt. tolerated procedure well, no adverse reactions. Wound care instructions given verbally and written. No need to dress wound per Dr. Smith. _____ J. Jimenez, CMA

Procedure 7-17

Prepare Patient For and Assist With Procedures, Treatments and Minor Office Surgeries: Perform Dressing Change

PURPOSE

When a patient's wound has not yet fully healed and needs to remain covered, the medical assistant removes the existing dressing from the wound and applies a new sterile one.

EQUIPMENT/SUPPLIES

- sterile field
- sterile sponge forceps
- sterile gauze
- sterile bowl of Betadine or other cleansing solution
- side tray of supplies
- bandaging materials

- antibacterial ointment
- sterile gloves
- sterile water
- wound care instructions
- patient chart
- pen

STANDARD PRECAUTIONS

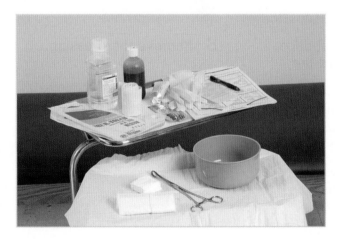

1. Gather all supplies.

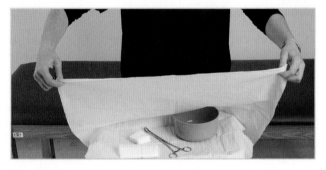

2. Set up sterile field and cover.

WHY? *Dressing change is a sterile procedure as the dressing will be placed on a site with an open wound. Unnatural openings into the body must be protected from microorganisms that can cause infection.*

This may be done ahead of time before the patient enters the room if you know the patient is coming in for this procedure. Always follow office protocol regarding advance set up for sterile fields; determine if it may be left in the room unattended.

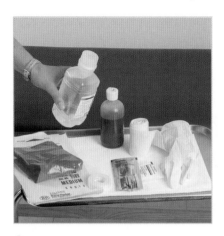

3. Set up side tray.

⫸ Include biohazard water-proof bag or container.

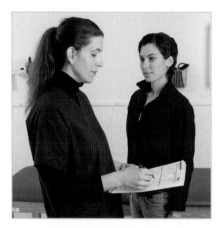

4. Identify the patient.

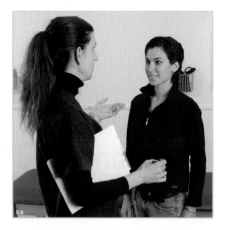

5. Explain the procedure.

⫸ Comfort the patient and obtain vitals as needed.

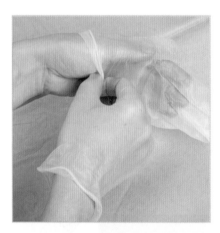

6. Apply regular gloves.

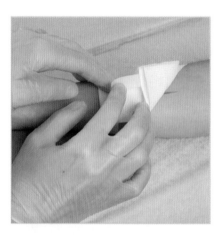

7. Loosen the bandage, pulling toward the wound.

WHY❓ *Pulling away from the wound may cause the healing edges of the wound to come apart.*

⫸ Cut off the bandage if necessary with bandage scissors; dispose in biohazard container if body fluid is present. Always inspect the bandage for signs of blood and/or other discharge.

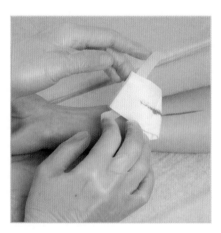

8. Remove the dressing.

⫸ Soak dressing if necessary with sterile water or 50/50 hydrogen peroxide as per office protocol or provider instructions. Dispose in biohazard container.

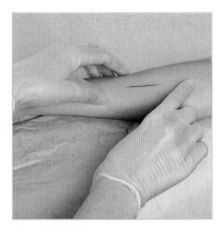

9. Examine the wound for signs of infection or drainage.

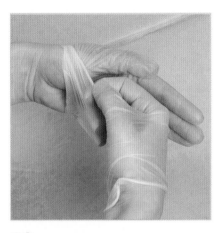

10. Remove gloves.

WHY? *The gloves are contaminated and cannot be worn when applying the new dressing; sterile gloves must be used.*

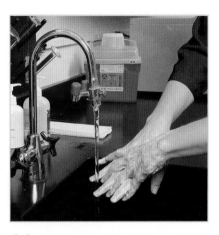

11. Wash hands.

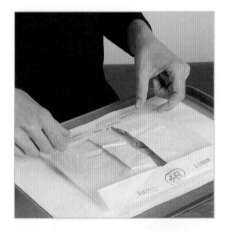

12. Open the package of sterile gloves on clean countertop.

TIP Inspect the package for tears or signs of disrepair.

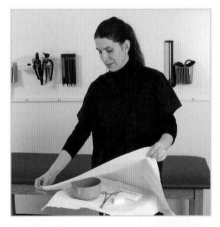

13. Remove cover of sterile field.

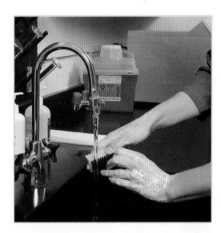

14. Perform a surgically aseptic handwash.

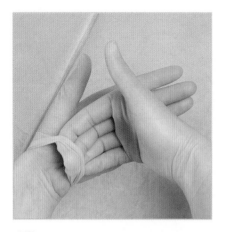

15. Apply sterile gloves.

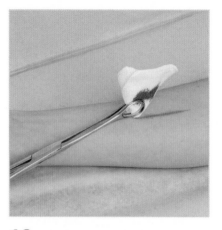

16. Clean the wound with Betadine scrub, rinse, and dispose of used gauze in the biohazard container.

WHY❓ *The wound must be cleaned before applying a new dressing.*

▷ Use whatever solution the provider dictates as per office protocol; some offices may just want the wound rinsed with sterile water.

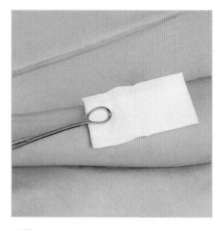

17. Using sterile forceps, place a sterile dressing over the wound.

▷ Apply anti-bacterial ointment only as dictated by the provider.

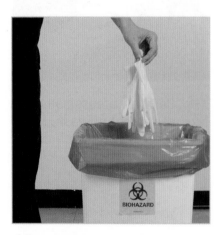

18. If gloves are soiled, remove, dispose in biohazard container and replace with regular gloves. If gloves are not soiled, continue.

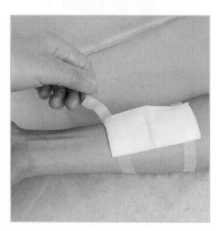

19. Secure the dressing with a bandage or adhesive tape as per office protocol.

▷ Use critical thinking to decide if the bandage needs a more secure dressing: Is it on a joint? Is it on an area that is used often and has movement? Is this a child? Does it need air to circulate and promote healing?

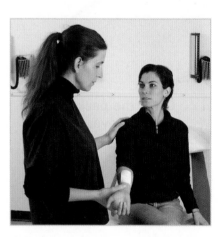

20. Assess the patient as necessary, including vitals.

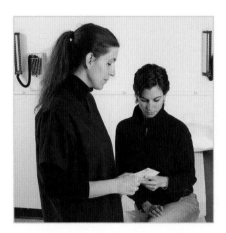

21. Give the patient both oral and written wound care instructions and make follow-up appointment as necessary.

WHY? *Providing instructions orally and in writing helps promote patient understanding and cooperation.*

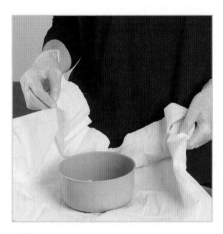

22. Clean and dispose of all supplies, as per OSHA guidelines.

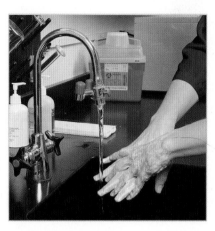

23. Wash hands.

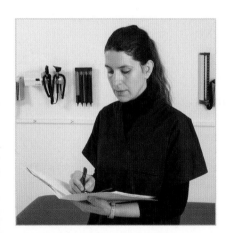

24. Document in the patient's chart, being sure to include wound appearance.

 As with any procedure, constantly assess the patient by checking skin color and reactions and asking how the patient feels. Stop any procedure if the patient has an adverse reaction and notify the provider.

Charting Example

6/7/07 3:00 p.m. Performed dressing change on 3cm wound on right forearm. No signs of infection, wound healing well. Applied antibacterial oint. Per Dr. Jones. Pt tol. proc. well, no adverse reactions. Oral and written wound care instructions given. F/U appt. scheduled for 6/14/07. _____ H. Lewinski, CMA

Procedure **7-18**

Prepare Patient For and Assist With Procedures, Treatments and Minor Office Surgeries: Set Up and Assist with Minor Surgery

PURPOSE

One of the medical assistant's key clinical duties is to set up and assist the provider with minor surgical procedures. In performing this task, the medical assistant must take care to maintain sterile technique, anticipate the provider's needs, reassure the patient, and observe for potential adverse reactions.

EQUIPMENT/SUPPLIES

- sterile field (sterile drapes) with sponge forceps
- gauze and bowl of Betadine scrub or other cleansing solution
- instruments the provider will need depending on procedure to be performed
- suture materials
- scissors
- extra instruments
- side tray of supplies
- Betadine solution (not cleanser)
- sterile gauze
- bandaging materials
- antibacterial ointment
- sterile gloves
- sterile water
- wound care instructions
- formalin container
- medication
- lidocaine drawn up in syringe(s)
- consent form
- fenestrated sterile drapes
- lab slip
- silver nitrate sticks
- electric cauterizer
- patient chart
- pen
- sphygmomanometer
- stethoscope
- biohazard container
- sharps container

STANDARD PRECAUTIONS

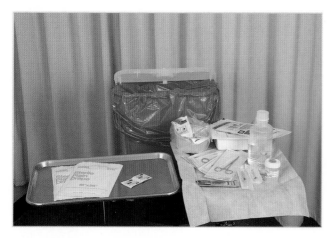

1. Gather all supplies.

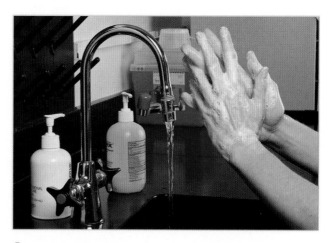

2. Wash hands.

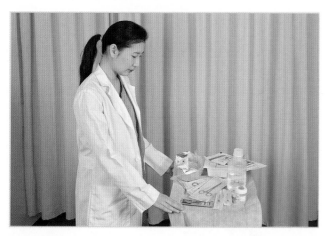

3. Set up side tray on a clean counter or tray.

▷ This may include many things depending on the procedure to be performed: extra gauze and bandaging supplies, extra instruments, Betadine scrub and solution, sterile gloves, regular gloves, consent form, medications, patient instructions, lab slip, tissue sample container with Formalin, 1cc syringes with lidocaine, or lidocaine with epinephrine drawn up, biohazard bag or container, silver nitrate sticks, electric disposable cauterizer, etc.

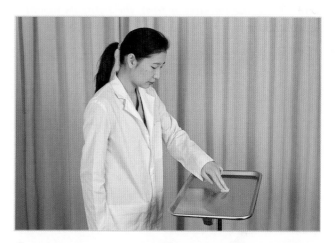

4. Clean Mayo stand with alcohol.

WHY? *This reduces microorganisms by sanitization and disinfection, but the Mayo stand is not sterile.*

▷ Use alcohol or sterilization solution as per office protocol, being sure to clean in a circular motion from center to outer edges.

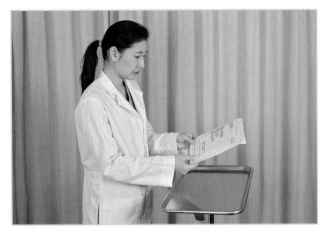

5. Select appropriate disposable sterile field package and inspect for tears.

WHY? *If the package is torn, the contents would be contaminated.*

TIP Some offices may use sterile towels fanfolded in a canister. Use whatever your office uses.

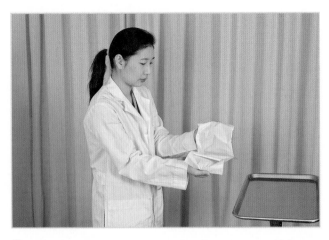

6. Open package exposing the fanfolded drape, being sure the corners are toward you; if not, turn the package as necessary.

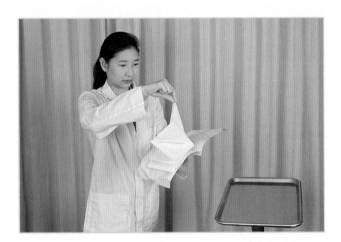

7. Grasp the corner of the drape carefully with thumb and forefinger, without touching the center of the drape, and lift it away from the package, allowing it to unfold naturally. Lift it high enough so that it doesn't touch any non-sterile area and is above waist level. You can let the package drop to the floor if you are holding it; you can clean up later.

WHY? *This method ensures that sterility is maintained.*

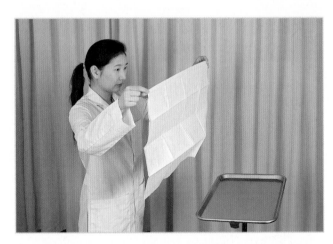

8. Grasp the opposing corner so that both corners along the long edge of the drape are being held; keep it above waist level so as not to breach sterility.

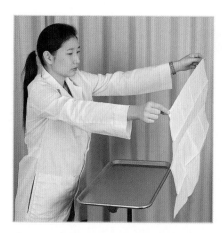

9. Keeping the drape above waist level and away from the body, reach over the Mayo stand with the drape.

TIP Take great care that the drape does not touch or drag on the Mayo stand.

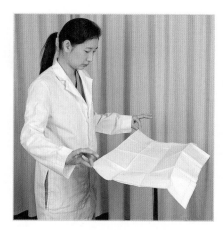

10. Gently pull the drape toward you as you lay it onto the tray. If adjustment is needed to center the drape, do not reach over the sterile field or touch the center, walk around, or reach underneath.

WHY? *Reaching over the sterile field or touching the center can cause contamination.*

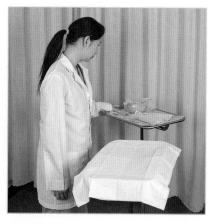

11. Prepare necessary instruments and supplies for the sterile tray.

TIP This will depend on the procedure you are going to perform and provider preference.

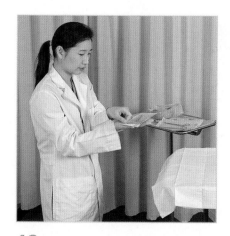

12. Position the first package of surgical instruments on the palm of your non-dominant hand with the opening on top.

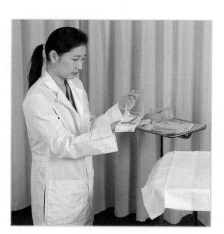

13. Open the package away from you, being sure not to cross over the sterile field. Avoid touching the inside of the package or the instruments.

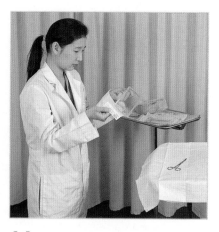

14. Flip the instruments onto the sterile tray.

TIP Some offices want you to flip, while others approve of dropping from 12 inches above the tray. If anything falls, leave it and clean it later; replace any fallen instruments with new. You can drop the empty package on the floor and clean it later if you wish. If you are using instruments in blue paper, open the package so that your non-dominant hand is covered with the blue paper and carefully drop the instruments onto the tray.

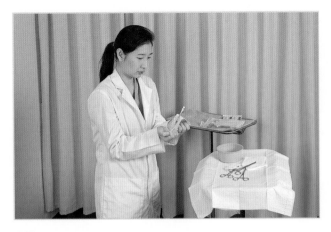

15. Repeat the process until all needed instruments and supplies are on the sterile tray.

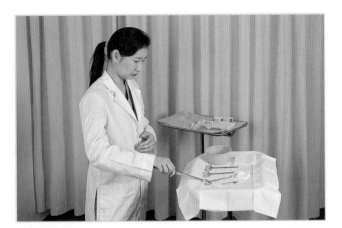

16. Use a sterile forceps to arrange the instruments on the tray, usually in order of use, with handles to the outside, being careful not to cross over the sterile field; walk around if you have to.

WHY❓ *This methods prevents contaminating the sterile field while you organize the items on the tray.*

TIP Again, this will depend on office protocol and provider preference. Whichever method you use, always be careful not to breach the sterile field and follow office protocol with all set ups.

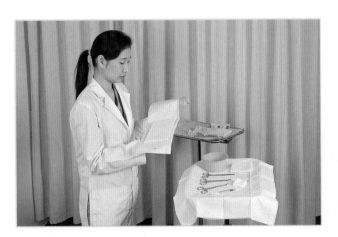

17. Open a second sterile drape in the same manner as above.

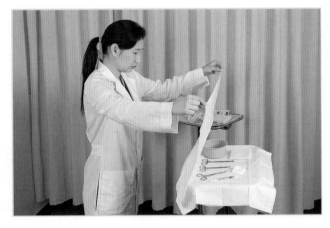

18. Once you have the two corners of the lengthwise drape grasped in your fingertips and above your waist, cover the sterile field by holding it up in front of the field of instruments, adjusting the lower edge so it is even with the lower edge of the bottom drape, and with a forward motion, carefully lay the cover over the sterile field.

WHY❓ *Cover the field away from you rather than towards you so as not to reach over the sterile field and do not drag the drape once the bottom edge touches the sterile field.*

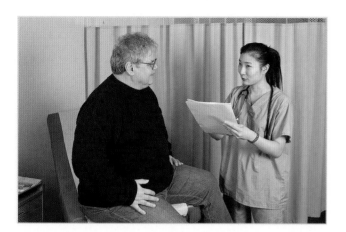

19. Identify the patient.

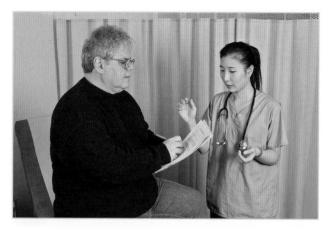

20. Explain the procedure, being sure to get a signed consent.

WHY? *Obtaining informed consent is critical for any surgical procedure, no matter how minor. The medical assistant may be required to explain the procedure in detail so the patient understands, or the provider may do this.*

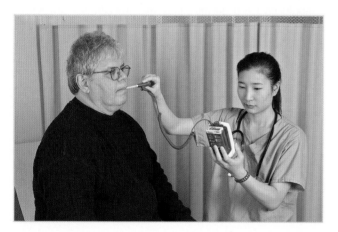

21. Obtain vitals signs and prepare the patient.

TIP Preparing the patient might include asking the patient to undress, preparing the skin, or applying a fenestrated sterile drape, depending on the procedure to be performed.

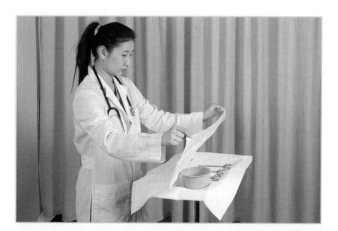

22. Remove the cover from the sterile field by reaching across, grasping the corners, and pulling toward you.

TIP Be careful not to cross the sterile field. The provider will apply sterile gloves at this time.

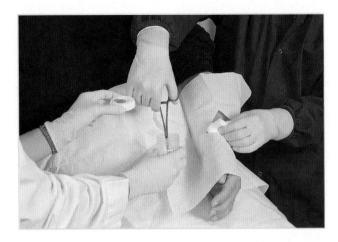

23. Assist the provider as necessary, following the principles of surgical asepsis whether you are in a sterile role or a non-sterile role of assisting.

The tasks you will perform will depend on whether you are sterile or non-sterile when you assist and what the physician requires (Box 7-6).

Box 7•6	**Sterile and Non-Sterile Assisting: Commonly Performed Tasks**

Sterile Assistant	*Non-sterile Assistant*
Dress and bandage wound following procedure	Adjust tray or light source
Hold retractors or other instruments	Comfort and assess patient during procedure
Use gauze or suction to clear blood from surgical site	Hold medication vial while physician draws up (see Tip below)
Cut sutures as they are put in	Hold biopsy container
	Provide new instruments or supplies as needed

It is up to your physician to determine what PPE should be worn during tasks and procedures—always follow the employer's guidelines.

When drawing up lidocaine without epinephrine or lidocaine with epinephrine (if the provider orders you to prepare the local anesthetic), remember the saying: "Penis, nose, fingers, toes, no epi." The reason for this is that you do not want to inject epinephrine, a vasoconstrictor, into appendages as it may cut off blood supply to that area.

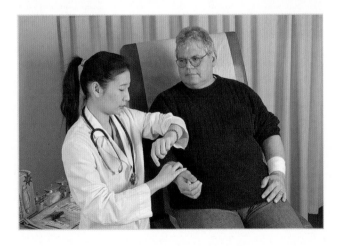

24. Assess the patient, obtaining vital signs as necessary and following provider's instructions for the recovery time.

Watch for vasovagal reaction or orthostatic hypotension. If patient is required to disrobe, have the patient lie or sit for awhile before getting dressed.

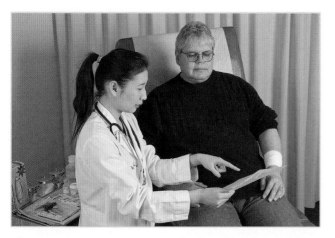

25. Provide the patient with oral and written post-surgical or wound care instructions.

ᴡʜʏ❓ *Giving instructions orally and in writing promotes patient understanding and promotes patient cooperation .*

▷ You may be giving the patient medications to take home, or possibly Tylenol to take now, or you may need to schedule a follow up appointment for the patient. Do this yourself, confirming that it is convenient for the patient, so the patient does not have to stand around in the reception area.

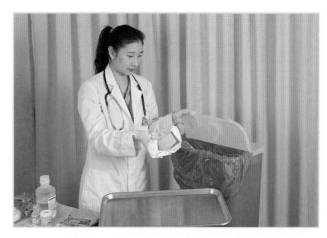

26. After the patient leaves the room, clean up and dispose of used items or instruments according to OSHA guidelines.

▷ When first removing the cover of the sterile field for the provider, save it on the side so that you can use it to cover the tray so the patient is not discomforted by the sight of used instruments and any blood. Wear proper PPE when cleaning the room.

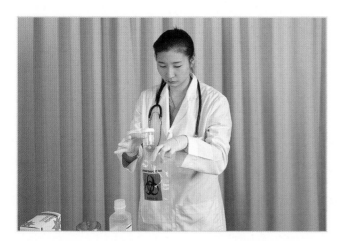

27. Send any specimens to the lab with a completed lab slip. Tightly secure the lid on the formalin container and properly label the container with patient identification and tissue source.

▷ The medical assistant should always wear gloves when handling specimens.

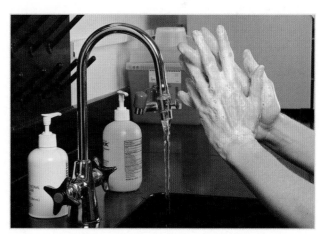

28. Wash hands.

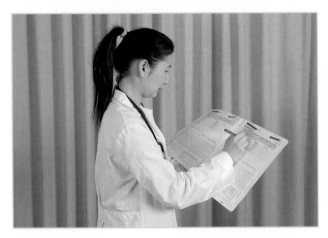

29. Document as necessary, including instructions or medications given, and put a copy of any lab slips in the chart. Document any adverse patient reactions occurring after the provider has left the room and inform the provider immediately.

 The provider will document the procedure.

 Charting Example

9/7/07 10:45 a.m. T 98.8 F, P 68, R 20, BP 136/82 surgical site was dressed and bandaged per Dr. Quintana, post-op instructions were given to the patient both orally and in writing. Patient to return for suture removal in one week. Appt. made for 9/14/07 at 1:00 pm, patient given appt. card. _____ R. Winkowski, CMA

Procedure **7-19**

Apply Pharmacology Principles to Prepare and Administer Oral and Parenteral (Excluding IV) Medications: Withdraw (Aspirate) Medication From a Vial

PURPOSE

Parenteral medications must be prepared correctly before they can be used for injections. By following the appropriate steps for withdrawing medication from a vial, the medical assistant protects patient safety and reduces the risk of infection.

EQUIPMENT/SUPPLIES

- medication vial
- syringe
- needle
- alcohol wipes
- pen
- medication order
- patient chart

STANDARD PRECAUTIONS

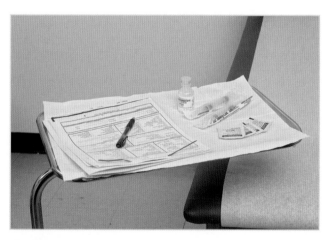

1. Gather all supplies.

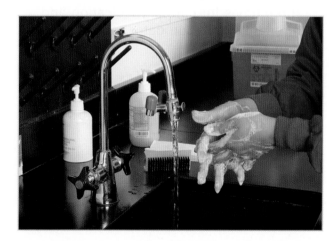

2. Wash hands. Apply gloves as per office protocol.

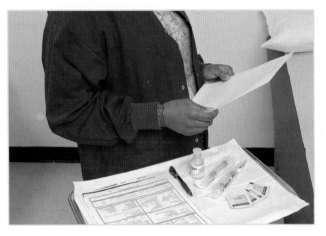

3. Read the medication order. Follow the six rights (Box 7-7).

TIP Many practices also include a seventh right: right technique.

Box 7•7   **"SIX RIGHTS"**

Right Drug
Right Dose
Right Route
Right Time
Right Patient
Right Documentation

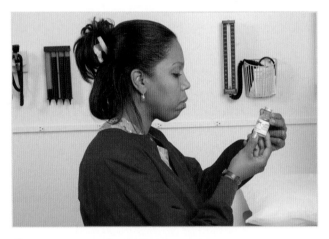

4. Read the vial label. This will be checked three times for correct medication and strength, expiration date, and medication appearance.

WHY? *This prevents errors of the wrong drug or strength and ensures that expired medication is not administered.*

TIP Be sure to read the medication strength on the labels as well as the name to further prevent errors; there may be more than one vial of the same drug but in different strengths.

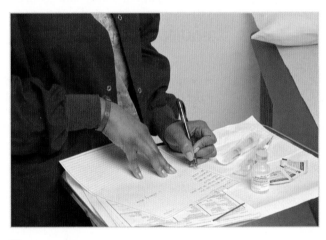

5. Calculate dosage if necessary.

TIP Some offices purchase single dose pre-filled syringes of certain medications; if so, check this label instead of the vial.

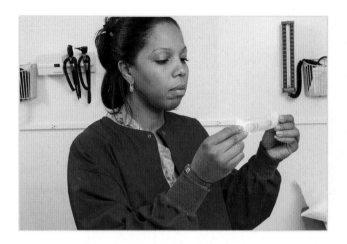

6. Select proper needle and syringe for medication type, patient size, and route (Box 7-8).

Box 7·8	Route	Typical Syringe/Needle Combinations*
	Intradermal	1cc syringe/25g-5/8 needle
	Subcutaneous	1cc syringe/25g-5/8 needle
	IM Deltoid	1-3cc syringe/23g-1 needle
	IM Vastus	1-3cc syringe/23g-1 needle
	IM Gluteus	1-3cc syringe/22g-1½ needle
	Z-Track	1-3cc syringe/21g-1½ needle
	Insulin	U-100 26g-½ needle

*Needle gauge will depend on the thickness of the medication being administered. Needle length will depend on the body mass of the patient.

Pharmacological principles and medication administration are critical aspects of the medical assistant's duties. Knowledge of medications, their actions on the body, safety measures, and accurate medication calculation is critical. OSHA guidelines, safety precautions, needlestick protocol, and proper site selection are also critical. A medical assistant must know, understand, and utilize all precautions and risk management guidelines when dealing with medications.

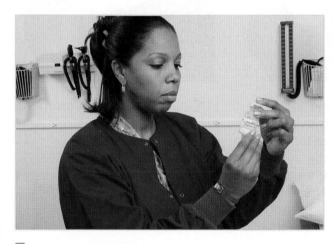

7. Check vial label.

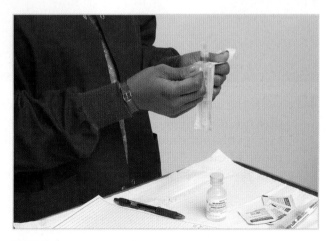

8. Assemble or prepare syringe.

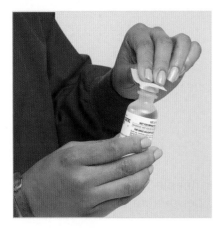

9. Clean the vial top with alcohol, even if opening new vial. If using a new vial, initial and date that you opened it.

WHY? *This prevents microorganisms from entering the medication when the needle pierces the rubber stopper.*

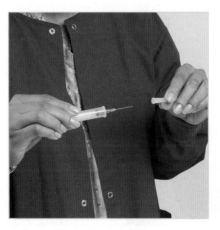

10. Remove needle cover by pulling it straight off.

TIP Do not throw the needle cap away yet—you will need to cover the needle by the scoop method or by using a recapping device after filling the syringe. The cap sitting upside down in the middle of a roll of 1 inch tape is an effective way as well.

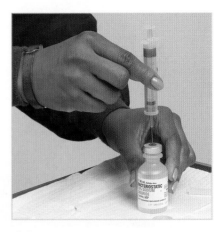

11. Inject air into the vial in the amount of medication you want to draw up. For example, if drawing up 1cc, inject 1cc of air.

WHY? *This keeps the pressure equalized by replacing the medication with air inside the airtight vial.*

TIP Try not to inject the air into the medication if possible—this will help prevent air bubbles in thicker medications.

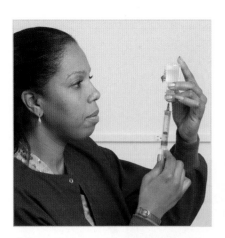

12. With the vial upside down and held at eye level, withdraw medication.

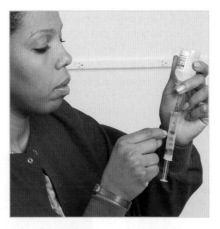

13. Check syringe for air bubbles; remove if necessary by tapping sharply on the syringe. Do not draw up more medication than necessary and expel it to remove bubbles; this is a waste of medication and a costly habit.

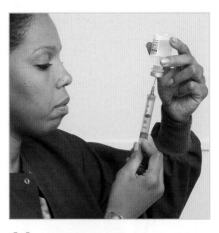

14. Check for measurement accuracy.

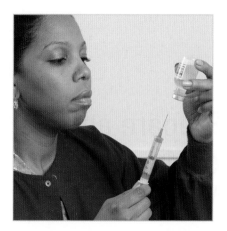

15. Remove needle from vial.

TIP Some offices will always have you change needles for any medication administration. If medication is caustic, be sure to change the needle.

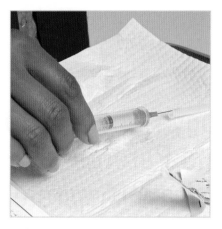

16. Recap by scoop method or with cap holder or tape.

WHY? *Recapping maintains sterility until the medication is given. Never recap by holding the sterile cover to avoid needle sticks!*

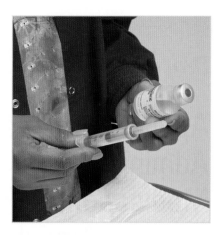

17. Check vial label for third time.

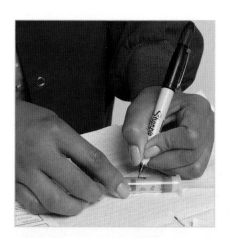

18. Label your syringe!

WHY? *To prevent administering the wrong drug, never give medication in an unlabeled syringe. Use paper tape or indelible ink pen to label.*

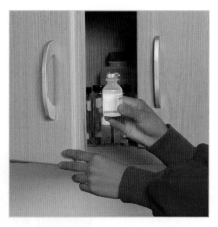

19. Return all medications and supplies to proper place. Discard used vials per OSHA guidelines.

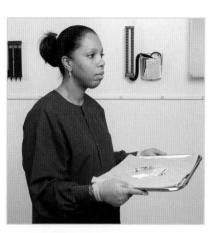

20. Transport medication properly, as per office protocol, to patient for administration.

LEGAL ALERT! Never give a medication you have not drawn up! Document all needlesticks, medication usage, medication discarding, and medication administration as per office protocol.

Procedure **7-20**

Apply Pharmacology Principles to Prepare and Administer Oral and Parenteral (Excluding IV) Medications: Withdraw (Aspirate) Medication From an Ampule

PURPOSE

Parenteral medications must be prepared correctly before they can be used for injections. By following the appropriate steps for withdrawing medication from an ampule, the medical assistant protects patient safety and reduces the risk of infection.

EQUIPMENT/SUPPLIES

- medication ampule
- syringe
- needle
- alcohol
- gauze
- pen
- medication order
- patient chart
- tape
- sharps container
- gloves

STANDARD PRECAUTIONS

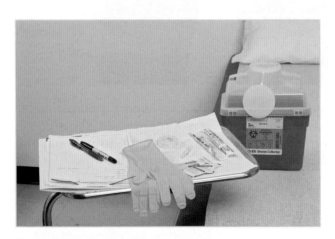

1. Gather all supplies.

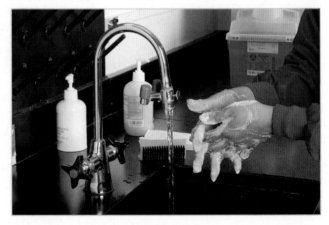

2. Wash hands. Apply gloves as per office protocol.

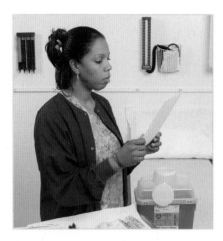

3. Read the medication order. Follow the six rights (see Box 7-7).

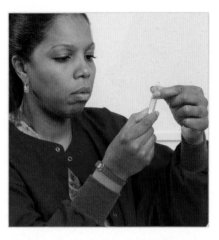

4. Read the ampule label. This will be checked three times for correct medication, expiration date, and medication appearance.

WHY? *This prevents errors and ensures that expired medication is not administered.*

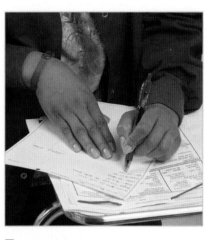

5. Calculate dosage if necessary.

TIP Some offices purchase single-dose pre-filled syringes of certain medications; if so, check this label instead of vial.

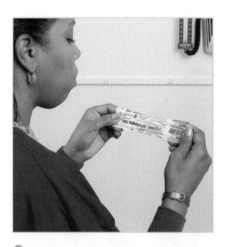

6. Select proper needle and syringe for medication type, patient size, and route (see Box 7-8).

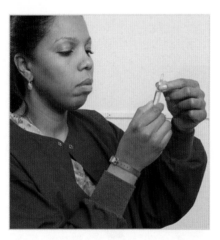

7. Check ampule label.

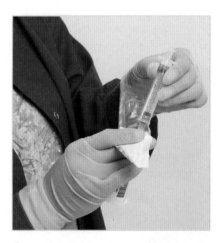

8. Assemble or prepare syringe.

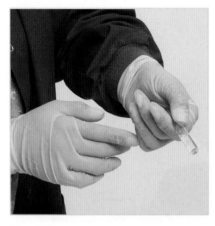

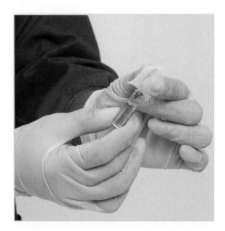

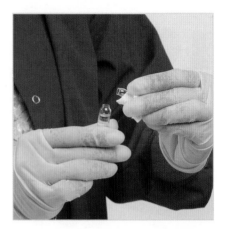

9. Hold ampule and flick in a downward motion to bring all medication into the bottom.

ᴡʜʏ❓ *Medication shifts in transport and may get trapped in the top of the ampule due to its shape.*

10. Disinfect the neck of the ampule with alcohol.

ᴡʜʏ❓ *This removes microorganisms.*

11. Using sterile gauze to surround the neck of the ampule, snap off the top, being sure to snap away from you.

ᴡʜʏ❓ *This prevents an accidental cut to your fingers when the glass snaps.*

TIP➤ Be sure to discard the top of the ampule in the sharps container.

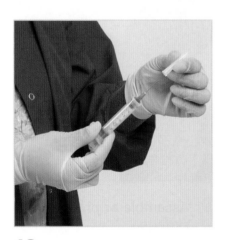

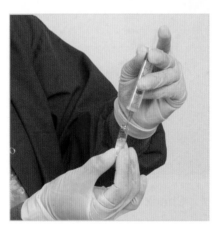

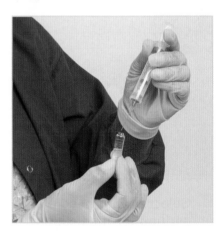

12. Remove needle cover by pulling it straight off.

13. Aspirate medication from the ampule with prepared syringe/needle.

TIP➤ Use filtered needle as per office protocol; most ampules are made of shatterproof glass where pieces do not break off.

14. Remove needle from ampule.

TIP➤ Always change needles when withdrawing from an ampule. Never inject medication into a patient with a filtered needle.

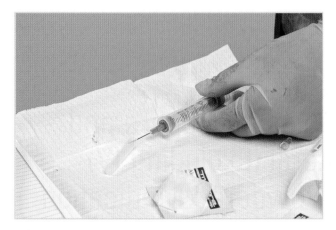

15. Recap by scoop method or with cap holder or tape.

WHY? *Recapping maintains sterility and safety until the medication is given.*

TIP Never recap by holding the sterile cover to avoid needle sticks!

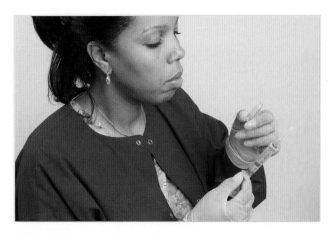

16. Check ampule label for third time.

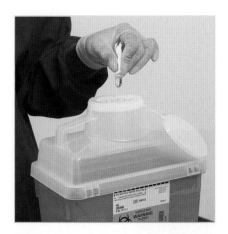

17. Discard used ampule and its top in sharps container.

TIP Be sure you have documented the medication's expiration date, lot number, and manufacturer before discarding the ampule.

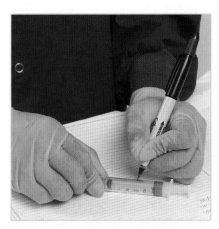

18. Label your syringe.

WHY? *To avoid administering the wrong drug, never give medication in an unlabeled syringe; use paper tape or indelible ink pen.*

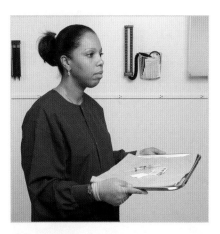

19. Transport medication properly, as per office protocol, to patient for administration.

LEGAL ALERT! Never give a medication you have not drawn up! Document all needlesticks, medication usage, medication discarding, and medication administration as per office protocol.

Procedure **7-21**

Apply Pharmacology Principles to Prepare and Administer Oral and Parenteral (Excluding IV) Medications: Reconstitute Powdered Medication

PURPOSE

Some parenteral medications are supplied in powdered form and must be properly reconstituted before being used for injections. The medical assistant must use the appropriate amount and type of diluent in order to ensure patient safety.

EQUIPMENT/SUPPLIES

- medication vial
- diluent
- syringe
- needle
- alcohol
- pen
- medication order
- patient chart
- gloves

STANDARD **PRECAUTIONS**

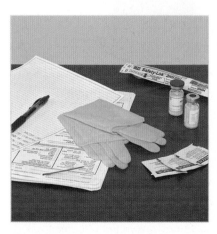

1. Gather all supplies.

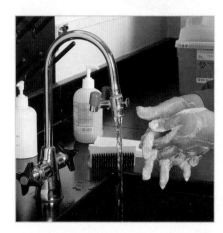

2. Wash hands. Apply gloves as per office protocol.

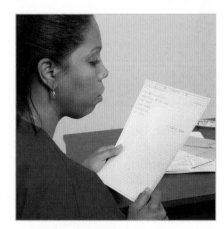

3. Read the medication order. Follow the six rights (see Box 7-7).

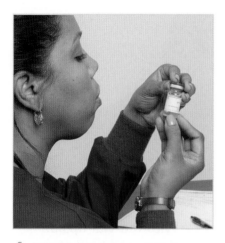

4. Read the vial label. This will be checked three times for correct medication, expiration date, and medication appearance.

WHY❓ *This prevents errors and ensures that expired medication is not administered.*

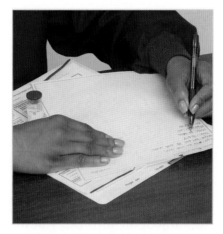

5. Calculate dosage if necessary. When checking vial of powder and vial of diluent, use the correct diluent as per provider order or medication manufacturer, and calculate for the correct strength of reconstitution.

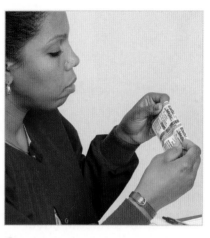

6. Select proper needle and syringe for medication type, patient size, and route (see Box 7-8).

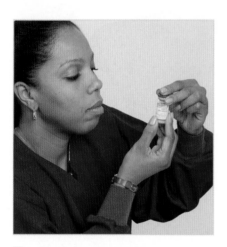

7. Check vial label.

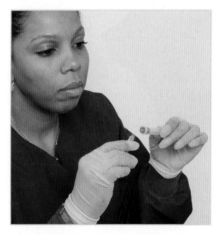

8. Assemble or prepare syringe.

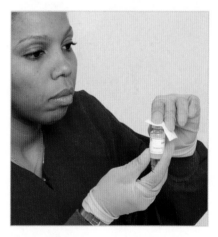

9. Clean the diluent vial top with alcohol, even if opening a new vial. If using a new vial, initial and date that you opened it.

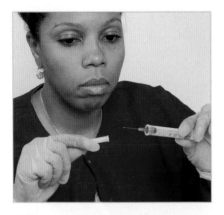

10. Remove needle cover by pulling it straight off.

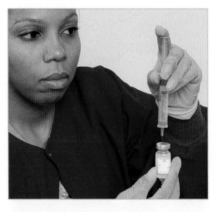

11. Inject air into the vial in the amount of medication you want to draw up. For example, if you are drawing up 1cc, inject 1cc of air.

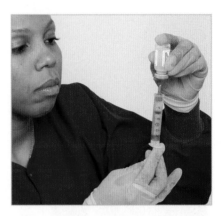

12. With the vial upside down and held at eye level, withdraw diluent.

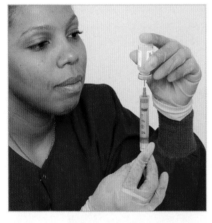

13. Check for measurement accuracy.

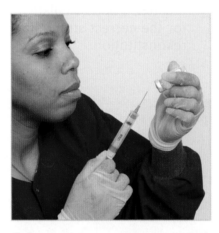

14. Remove needle from diluent vial.

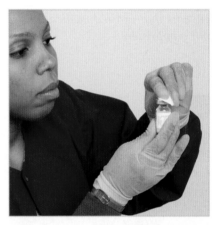

15. Clean top of medication vial.

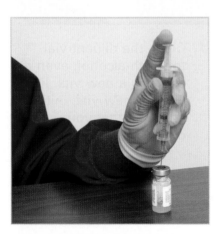

16. Inject diluent into medication.

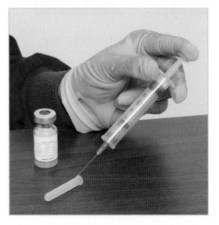

17. Remove needle from vial and recap with scoop method.

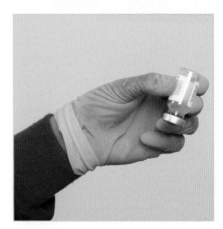

18. Gently rock medication vial to mix diluent with powder.

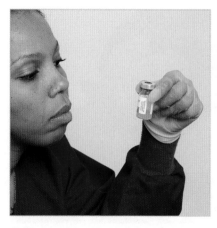

19. Check medication label the third time.

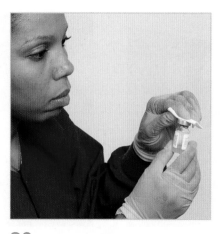

20. Clean top of vial again with alcohol.

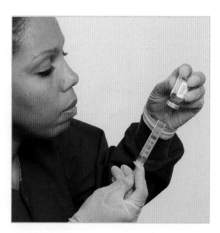

21. Insert needle into vial of mixed medication and withdraw the proper amount (this may be all of it).

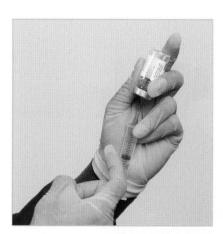

22. Check syringe for air bubbles. Remove if necessary by tapping sharply on the syringe. Do not draw up more medication than necessary and expel it to remove bubbles; this is a waste of medication and a costly habit.

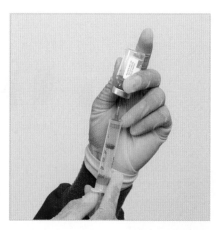

23. Check for measurement accuracy.

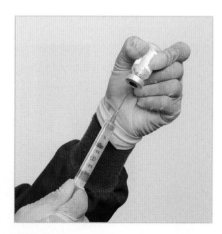

24. Remove needle from vial.

⏵ *Some offices will always have you change needles for any medication administration. If medication is caustic, be sure to change the needle.*

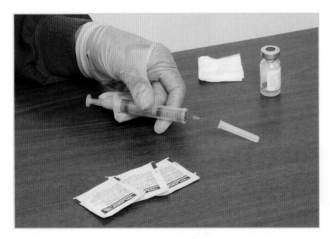

25. Recap by scoop method or with cap holder or tape.

WHY? *Recapping maintains sterility until the medication is given. Never recap by holding the sterile cover to avoid needle sticks!*

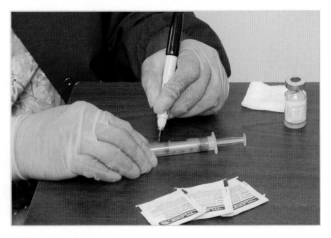

26. Label your syringe.

WHY? *To avoid administering the wrong drug, never give medication in an unlabeled syringe; use paper tape or indelible ink pen to label.*

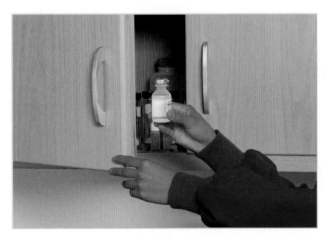

27. Return all medications and supplies to the proper place. Discard used vials as per OSHA guidelines.

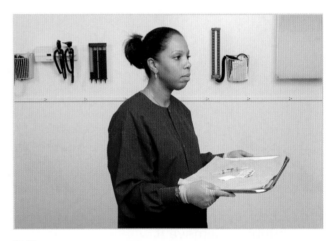

28. Transport medication properly, as per office protocol, to patient for administration.

LEGAL ALERT! Never give a medication you have not drawn up! Document all needlesticks, medication usage, medication discarding, and medication administration as per office protocol.

Procedure **7-22**

Apply Pharmacology Principles to Prepare and Administer Oral and Parenteral (Excluding IV) Medications: Administer Intradermal Injection

PURPOSE

Intradermal injections, which are administered into the skin's dermal layer, are commonly used for PPD or allergy testing.

EQUIPMENT/SUPPLIES

- medication vial
- syringe
- needle
- alcohol
- gauze or cotton
- Band-Aid
- sharps container
- medication tray
- pen
- medication order
- patient chart
- gloves

STANDARD PRECAUTIONS

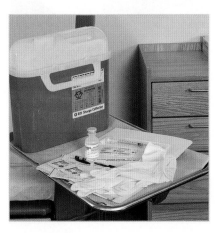

1. Gather all supplies.

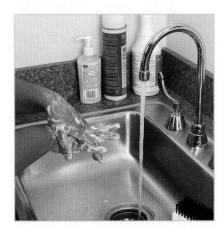

2. Wash hands. Apply gloves as per office protocol.

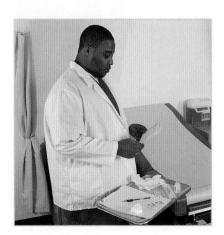

3. Read the medication order. Follow the six rights (see Box 7-7).

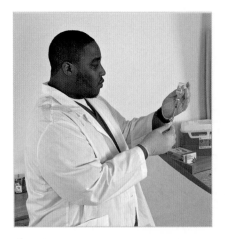

4. Correctly prepare medication (as per procedure 7-19, 7-20, or 7-21).

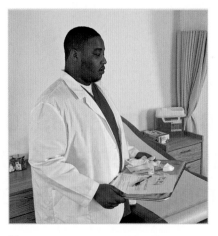

5. Transport medication properly, as per office protocol, to patient for administration.

LEGAL ALERT ! Never give a medication you have not drawn up! Document all needlesticks, medication usage, medication discarding, and medication administration as per office protocol.

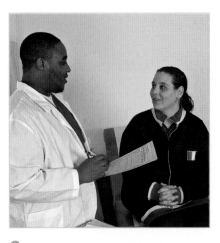

6. Identify the patient.

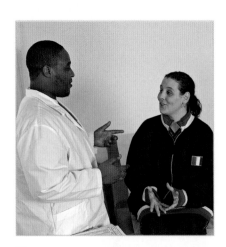

7. Explain the procedure.

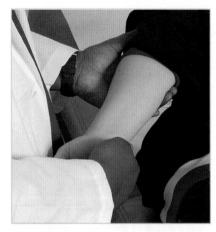

8. Assess the patient, including appropriate site selection, allergies to medications, latex allergies, medication specific questions, previous reactions to injections, etc.

TIP Note areas to avoid for injections (Box 7-9).

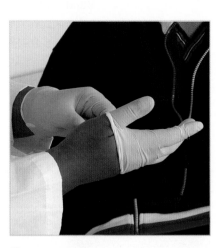

9. Apply gloves.

Box 7·9	**Areas to Avoid When Injecting Medications**

- Scars, tattoos (if possible), excessive hair
- Edematous areas, paralyzed areas
- Moles, warts, birthmarks, tumors, lumps, nodules
- Rashes, inflamed areas
- Wounds, lesions, burns
- Bones, joints, blood vessels, nerves
- Arm on same side as mastectomy
- Traumatized areas, cyanotic areas
- Previous injection sites

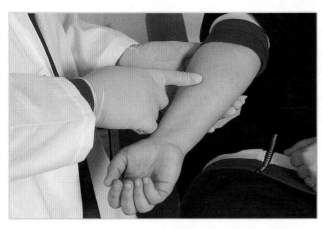

10. Select appropriate site.

TIP Intradermal injections may be performed on the anterior mid forearm or for numerous intradermals such as in allergy testing, the back on either side of the spine. Avoid injecting near the elbow and wrist joints as well.

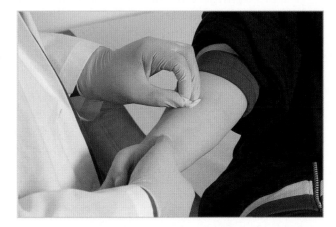

11. Clean site with alcohol. Use a circular motion going from the center out; let air dry for maximum destruction of microorganisms.

WHY? *The site must be cleaned before giving the injection. The circular technique moves microorganisms away from the site.*

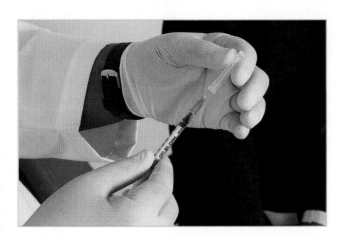

12. Remove needle guard.

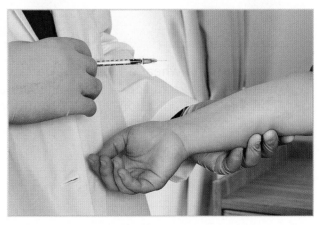

13. Pull forearm skin taut.

WHY? *This helps the needle enter the skin more easily.*

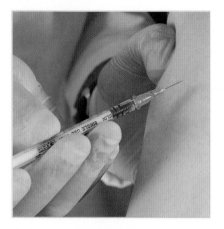

14. Hold syringe with bevel up so that you can inject with one hand as you are holding the skin of the arm taut.

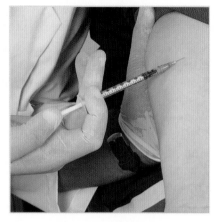

15. Insert needle at a 5–10 degree angle in between the first layers of skin, making sure the bevel is fully inserted.

WHY? *This ensures that the needle enters shallowly within the skin layers and not the subcutaneous tissue directly below.*

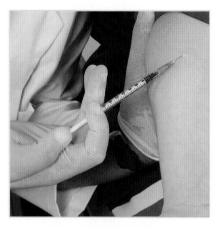

16. Slowly and steadily, inject the medication. Do not aspirate with intradermal medication!

WHY? *Since the injection is given within the layers of skin, there are no blood vessels to worry about injecting into.*

TIP The injections may be for PPD or allergy testing.

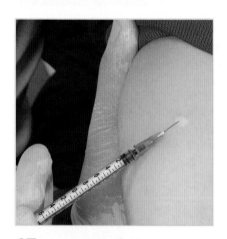

17. Watch for the wheal or bleb, which is a raised "bubble" of medication.

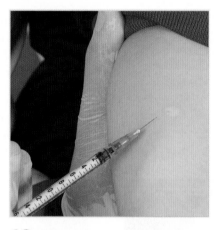

18. Quickly withdraw needle straight out from the patients arm.

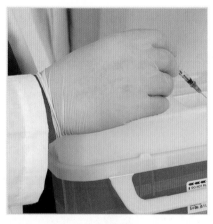

19. Discard needle immediately into sharps container. Use of safety needles is required by OSHA; close the safety feature first.

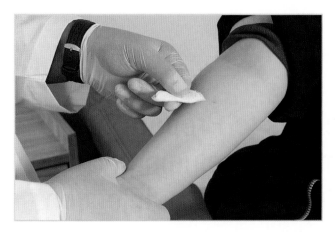

20. Blot site.

WHY? *Do not massage because doing so can cause the medication to move into the tissues. Do not cover.*

TIP If the site bleeds a very small amount, you can gently touch the corner of a gauze square to soak it up until it clots or you can place a Band-Aid with the adhesive portions close to the injection site so that the dressing portion is hovering above the site. This will avoid any blood soiling the patient's clothing but does not touch the site and therefore does not alter the results.

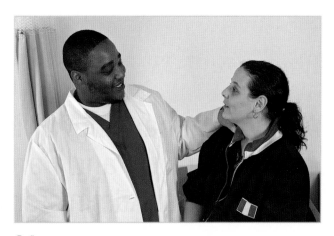

21. Observe patient reaction.

TIP The patient must wait at least 20 minutes after any injection of medications. Make sure the patient has a ride home if necessary, e.g., after narcotic administration.

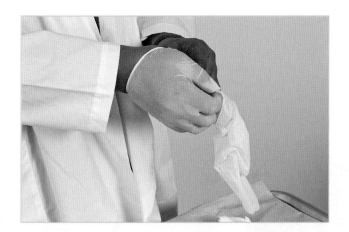

22. Remove gloves and wash hands.

Charting Example
4/25/07 9:45 a.m. Administered PPD, left anterior forearm, pt tol. well, no adv. react. RTC 48-72 hrs for reading. (lot #1234, Merck, exp. 4/08) _____ H. Lee, CMA

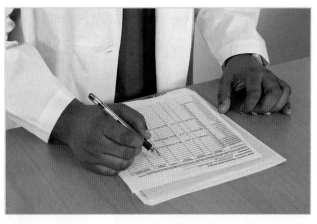

23. Document the procedure.

TIP If the patient was asked to remain for 20 minutes but chooses to leave anyway, be sure to chart that as well. Be sure to document patient reaction even if there is none.

TIP Allergy testing requires the patient to wait so that induration (elevation + redness) can be observed and documented. PPD testing requires the patient to return to the medical office between 48–72 hours for "reading" the induration and possible administration of a second dose. Follow all medication guidelines and office protocol for these types of medications.

Procedure 7-23

Apply Pharmacology Principles to Prepare and Administer Oral and Parenteral (Excluding IV) Medications: Administer Subcutaneous Injection

PURPOSE

The subcutaneous route is used when medication needs to be absorbed at a slower rate than if given intramuscularly.

EQUIPMENT/SUPPLIES

- medication vial
- syringe
- needle
- alcohol
- gauze or cotton
- Band-Aid

- sharps container
- medication tray
- pen
- medication order
- patient chart
- gloves

STANDARD PRECAUTIONS

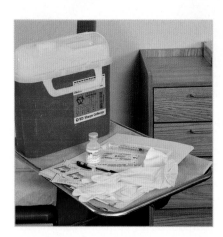

1. Gather all supplies.

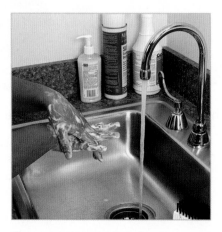

2. Wash hands. Apply gloves as per office protocol.

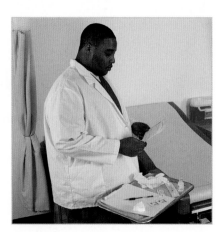

3. Read the medication order. Follow the six rights (see Box 7-7).

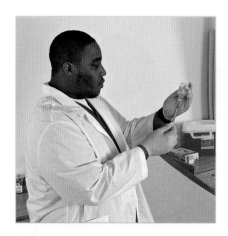

4. Correctly prepare medication (as per procedure 7-19, 7-20, or 7-21).

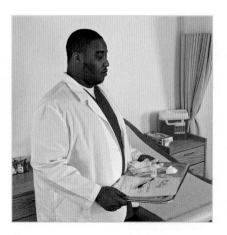

5. Transport medication properly, as per office protocol, to patient for administration.

LEGAL ALERT *!* Never give a medication you have not drawn up! Document all needlesticks, medication usage, medication discarding, and medication administration as per office protocol.

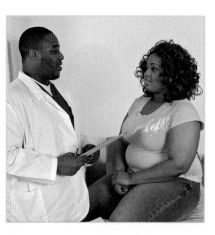

6. Identify patient.

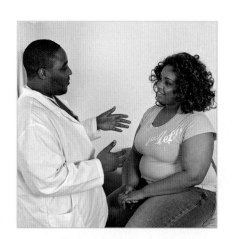

7. Explain the procedure.

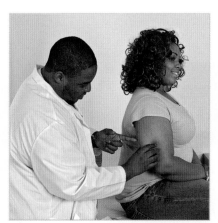

8. Assess the patient, including appropriate site selection, allergies to medications, latex allergies, medication specific questions, previous reactions to injections, etc.

TIP Note areas to avoid for injections (see Box 7-9).

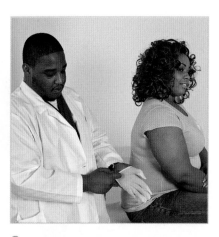

9. Apply gloves.

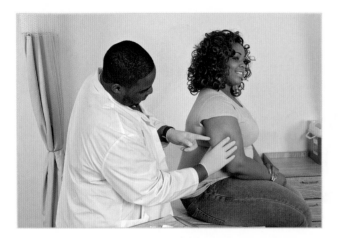

10. Select appropriate site.

TIP A subcutaneous injection is performed most commonly on the posterior mid upper arm, although the fatty tissue around the waist anteriorly and the lateral upper thigh where there is usually some subcutaneous tissue may also be used. Avoid selecting a site near the elbow and shoulder joints.

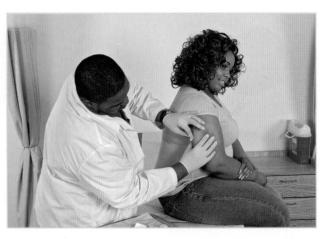

11. Clean site with alcohol. Use a circular motion going from the center out; let air dry for maximum destruction of microorganisms.

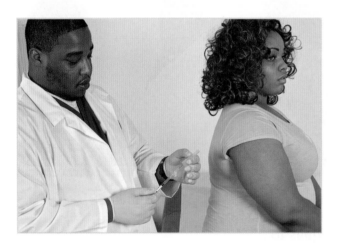

12. Remove needle guard.

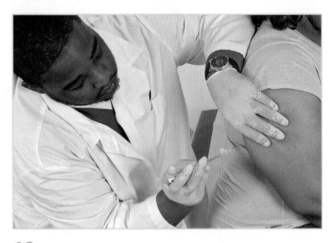

13. Gently pinch skin, gathering about an inch of subcutaneous tissue.

WHY? If you pinch too hard it will hurt the patient and possibly leave a bruise, and the medication will be forced back out when the needle is removed from the arm.

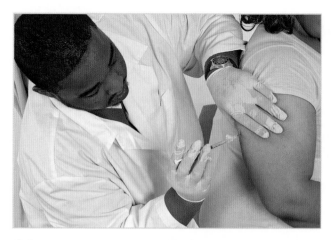

14. Insert needle quickly using a darting motion at a 45-degree angle.

WHY? Quick insertion helps lessen patient discomfort.

TIP Some providers prefer that you inject upward toward the shoulder for proper medication disbursement and to avoid medication from pooling toward the elbow joint.

TIP Always remember that although insulin is given subcutaneously, it requires administration at a 90-degree angle and site rotation.

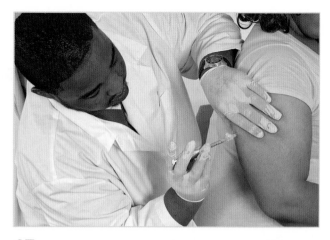

15. Aspirate to make sure you are not in a blood vessel.

WHY? If the medication were injected into this site, it would be injected intravenously, which is not correct and could be life-threatening.

TIP If you should draw some blood into the hub of the needle, withdraw and follow office policy regarding giving the injection in another site. You may need to simply change the needle or you may be required to discard the entire set up and medication and begin again.

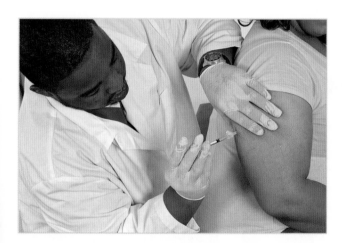

16. Slowly and steadily, inject the medication.

WHY? This prevents patient discomfort and avoids potential damage to tissues.

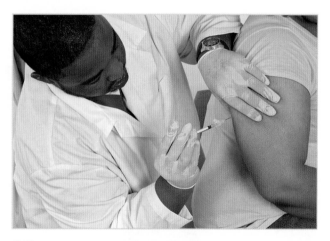

17. Quickly withdraw needle straight out from the patient's arm.

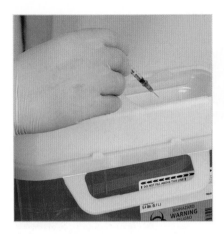

18. Discard needle immediately into sharps container. Use of safety needles is required by OSHA; close the safety feature first.

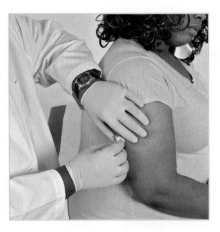

19. Massage the site unless contra-indicated by gently pressing the gauze/cotton ball to the site and moving in a circular motion for a moment.

WHY? *This helps to distribute the medication into the surrounding tissues, promoting better absorption and minimizing discomfort to the patient.*

TIP Insulin, Imferon, and heparin are examples of medications that should NOT be massaged.

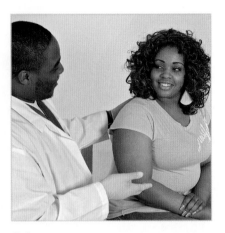

20. Observe patient reaction.

TIP The patient must wait at least 20 minutes after any injection of medications. Make sure the patient has a ride home if necessary, e.g., after narcotic administration.

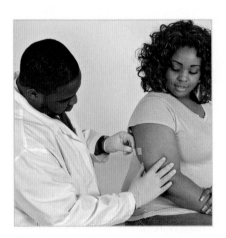

21. Apply Band-Aid.

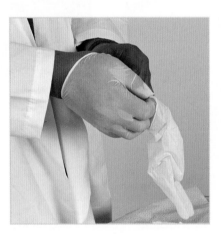

22. Remove gloves and wash hands.

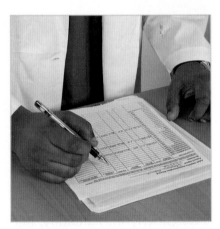

23. Document the procedure.

TIP Be sure to document patient reaction even if there is none.

✎ *Charting Example*

2/18/07 10:20 a.m. Administered 15U Humulin Insulin, LA, subcutaneously, per Dr. Jones, pt tolerated well, no adv. reactions. Pt waited 30 minutes, left fine. (lot #3455, Merck, exp 5/09) _____ C. Andrews, CMA

Procedure 7-24

Apply Pharmacology Principles to Prepare and Administer Oral and Parenteral (Excluding IV) Medications: Administer Intramuscular Injection in the Deltoid Area

PURPOSE

When medication needs to be absorbed rapidly, the intramuscular (IM) route is used. The deltoid area is one of several sites recommended for IM injections.

EQUIPMENT/SUPPLIES

- medication vial
- syringe
- needle
- alcohol
- gauze or cotton
- Band-Aid

- sharps container
- medication tray
- pen
- medication order
- patient chart
- gloves

STANDARD PRECAUTIONS

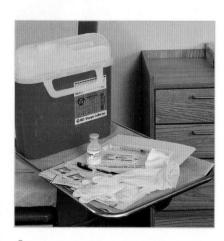

1. Gather all supplies.

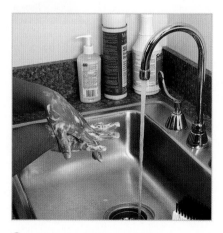

2. Wash hands. Apply gloves as per office protocol.

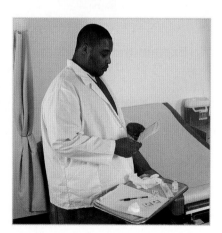

3. Read the medication order. Follow the six rights (see Box 7-7).

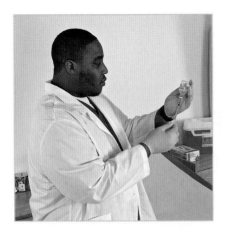

4. Correctly prepare medication (as per procedure 7-19, 7-20, or 7-21).

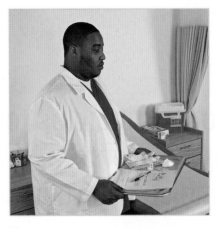

5. Transport medication properly, as per office protocol, to patient for administration.

LEGAL ALERT! *Never give a medication you have not drawn up! Document all needlesticks, medication usage, medication discarding, and medication administration as per office protocol.*

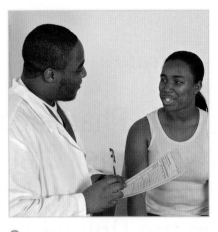

6. Identify patient.

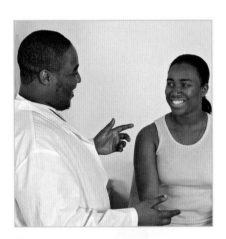

7. Explain the procedure.

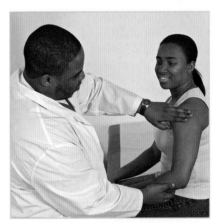

8. Assess the patient, including appropriate site selection, allergies to medications, latex allergies, medication specific questions, previous reactions to injections, etc.

TIP *Note areas to avoid for injections (see Box 7-9).*

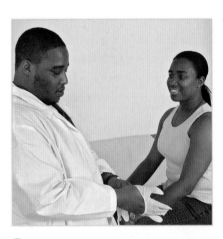

9. Apply gloves.

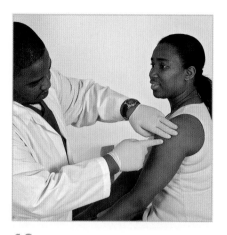

10. Select appropriate site.

WHY? *It is important to select the correct site to avoid damaging nearby blood vessels or nerves.*

TIP Use the upper outer aspect of the arm below the lower edge of the acromion process. This is sometimes measured by using three fingers down from the acromion. (See illustration at the end of this procedure.)

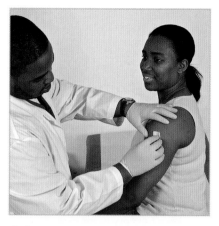

11. Clean the site with alcohol. Use a circular motion going from the center out, let air dry for maximum destruction of microorganisms.

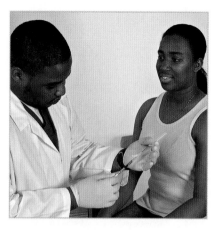

12. Remove the needle guard.

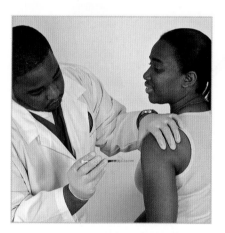

13. Gently grasp deltoid muscle.

TIP Some providers recommend spreading skin here with one hand. If you grasp, be sure to grasp the muscle and not just the subcutaneous tissue above the muscle.

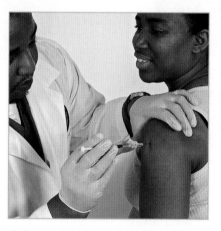

14. Insert needle quickly using a darting motion at a 90-degree angle.

WHY? *A quick motion helps prevent patient discomfort.*

TIP Be sure you get the middle of the deltoid and avoid the nerves and blood vessels in that area.

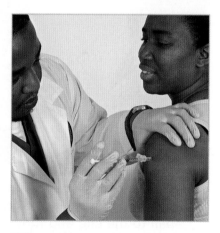

15. Aspirate to make sure you are not in a blood vessel.

WHY? *If the medication were injected into this site, it would be injected intravenously, which is not correct and could be life-threatening.*

TIP If you should draw some blood into the hub of the needle, withdraw and follow office policy regarding giving the injection in another site. You may need to simply change the needle or you may be required to discard the entire set up and medication and begin again.

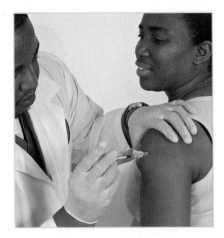

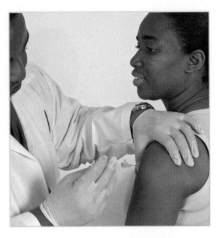

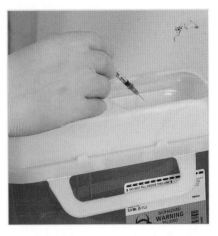

16. Slowly and steadily, inject the medication.

WHY? *This lessens patient discomfort and avoids potential damage to tissues.*

17. Quickly withdraw needle straight out from the patient's arm.

18. Discard needle immediately into sharps container. Use of safety needles is required by OSHA; close the safety feature first.

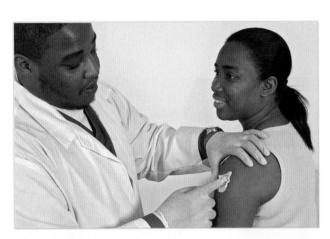

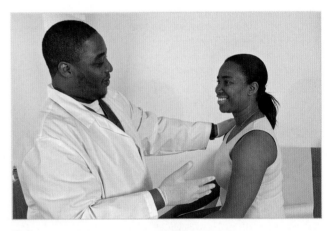

19. Massage site, unless contra-indicated, by gently pressing the gauze/cotton ball to the site and moving in a circular motion for a moment.

WHY? *This helps to distribute the medication into the surrounding tissues, promoting better absorption and minimizing discomfort to the patient.*

TIP> Insulin, Imferon, and heparin are examples of medications that should NOT be massaged.

20. Observe the patient's reaction.

TIP> The patient must wait at least 20 minutes after any injection of medications. Make sure the patient has a ride home if necessary, e.g., after narcotic administration.

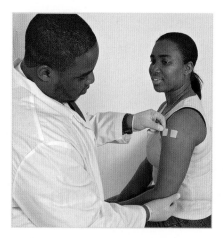

21. Apply Band-Aid.

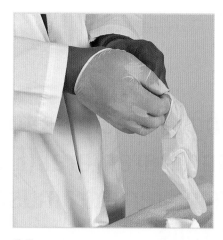

22. Remove gloves and wash hands.

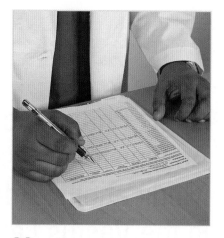

23. Document the procedure.

⏩ Be sure to document patient reaction even if there is none.

⏩ Following the six rights of medication administration, checking the medication label three times, using proper needle sizes and body location, and proper documentation are critical skills.

✎ *Charting Example*

2/4/07 2:45 p.m. Administered 1gm Rocephin L Delt. Per Dr. Smith, pt. tol. well, no adv. react. Pt waited 30 mins, left fine. (lot #12345, Merck, exp 5/09) _____ I. Proknaw, CMA

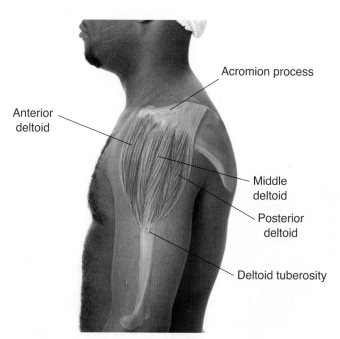

Acromion process

Anterior deltoid

Middle deltoid

Posterior deltoid

Deltoid tuberosity

Deltoid anatomy.

Procedure **7-25**

Apply Pharmacology Principles to Prepare and Administer Oral and Parenteral (Excluding IV) Medications: Administer Intramuscular Injection in the Vastus Lateralis

PURPOSE

When medication needs to be absorbed rapidly, the intramuscular route is used. The vastus lateralis is one of several sites recommended for IM injections.

EQUIPMENT/SUPPLIES

- medication vial
- syringe
- needle
- alcohol
- gauze or cotton
- Band-Aid
- sharps container
- medication tray
- pen
- medication order
- patient chart
- gloves

STANDARD PRECAUTIONS

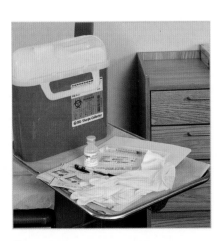

1. Gather all supplies.

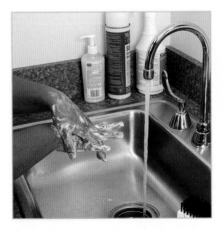

2. Wash hands. Apply gloves as per office protocol.

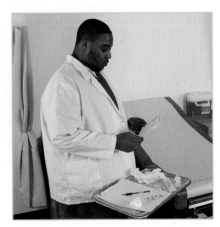

3. Read the medication order. Follow the six rights (see Box 7-7).

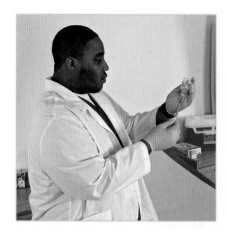

4. Correctly prepare medication (as per procedure 7-19, 7-20, or 7-21).

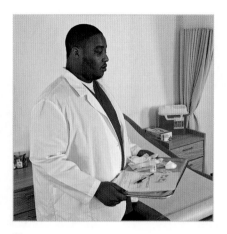

5. Transport medication properly, as per office protocol, to patient for administration

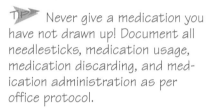 Never give a medication you have not drawn up! Document all needlesticks, medication usage, medication discarding, and medication administration as per office protocol.

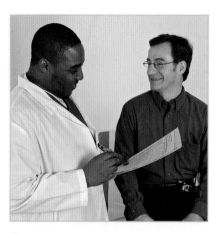

6. Identify patient.

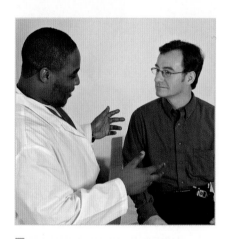

7. Explain the procedure.

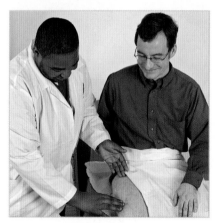

8. Assess the patient, including appropriate site selection, allergies to medications, latex allergies, medication specific questions, previous reactions to injections, etc.

 Note areas to avoid for injections (see Box 7-9).

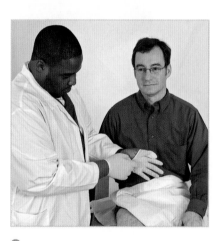

9. Apply gloves.

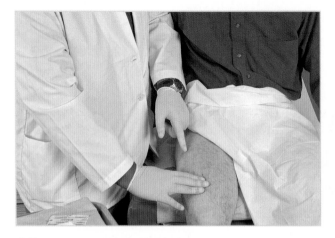

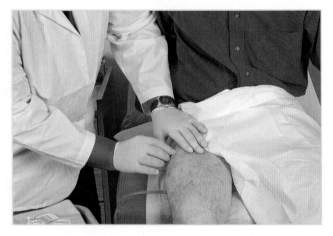

10. Select appropriate site.

WHY? *It is important to select the correct site to avoid damaging nearby blood vessels or nerves.*

TIP Palpate for vastus lateralis muscle. Divide leg into thirds, and administer into middle third of area. (See illustration at the end of this procedure.)

11. Clean site with alcohol. Use a circular motion going from the center out, and let air dry for maximum destruction of microorganisms.

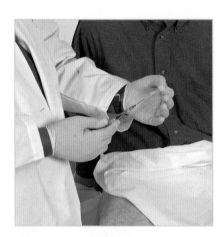

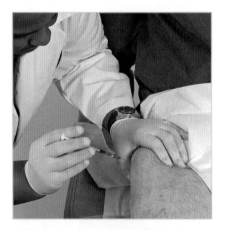

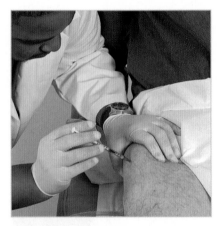

12. Remove needle guard.

13. Gently grasp vastus muscle.

TIP Some providers recommend spreading skin here with one hand.

14. Insert needle quickly using a darting motion at a 90-degree angle.

WHY? *A quick motion helps lessen patient discomfort.*

TIP Be sure you get the middle of the vastus and avoid the nerves and blood vessels in that area.

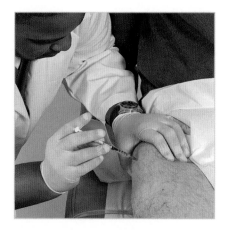

15. Aspirate to make sure you are not in a blood vessel.

WHY❓ *If the medication were injected into this site, it would be injected intravenously, which is not correct and could be life-threatening.*

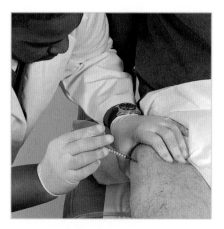

16. Slowly and steadily, inject the medication.

WHY❓ *This lessens patient discomfort and avoids potential damage to tissues.*

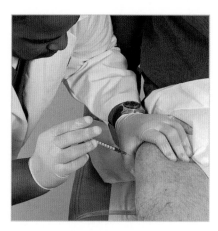

17. Quickly withdraw needle straight out from the patient's leg.

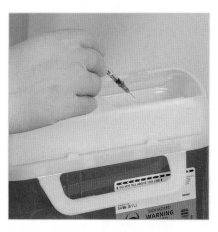

18. Discard needle immediately into sharps container. Use of safety needles is required by OSHA; close the safety feature first.

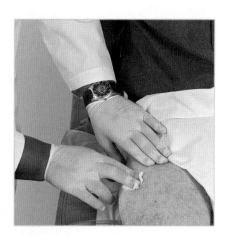

19. Massage the site unless contra-indicated by gently pressing the gauze/cotton ball to the site and moving in a circular motion for a moment.

WHY❓ *This helps to distribute the medication into the surrounding tissues, promoting better absorption and minimizing discomfort to the patient.*

TIP▶ Insulin, Imferon, and heparin are examples of medications that should NOT be massaged.

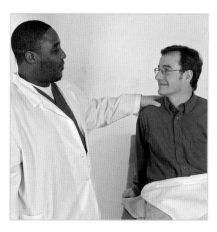

20. Observe the patient's reaction.

TIP▶ The patient must wait at least 20 minutes after any injection of medications. Make sure the patient has a ride home if necessary, e.g, after narcotic administration.

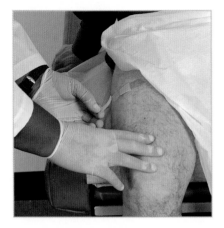

21. Apply Band-Aid.

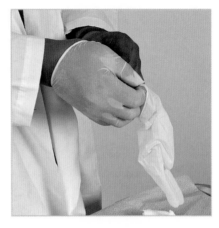

22. Remove gloves and wash hands.

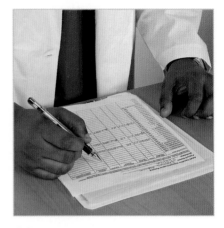

23. Document the procedure.

🔺 *Be sure to document patient reaction even if there is none.*

✎ **Charting Example**

4/5/07 3:15 p.m. Administered 1gm Rocephin L Vastus per Dr. Smith, pt. tol. well, no adv. react. Pt waited 30 mins, left fine. (lot #12345, Merck, exp 5/09)
_____ L. Tanaka, CMA

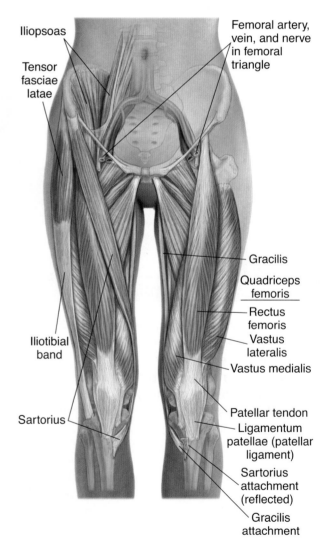

Muscles of the thigh. Note the location of the vastus lateralis.

Procedure **7-26**

Apply Pharmacology Principles to Prepare and Administer Oral and Parenteral (Excluding IV) Medications: Administer Intramuscular Injection in the Dorsal or Ventral Gluteus

PURPOSE

When medication needs to be absorbed rapidly, the intramuscular route is used. The dorsal and ventral gluteus are one of several sites recommended for IM injections.

EQUIPMENT/SUPPLIES

- medication vial
- syringe
- needle
- alcohol
- gauze or cotton
- Band-Aid

- sharps container
- medication tray
- pen
- medication order
- patient chart
- gloves

STANDARD PRECAUTIONS

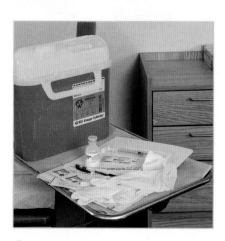

1. Gather all supplies.

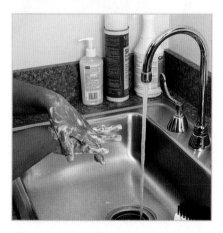

2. Wash hands. Apply gloves as per office protocol.

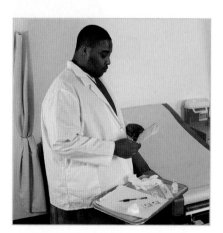

3. Read the medication order. Follow six rights (see Box 7-7).

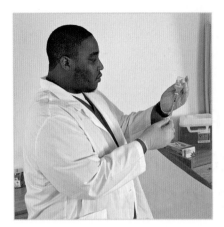

4. Correctly prepare medication (as per procedure 7-19, 7-20, or 7-21).

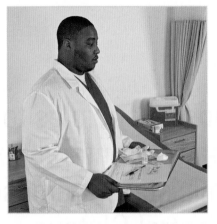

5. Transport medication properly, as per office protocol, to patient for administration.

LEGAL ALERT! *Never give a medication you have not drawn up! Document all needlesticks, medication usage, medication discarding, and medication administration as per office protocol.*

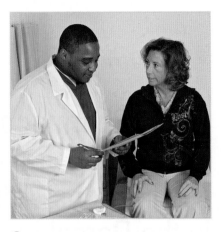

6. Identify the patient.

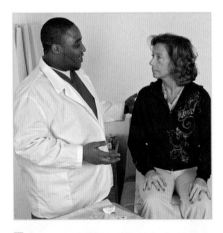

7. Explain the procedure.

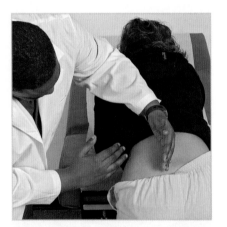

8. Assess the patient, including appropriate site selection, allergies to medications, latex allergies, medication specific questions, previous reactions to injections, etc.

Note areas to avoid for injections (see Box 7-9).

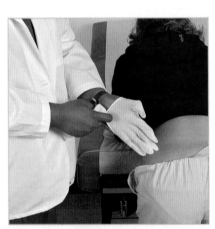

9. Apply gloves.

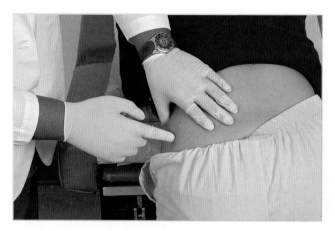

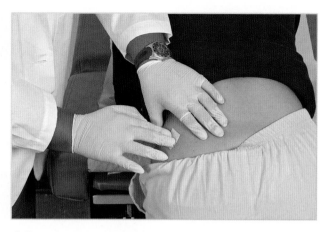

10. Select the appropriate site. Palpate for dorsal gluteus in the upper outer aspect of the patient's buttock. Palpate for ventral gluteus by placing the palm of the hand on the greater trochanter and the index finger on the anterior superior iliac spine. Spread the middle finger along the iliac crest posteriorly as far as possible to form a "v," and the injection is given in the middle of the "v."

WHY？ *It is important to select the correct site to avoid nearby blood vessels and nerves.*

TIP *See illustration at the end of this procedure.*

11. Clean site with alcohol. Use a circular motion going from the center out, let air dry for maximum destruction of microorganisms.

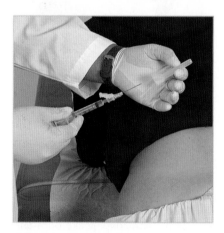

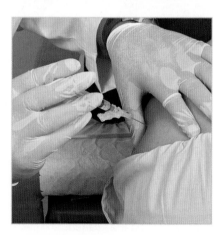

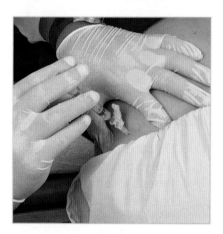

12. Remove needle guard.

13. Spread the patient's skin with one hand.

14. Insert needle quickly using a darting motion at a 90-degree angle.

WHY？ *A quick motion helps lessen patient discomfort.*

TIP *Avoid the sciatic nerve and blood vessels in the dorsal gluteal area.*

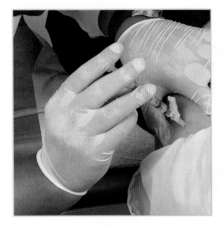

15. Aspirate to make sure you are not in a blood vessel.

WHY? *If the medication were injected into this site, it would be injected intravenously, which is not correct and could be life-threatening.*

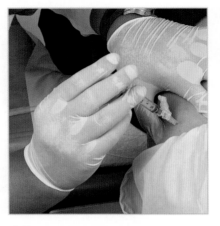

16. Slowly and steadily, inject the medication.

WHY? *This lessens patient discomfort and avoids potential damage to tissues.*

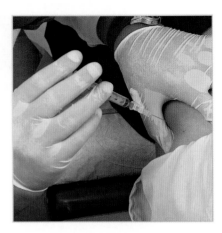

17. Quickly withdraw needle straight out from the patient's buttock/hip.

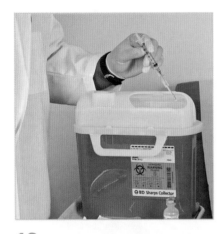

18. Discard needle immediately into sharps container. Use of safety needles is required by OSHA; close the safety feature first.

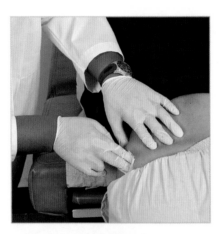

19. Massage the site unless contra-indicated.

TIP Insulin, Imferon, and heparin are examples of medications that should NOT be massaged.

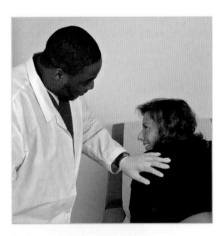

20. Observe the patient's reaction.

TIP The patient must wait at least 20 minutes after any injection of medications. Make sure the patient has a ride home if necessary, e.g., after narcotic administration.

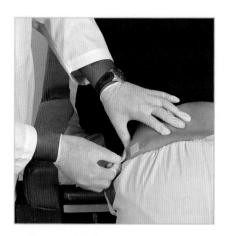

21. Apply Band-Aid.

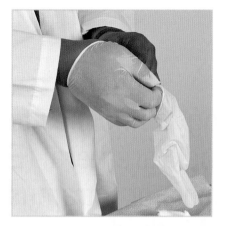

22. Remove gloves and wash hands.

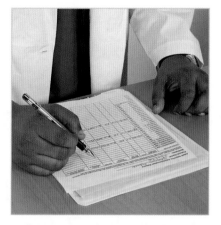

23. Document the procedure.

Be sure to document patient reaction even if there is none.

Charting Example

10/12/07 10:00 a.m. Administered 1gm Rocephin L Glut. per Dr. Smith, pt. tol. well, no adv. react. Pt waited 30 mins, left fine. (lot #12345, Merck, exp 5/09)

_____ D. Win, CMA

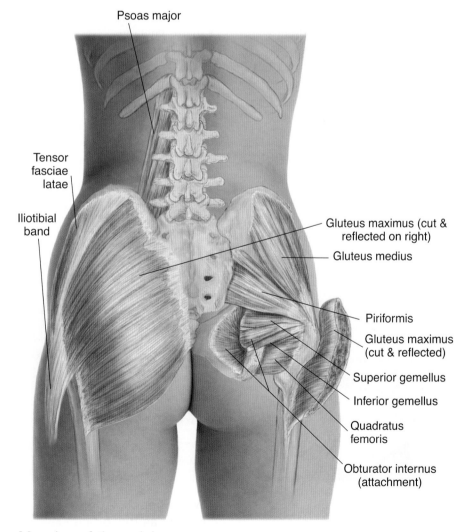

Psoas major

Tensor fasciae latae

Iliotibial band

Gluteus maximus (cut & reflected on right)

Gluteus medius

Piriformis

Gluteus maximus (cut & reflected)

Superior gemellus

Inferior gemellus

Quadratus femoris

Obturator internus (attachment)

Muscles of the pelvis.

Procedure 7-27

Apply Pharmacology Principles to Prepare and Administer Oral and Parenteral (Excluding IV) Medications: Administer Intramuscular Injection Using the Z-track Method

PURPOSE

Certain medication can irritate or damage tissue if it leaks back into the tissues. The Z-track method of IM injection can prevent this.

EQUIPMENT/SUPPLIES

- medication vial
- syringe
- needle
- alcohol
- gauze or cotton
- Band-Aid
- sharps container
- medication tray
- pen
- medication order
- patient chart
- gloves

STANDARD PRECAUTIONS

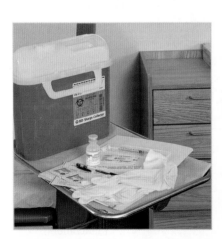

1. Gather all supplies.

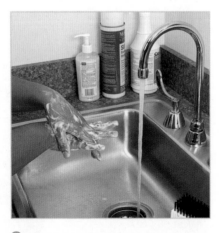

2. Wash hands. Apply gloves as per office protocol.

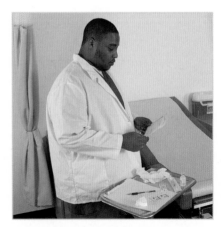

3. Read the medication order. Follow the six rights (see Box 7-7).

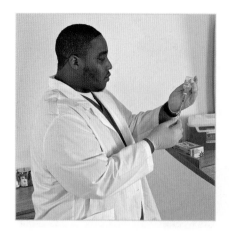

4. Correctly prepare medication (as per procedure 7-19, 7-20, or 7-21).

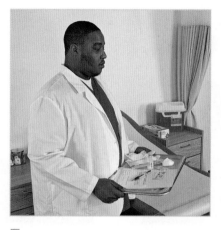

5. Transport medication properly, as per office protocol, to patient for administration.

LEGAL ALERT! Never give a medication you have not drawn up! Document all needlesticks, medication usage, medication discarding, and medication administration as per office protocol.

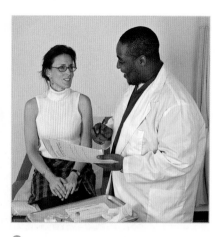

6. Identify the patient.

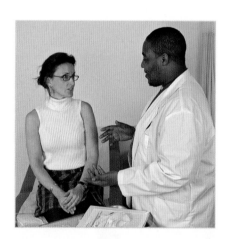

7. Explain the procedure.

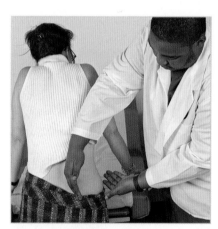

8. Assess the patient, including appropriate site selection, allergies to medications, latex allergies, medication specific questions, previous reactions to injections, etc.

TIP Note areas to avoid for injections (see Box 7-9).

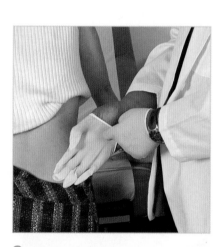

9. Apply gloves.

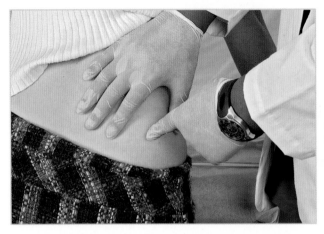

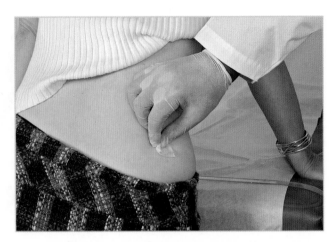

10. Select appropriate site. Palpate for dorso gluteus in the upper outer aspect of the patient's buttock. Palpate for ventral gluteus by placing the palm of the hand on the greater trochanter and the index finger on the anterior superior iliac spine. Spread the middle finger along the iliac crest posteriorly as far as possible to form a "v," and the injection is given in the middle of the "v."

 See illustration at the end of this procedure.

11. Clean site with alcohol. Use a circular motion going from the center out, and let air dry for maximum destruction of microorganisms.

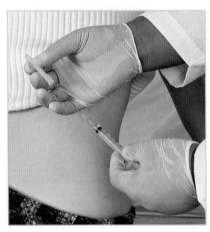

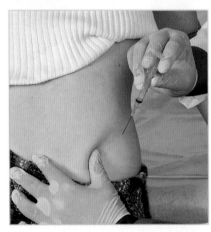

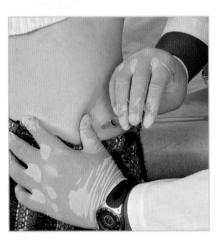

12. Remove needle guard.

13. Firmly displace or pull the patient's skin laterally 1 to 2 inches away from the injection site with one hand.

14. Insert needle quickly using a darting motion at a 90-degree angle.

WHY? *A quick motion helps lessen patient discomfort.*

Avoid the sciatic nerve and blood vessels in the dorso gluteal area.

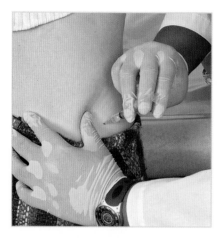

15. Aspirate to make sure you are not in a blood vessel.

WHY? *If the medication were injected into this site, it would be injected intravenously, which is not correct and could be life-threatening.*

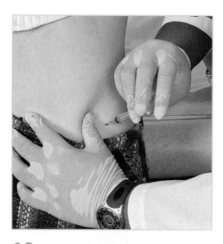

16. Slowly and steadily, inject the medication.

WHY? *This lessens patient discomfort and avoids potential damage to tissues.*

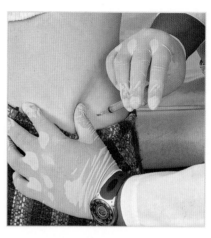

17. Wait 10 seconds after fully injecting medication before withdrawing needle.

WHY? *This allows the medication to be absorbed.*

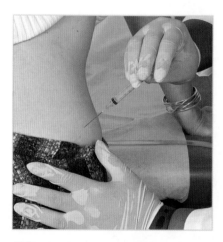

18. Quickly withdraw needle straight out from the patient's buttock/hip, then release your hold on the patient's skin.

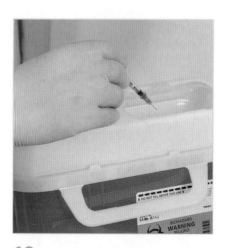

19. Discard needle immediately into sharps container. Use of safety needles is required by OSHA; close the safety feature first.

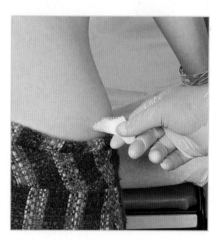

20. Do not massage!

WHY? *The z-track method is used to insert medication into deep muscle tissue without a route for the medication to ooze back out once the needle is withdrawn. Massaging with this injection technique would likely cause some medication to seep out which could damage the fatty tissue or skin above the muscle.*

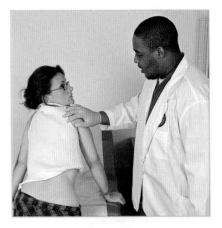

21. Observe patient reaction.

TIP The patient must wait at least 20 minutes after any injection of medications. Make sure the patient has a ride home if necessary, e.g., after narcotic administration.

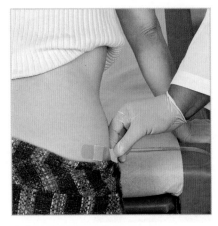

22. Apply Band-Aid.

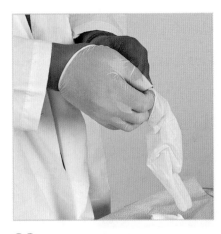

23. Remove gloves and wash hands.

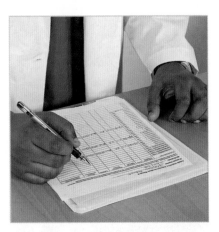

24. Document the procedure.

TIP Be sure to document patient reaction even if there is none.

✎ **Charting Example**

5/14/07 11:15 a.m. Administered 1gm Rocephin L Glut. Using Z-Track method, Per Dr. Smith, pt. tol. well, no adv. react. Pt waited 30 mins, left fine. (lot #12345, Merck, exp 5/09) _____ M. Nguyen, CMA

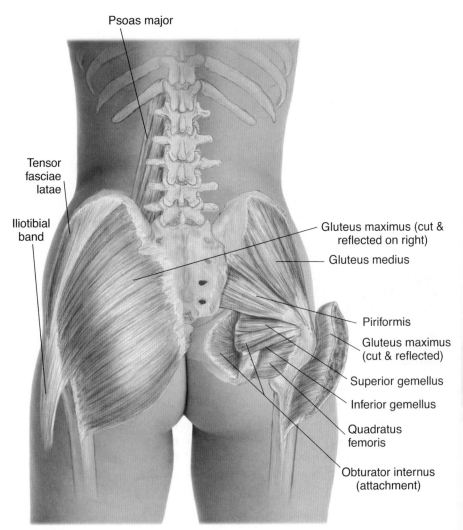

Muscles of the pelvis.

Labels: Psoas major, Tensor fasciae latae, Iliotibial band, Gluteus maximus (cut & reflected on right), Gluteus medius, Piriformis, Gluteus maximus (cut & reflected), Superior gemellus, Inferior gemellus, Quadratus femoris, Obturator internus (attachment)

Procedure **7-28**

Apply Pharmacology Principles to Prepare and Administer Oral and Parenteral (Excluding IV) Medications: Prepare and Administer Oral Medication

PURPOSE

Medications that can be swallowed and are absorbed through the gastrointestinal tract are administered orally.

EQUIPMENT/SUPPLIES

- medication bottle
- medication cup
- water or juice
- drinking cup
- medication tray
- pen
- medication order
- patient chart
- gloves

STANDARD PRECAUTIONS

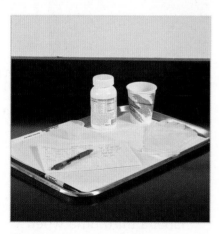

1. Gather all supplies.

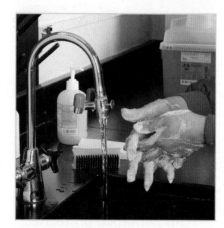

2. Wash hands. (Apply gloves as per office protocol.)

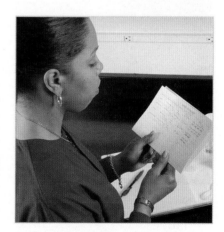

3. Read the medication order, following the six rights (see Box 7-7).

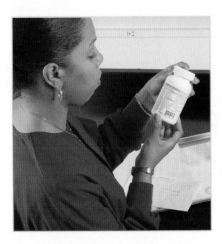

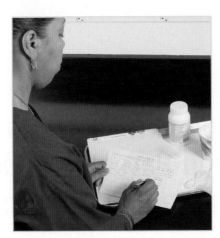

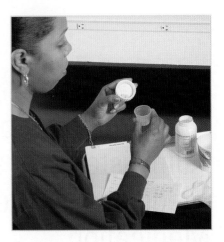

4. Read the medication label. This will be checked three times for correct medication, expiration date, and medication appearance.

ᴡʜʏ❓ *This prevents errors and ensures that outdated medication is not administered.*

5. Calculate dosage if necessary.

6. Correctly prepare medication (multiple dose solid, unit dose, or liquid) by putting it into a medicine cup. Measure liquids carefully using a syringe if necessary and be sure to LABEL! Do not touch solid medication with your hand; instead pour it into the medication bottle lid then tip into medicine cup.

ᴡʜʏ❓ *This prevents errors and avoids contaminating the medication.*

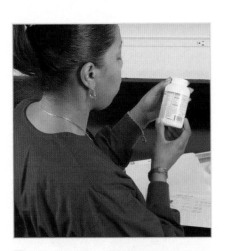

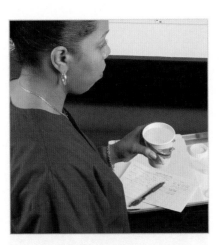

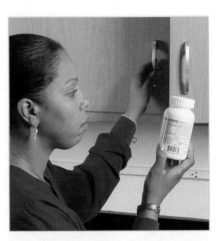

7. Check the medication label.

8. Prepare water or juice in cup per office protocol.

ᴡʜʏ❓ *This helps in swallowing the medication.*

9. Check the medication label a third time when putting away the medication bottle.

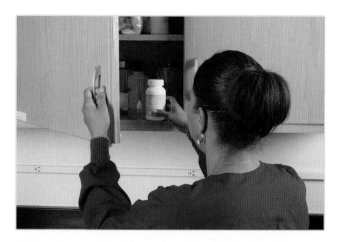

10. Return all medications and supplies to proper place. Discard used vials as per OSHA guidelines.

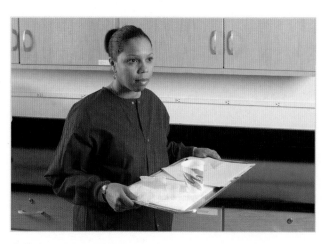

11. Transport medication properly, as per office protocol, to the patient for administration.

TIP Never give a medication you have not prepared! Document all needlesticks, medication usage, medication discarding, and medication administration as per office protocol.

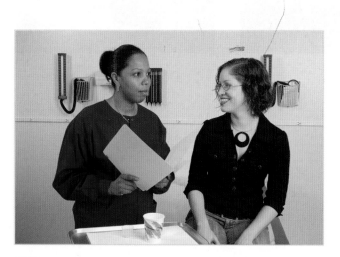

12. Identify the patient.

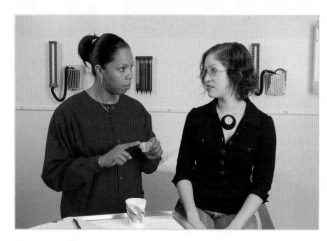

13. Explain the procedure.

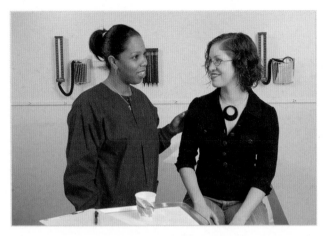

14. Assess the patient. Ask about allergies to medications, latex allergies, medication specific questions, previous reactions to oral medications, etc.

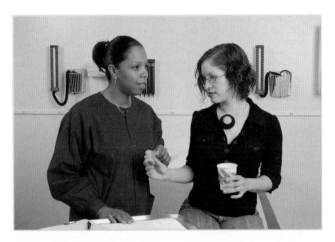

15. Give the patient the medication, being sure the patient takes it.

WHY❓ *You must observe the patient swallowing the medication in order to document that the patient has taken it.*

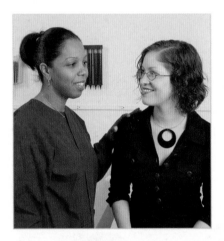

16. Observe the patient's reaction.

TIP▸ The patient must wait at least 20 minutes after any medication administration. Make sure patient has a ride home if necessary, e.g., after narcotic administration.

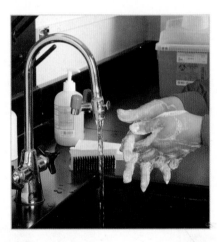

17. Wash hands.

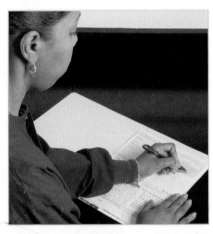

18. Document the procedure.

TIP▸ Be sure to document patient reaction even if there is none.

 Charting Example

7/28/07 11:00 a.m. Administered 800mg Tylenol p.o. per Dr. Jones, pt. swallowed all meds, tol. well, no adv. react. Exp 7/09, Merck, Lot #34792 _____ S. Kenny, CMA

Procedure 7-29

Maintain Medication and Immunization Records

PURPOSE

Proper documentation and record keeping is a critical task the medical assistant must perform. It is crucial for billing as well as patient safety. Medications are sometimes recalled, or patients may have an adverse reaction after leaving the medical office, and proper documentation of medication name, manufacturer, lot number, expiration date, site of injection, and medication dosage is critical. Patients need to be able to access immunization records for many reasons such as employment or school entrance for a child. The state health departments that supply child immunizations to the medical office require separate and accurate documentation of administration, as well as dispersal of proper immunization information.

EQUIPMENT/SUPPLIES

- patient chart
- pen
- medication order or refill request
- medication bottle
- medication list or immunization record
- tickler file
- other office record keeping charts/paperwork

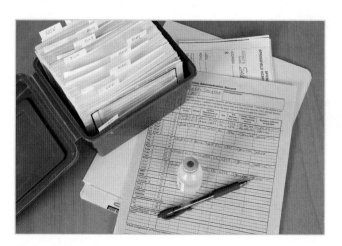

1. Gather all supplies.

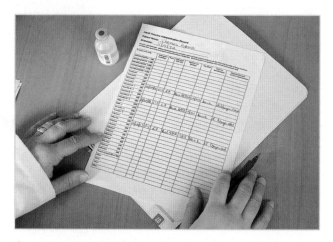

2. Access patient medication list or immunization record.

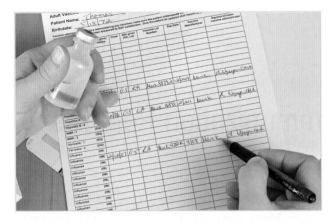

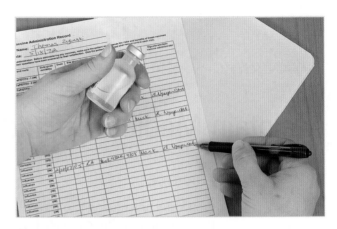

3. Properly document medication refills or administration.

LEGAL ALERT! *Always check with provider before refilling any medication; remember that medical assistants cannot prescribe. Always include manufacturer, lot #, and expiration date of any medication administered. Do not administer immunizations to children without parents' signatures; never say "I'll get it later."*

LEGAL ALERT! *Always chart "per so and so" (MD) when administering medication. This protects you.*

4. Sign document.

TIP *Many offices require adult medication administration (medications the office purchases) to be documented on some sort of medication flow sheet for office administration tracking use in addition to charting on the progress note.*

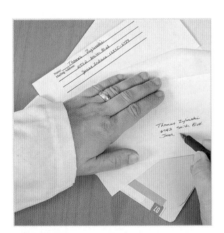

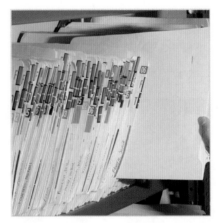

5. Prepare tickler file or reminder card for next dose per office protocol.

6. File chart.

LEGAL ALERT! *Clear, accurate, and complete medical record keeping is a legal issue. It is also important for the proper care of each patient. Proper record keeping by the medical assistant is also a way to observe risk management guidelines in the medical office and a way to protect your provider and yourself. If it isn't charted, it didn't happen.*

Charting Example

Adult Vaccine Administration Record
Patient Name: Thomas Zylinski
Birthdate: 5/18/72

Procedure 7-30

Screen and Follow Up Test Results

PURPOSE

Testing is a critical part of patient care and diagnosis. It is the medical assistant's responsibility to follow up on test results in a timely and accurate manner to ensure proper and accurate patient treatment.

EQUIPMENT/SUPPLIES

- patient chart
- pen
- test results
- tickler file
- telephone
- reminder/WNL cards

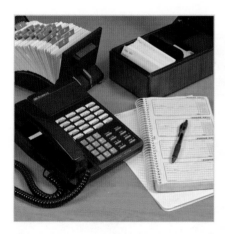

1. Gather all supplies.

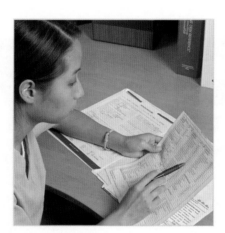

2. Review test results.

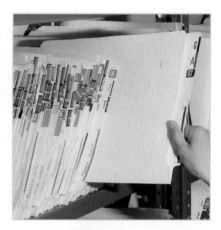

3. Pull the patient's chart.

TIP➤ Follow office protocol to alert the provider to any abnormal or urgent results ASAP.

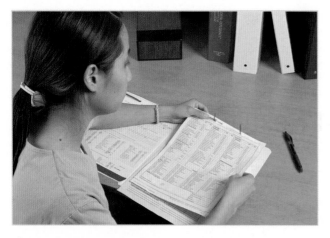

4. Attach test results to the patient's chart.

WHY? *If a patient is coming in for a follow-up exam based on testing, it is critical to have the results attached to the chart before the provider enters the room with the patient.*

Anticipate the provider's needs and get all documentation prepared before the patient arrives at the office. If necessary, call other offices or hospital record facilities to obtain these results.

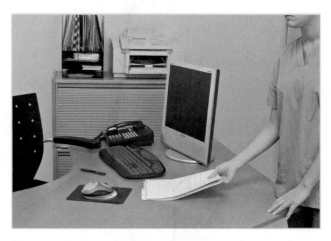

5. Place in provider's office.

Every office will have a spot for incoming labs and other test results to be placed for provider review; follow office protocol.

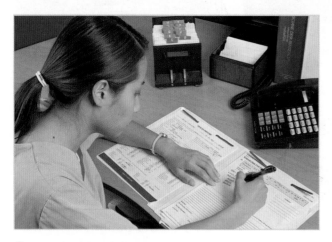

6. Follow provider orders upon provider's review and comments.

Providers often write on the results what needs to be done, such as medication refill or dosage change, new medication order, follow-up appointment, etc. If the results are within normal limits (WNL), place a tickler card in the file to remind the patient to return later for a follow-up visit. Results may also be shared with the patient via mail or phone; follow confidentiality guidelines when calling patients.

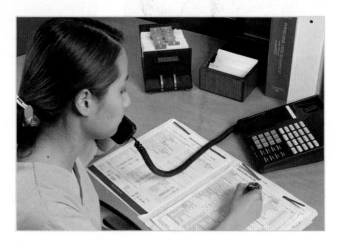

7. Inform the patient of test results.

WHY? *The provider often does not have time to contact every patient, so informing a patient about normal results is often delegated to the medical assistant.*

If the patient is not in for an appointment, either call or send results by mail, per office protocol, and be sure to document whether the patient was called or sent the information.

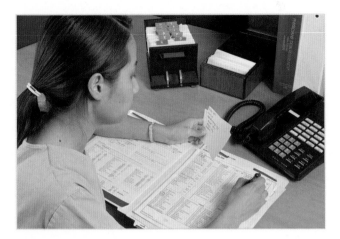

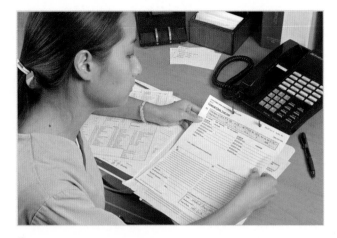

8. Document the procedure.

9. File the results in the patient's chart.

LEGAL ALERT ! Never file paperwork of any kind in the patient's chart unless the provider has first reviewed and signed it! You must do this for legal and administrative reasons, as well as to ensure patient safety. The provider needs to know all testing outcomes in order to diagnose and treat the patient correctly.

Charting Example

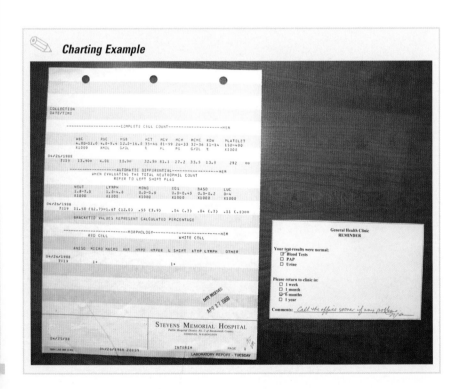

PART THREE

General Competencies

Chapter 11 Operational Functions

CHAPTER 8

Professional Communications

INTRODUCTION

Communication is the basis of all actions taken in the care and treatment of patients in the medical office. As a result, the ability to communicate well is a vital skill for medical assistants. Communication may be written, verbal, or non-verbal. In the medical office, communication occurs with patients, staff, providers, and other medical offices and personnel. Accuracy, professionalism, courtesy, empathy, and understanding are crucial to providing appropriate medical treatment and care. Proper documentation is also important, to make sure that key information is recorded correctly and to fulfill legal requirements.

PROCEDURES

8-1 Respond to and Initiate Written Communications: Prepare and Compose a Business Letter

8-2 Respond to and Initiate Written Communications: Address Envelopes

8-3 Respond to and Initiate Written Communications: Fold Letters for Envelopes

8-4 Respond to and Initiate Written Communications: Prepare and Send a Fax

8-5 Recognize and Respond to Verbal Communications

8-6 Recognize and Respond to Non-verbal Communications

8-7 Demonstrate Telephone Techniques: Answer Incoming Calls

8-8 Demonstrate Telephone Techniques: Handle Problem Calls

8-9 Demonstrate Telephone Techniques: Make Outgoing Calls

Procedure 8-1

Respond to and Initiate Written Communications: Prepare and Compose a Business Letter

PURPOSE

By handling written communications appropriately, the medical assistant ensures that information is communicated efficiently and accurately and promotes the professional image of the medical office.

EQUIPMENT/SUPPLIES

- computer and printer
- notes needed to prepare letter
- envelopes
- letterhead
- paperclip
- recipient's address

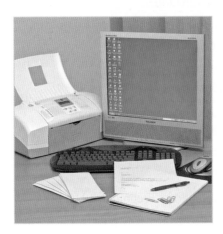

1. Gather all supplies.

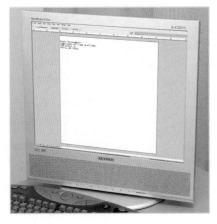

2. Choose appropriate letter format per office policy.

WHY? *Using the correct format ensures that the letter will have a professional appearance.*

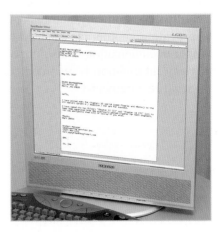

3. Prepare a rough draft of the letter using typewriter or computer.

TIP Be clear, concise, and courteous.

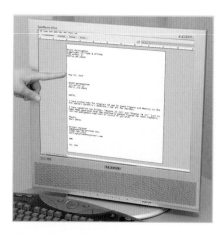

4. Key the date 2 to 4 spaces below the letterhead, writing out completely.

WHY❓ *The date tells the recipient when the letter was written.*

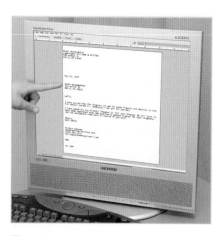

5. Key recipient's name and address 4 spaces below the date.

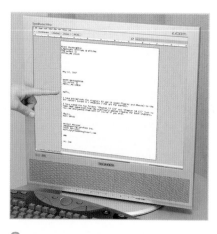

6. Key salutation line 3 lines below address.

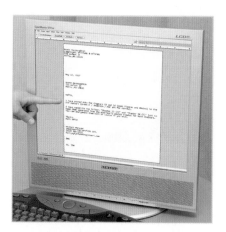

7. Key subject line 2 lines below salutation.

WHY❓ *A subject line allows the recipient to quickly determine the letter's main purpose.*

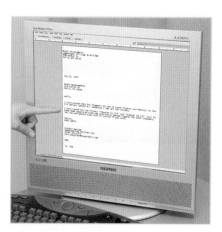

8. Begin the body of the letter 2 lines below subject line. Use single spacing between sentences and double spacing between paragraphs.

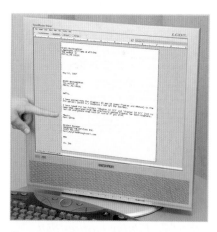

9. Key the complimentary closure 2 lines below the body of the letter.

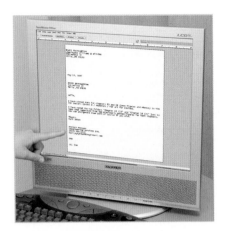

10. Key the signature 4 to 6 lines below the complimentary closure.

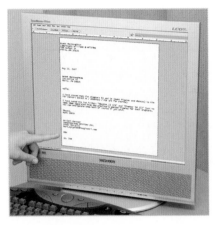

11. Key the reference initials 2 lines below the signature.

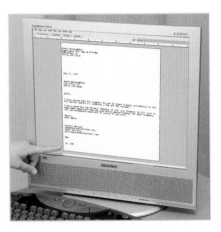

12. Key the enclosure or carbon copy line 2 lines below the reference initials.

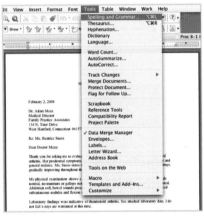

13. Edit the draft, using the computer grammar and spell check function.

WHY? *Editing ensures that the letter is free of mistakes and successfully communicates the intended message.*

As you review the draft, check that the language used is easy to understand and that all key points have been addressed. Keep in mind that computer spell checkers only catch misspelled words—not those that are spelled right but used incorrectly.

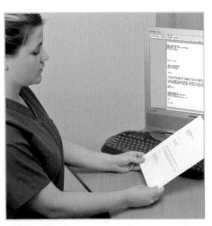

14. Make all corrections identified during the editing step, then print out the letter, either on regular computer paper or on the medical office's preprinted letterhead.

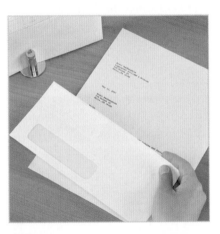

15. Prepare the envelope (see Procedure 8-2) and attach to letter with a paperclip and place on provider's desk to be signed.

Keep a copy of the letter and file it appropriately (e.g., patient correspondence should go in the medical record).

It is important that the medical assistant has knowledge and proficiency in business correspondence and also understands and applies confidentiality laws to any written communication or transmission of medical information. Legal guidelines must also be followed.

Procedure **8-2**

Respond to and Initiate Written Communications: Address Envelopes

PURPOSE

Correctly addressed envelopes ensure that business letters mailed through the U.S. Postal Service are properly sorted and delivered to the intended recipients.

EQUIPMENT/SUPPLIES

- computer and printer or typewriter
- envelopes
- recipient's address

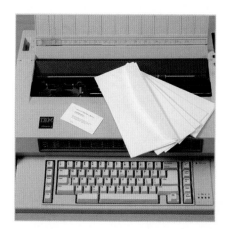

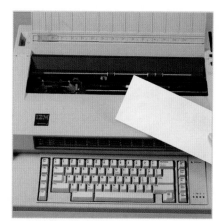

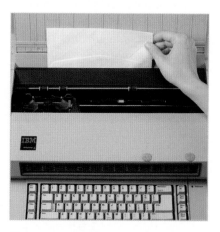

1. Gather all supplies.

2. Choose appropriate envelope size.

The most commonly used envelopes are number 10 and number 6 3/4. Number 10 is the most professional and is used for business letters. Number 6 3/4 is often used for small reminder notes or copies of the ledger sent to patients from small offices to remind them of their balance due. Follow office protocol when selecting envelopes for the type of correspondence to be sent. Window envelopes may also be used by your office; be sure the address shows through the window when typing or printing a letter to be inserted.

3. Choose the envelope or label format on the computer or the typewriter.

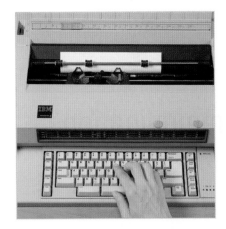

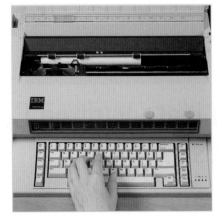

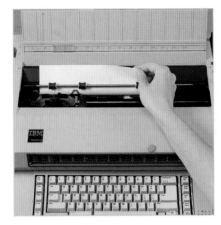

4. Using U.S. postal regulations, key the address using upper-case letters in the proper area, 5/8 to 2 inches from the bottom of the envelope with 1/2 inch on each side.

WHY? *The optical character reader at the post office prefers all upper-case lettering for fast and efficient mail sorting. Typing portrays a professional image; handwritten envelopes do not.*

TIP Be sure to maintain a uniform left margin. Include the Zip + 4 code if known.

5. If preprinted envelopes are not used, key in the return address in the top left corner of the envelope.

WHY? *This is the standard location for the return address on business letters.*

6. Proofread the envelope and make corrections as necessary.

TIP For a professional appearance, retype the envelope to correct any mistakes.

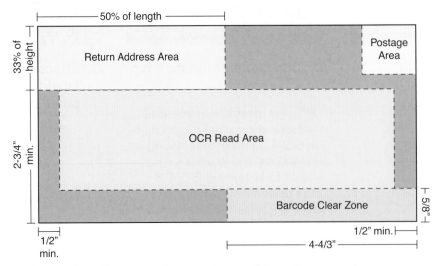

Refer to the diagram above when addressing envelopes.

Procedure 8-3

Respond to and Initiate Written Communications: Fold Letters for Envelopes

PURPOSE

Written communications must have a professional look. Correctly folded letters display a neat appearance and allow the recipient to open the letter easily.

EQUIPMENT/SUPPLIES

- envelopes
- letter to be mailed
- postage
- moistener

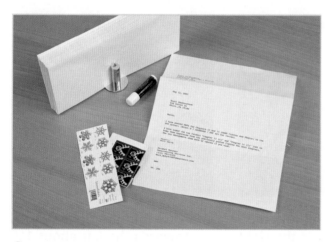

1. Gather all supplies.

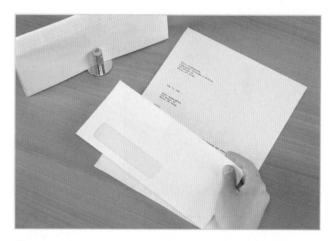

2. Choose the appropriate envelope.

For a No. 10 envelope:

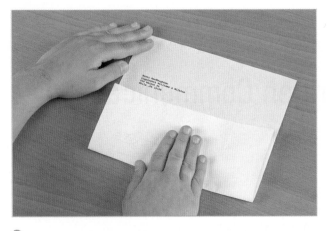

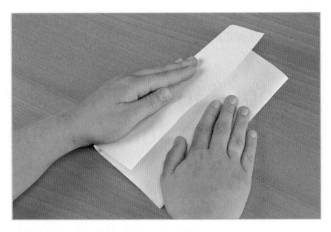

3. Place the letter face up and fold the bottom 1/3 of the letter up.

4. Fold the top 1/3 of the letter down.

For a No. 6 3/4 envelope:

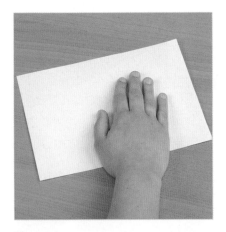

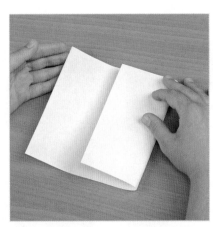

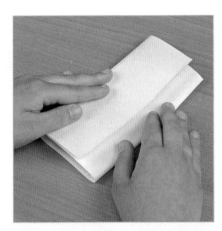

5. Place the letter face up and fold the bottom upwards, leaving about 1/2 inch at the top.

6. Lay this flat and fold the left side towards the right 1/3 of the way.

7. Now fold the right side towards the left about 1/3 of the way, leaving about 1/2 inch at the right side.

For a window envelope:

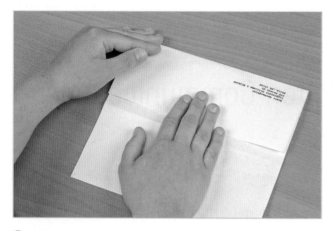

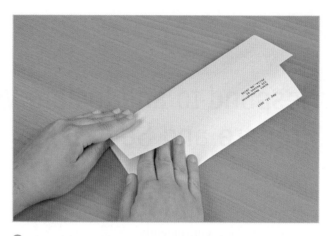

8. Place the letter face down and fold the top 1/3 of the letter down.

9. Fold the bottom 1/3 of the letter under, turning over to be sure that the address is showing.

For all envelope types:

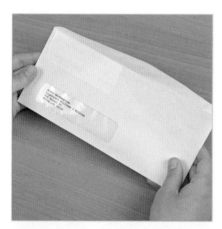

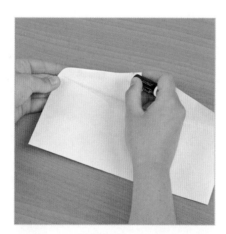

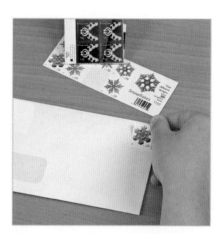

10. After folding, insert the letter into the envelope (make sure the address shows through a window envelope).

11. Seal the envelope with an envelope moistener.

WHY? *Licking an envelope is a bad habit and can transfer germs to you and to the envelope.*

TIP For multiple envelopes, stagger them backwards, and use an envelope moistener to moisten many at one time.

12. Affix proper postage to the envelope, either using stamps or office postage meter.

Procedure 8-4

Respond to and Initiate Written Communications: Prepare and Send a Fax

PURPOSE

Sending a fax allows the medical practice to transmit written communications quickly and conveniently.

EQUIPMENT/SUPPLIES

• fax machine
• documents to be faxed
• recipient's fax number
• pen

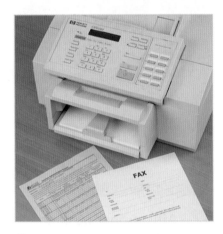

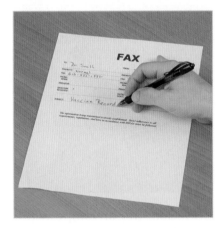

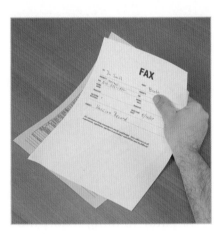

1. Gather all supplies.

2. Prepare a cover sheet, including the names of the sender and receiver as well as the number of pages, any notes, and a confidentiality statement (per HIPAA regulations).

WHY? *The cover sheet provides key information for the intended recipient.*

3. Gather the medical records or other information to be faxed, and place the cover sheet on top.

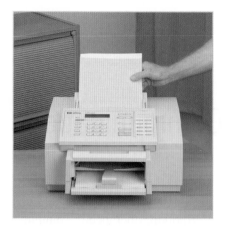

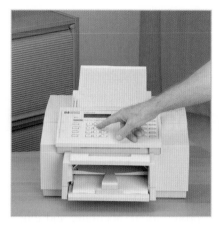

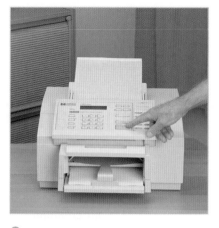

4. Place the documents appropriately in the fax machine.

5. Dial the number to which you are faxing.

6. Press send or start.

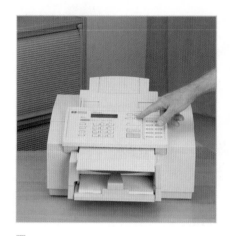

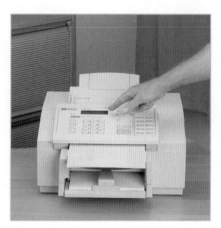

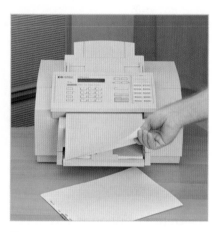

7. When the faxing is complete and all documents have passed through the fax, press the button that requests a receipt (some machines do this automatically).

why? *A receipt shows that the fax has been sent.*

8. Check the machine for the fax status (it should say ok and tell you how many pages were sent). Call the recipient to verify receipt as per office policy.

why? *It is important to ensure that the total number of pages to be faxed were sent as intended and that the correct person received them.*

9. Remove the documents from the machine and replace in the patient's chart, being sure to document as per HIPAA regulations in the chart.

why? *For privacy purposes, documents must be removed from the fax machine so that unauthorized individuals do not have access to them.*

 Charting Example

10/12/07 9:45 a.m. Faxed lab results and chart notes from 9/23/07 to Dr. Smith at NW Neurology. _ D. Rodriguez, CMA

Procedure 8-5

Recognize and Respond to Verbal Communications

PURPOSE

As the liaison between the provider and the patient, the medical assistant must make sure that all communication is professional, accurate, and empathetic. Applying therapeutic communication to every situation ensures that the patient is treated with dignity and respect.

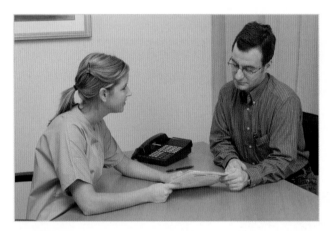

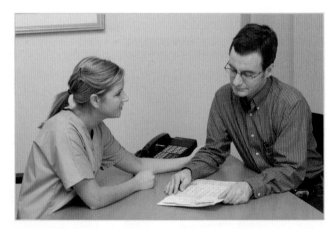

1. Sender encodes (creates) message.

Before sending the message, observe the receiver and assess the receiver's ability to understand verbal communications. Then determine the appropriate complexity level for the message.

EXAMPLE 1: *Patient/sender:* "I am very worried about the tests the doctor is having me do."

EXAMPLE 2: *Medical assistant/sender:* "Mr. Jones, the doctor would like you to take this new medication for your asthma. You will take one pill every day, in the morning."

2. Message is sent.

Make sure the message is complete, clear, concise, courteous, and cohesive.

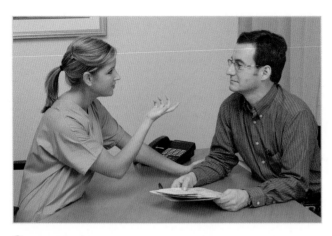

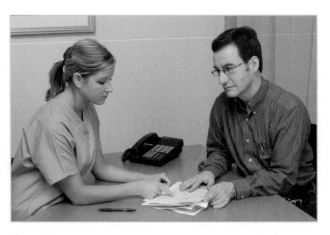

3. Receiver gets the message and decodes (interprets) it.

Use active listening to accurately decode the message.

EXAMPLE 1: *Medical assistant/receiver:* The patient is concerned about his health and is possibly fearful.

EXAMPLE 2: *Patient/receiver:* The doctor is giving me new asthma medication to take once a day in the morning.

4. Receiver gives feedback to the sender.

EXAMPLE 1: *Medical Assistant/receiver:* "I understand you are concerned. Can I answer any questions for you or give you any more information to help you feel more comfortable?"

EXAMPLE 2: *Patient/receiver:* "I need to take one of these blue pills every morning?"

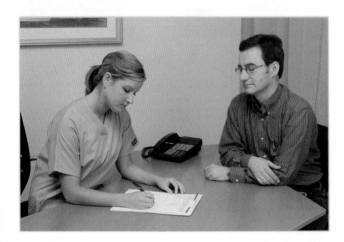

5. Document the conversation in the patient chart.

> **Charting Example**
>
> EXAMPLE 1
>
> 3/12/07 10:00 a.m. Clarified test procedures for patient. Patient very concerned. Answered all questions and referred patient to Dr. Smith for continued discussion.
> ———————————————— L. Hernandez, CMA
>
> EXAMPLE 2
>
> 3/12/07 10:20 a.m. Instructed pt. in asthma medication use and dosage. Pt. understood all instructions and was able to repeat. Verbal and written instructions given. ———————————————— M. Lee, CMA

Medical assistants have a professional and ethical duty to keep all bias, prejudice, and threatening behavior out of their communication.

Procedure **8-6**

Recognize and Respond to Non-verbal Communications

PURPOSE

An important part of communication with patients is to recognize non-verbal communication. Patients may not always say what they feel or mean, and it is crucial that the medical assistant knows how to recognize non-verbal cues.

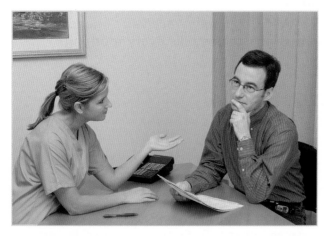

1. Observe the patient's facial expression.

WHY? *Emotions (e.g., sadness, fear, anger) may be revealed through facial expressions.*

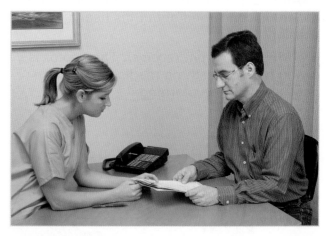

2. Maintain proper personal space (territoriality).

WHY? *This puts the patient at ease. Many people feel uncomfortable when their personal space is invaded.*

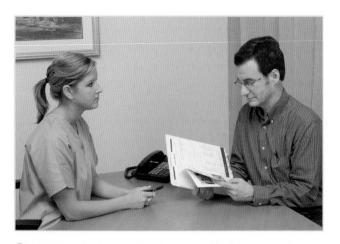

3. Observe the patient's posture.

WHY? *Body language can be a critical part of the message the patient is sending.*

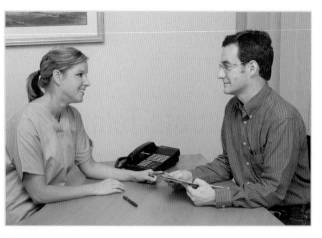

4. Maintain proper position. Always look the patient in the face, and remain at eye level.

TIP If the patient is sitting, the medical assistant should sit too, since standing might be interpreted as displaying dominance over the patient.

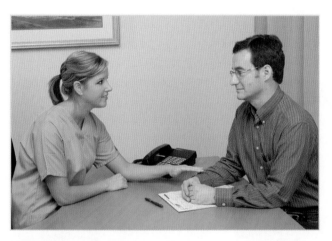

5. Use proper gestures and mannerisms.

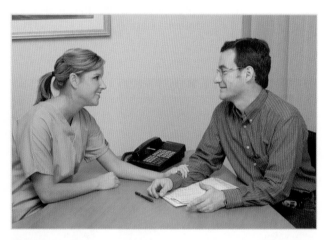

6. Use therapeutic touch, if appropriate.

WHY? *Before touching the patient, the MA should assess the patient's demeanor to determine if touch would likely be acceptable, since some patients dislike being touched.*

Procedure 8-7

Demonstrate Telephone Techniques: Answer Incoming Calls

PURPOSE

The telephone is often the first contact a patient has with the medical office. Patients often call to report symptoms or emergencies, as well as to obtain medication refills, schedule appointments, or ask general questions. Effective telephone communication allows patients to get the care and information they require.

EQUIPMENT/SUPPLIES

- telephone
- pen
- telephone message pad with carbonless copy
- patient chart

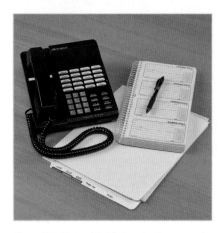

1. Gather all supplies.

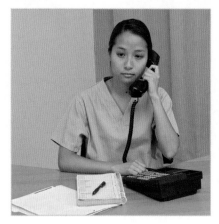

2. Answer the telephone promptly by the third ring, using the correct greeting as per office policy.

WHY? *Callers appreciate a prompt and professional response.*

TIP Be sure you speak directly into the mouthpiece and be clear and polite. Smile as you speak to convey warmth and reassurance over the phone.

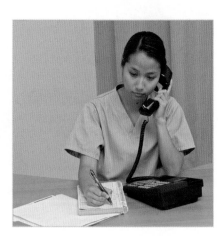

3. Ask the name of the caller and determine if it is an emergency call.

WHY? *You need to determine the nature of the call so that it can be handled appropriately.*

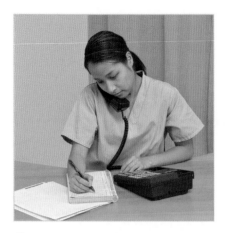

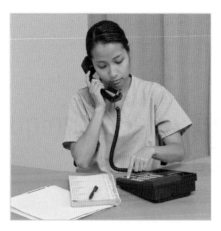

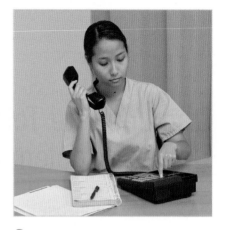

4. Write the message on the message pad, and repeat the information back to caller.

WHY? *This ensures accuracy and avoids miscommunication.*

TIP Be sure to get the caller's number in case you have multiple calls or get cut off, as well as the date and time the person called.

5. If it is necessary to put the caller on hold, always ask permission first.

WHY? *It is courteous to wait for an answer before putting a caller on hold.*

6. If it is necessary to transfer the caller, tell the caller before doing so.

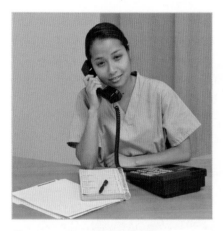

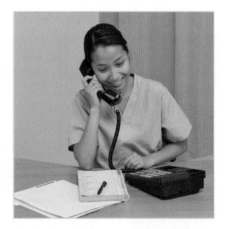

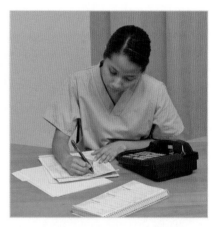

7. Prior to discontinuing the call, ask the caller if there are any other questions.

WHY? *This promotes good communication.*

8. End the call with a courteous "thank you" and "good-bye."

WHY? *It is important to be professional and polite when communicating with patients or other callers.*

TIP Always let the caller hang up first, which ensures that the caller's message is completely finished.

9. Document in the patient's chart and on the telephone message pad the call and any follow-up necessary.

TIP You must keep the carbon copy of the message on file just as you would a medical record.

TIP Medical assistants must always follow confidentiality regulations as they apply to telephone calls and messages.

 Charting Example

3/12/07 8:45 a.m. Pt. called with concerns regarding lab results. Scheduled f/u appt. with Dr. Jones for Thursday, 3/15/07. _____ H. Lee, CMA

Procedure 8-8

Demonstrate Telephone Techniques: Handle Problem Calls

PURPOSE

Occasionally, the medical office receives calls from patients who are distressed by their health situation or other matters. By handling these calls effectively, the medical assistant ensures that appropriate patient care is provided, while still projecting a professional demeanor.

EQUIPMENT/SUPPLIES

• telephone
• pen
• telephone message pad
• patient chart

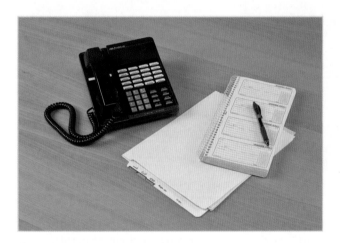

1. Gather all supplies.

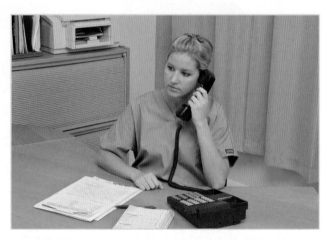

2. If the caller is angry or upset, remain calm and let the caller speak without interruption.

ᴡʜʏ❓ *Getting upset yourself only exacerbates the situation and is unprofessional. By letting the caller finish speaking, the caller can express what is bothersome and reduce anxiety.*

TIP▶ If this is an emergency call, interruption may be necessary to get help. Follow triage protocol, and have the caller repeat instructions if any are given to aid memory and understanding.

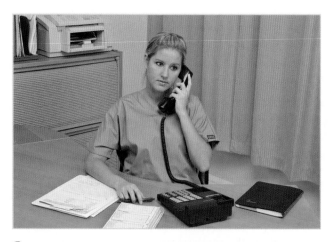

3. Lower your voice in both pitch and volume, and speak slowly if necessary.

WHY?   *This will calm the patient.*

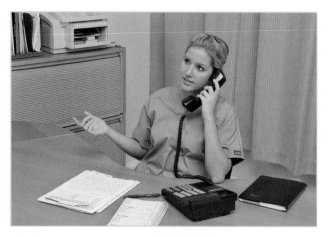

4. Use proper communication such as "I understand" and "What can I do to help you?"

WHY?   *This is considered therapeutic communication. It is also non-confrontational and can help reduce the patient's anxiety and/or anger.*

TIP   Do not take the call personally; it is not about you. Follow through with any assistance and avoid making empty promises.

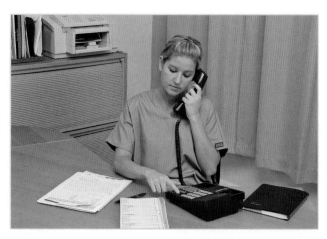

5. Transfer the caller to the office manager, if necessary, or per office protocol.

WHY?   *Many offices have the manager deal with angry callers, as the manager is trained in conflict resolution.*

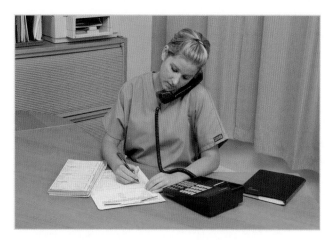

6. Document the conversation in the patient's chart and on the telephone message pad.

WHY?   *Proper documentation is a legal issue; all patient care must be documented.*

 Charting Example

3/12/07 11:20 a.m. Pt called with billing issues. Referred pt. to Mary Jones, Office Manager. _____ F. Napier, CMA

Procedure **8-9**

Demonstrate Telephone Techniques: Make Outgoing Calls

PURPOSE

Outgoing calls require the medical assistant to follow the same communication principles used for handling incoming calls. By effectively making outgoing calls, the medical assistant forges professional connections between the medical office and patients, physicians, hospitals, and others in the medical community.

EQUIPMENT/SUPPLIES

- telephone
- pen
- notepad
- patient chart

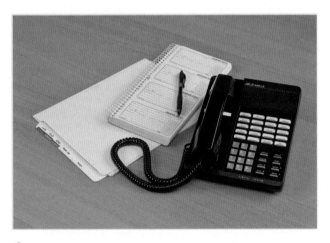

1. Gather all supplies.

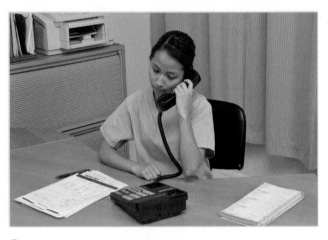

2. Use a quiet and private area.

TIP *Do not leave personal messages on answering machines per HIPAA and confidentiality laws.*

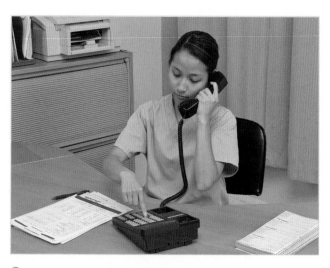

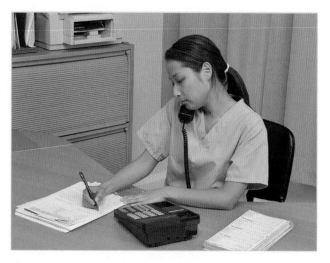

3. Use proper telephone techniques of professionalism, clarity, and courteousness.

 Identify yourself by giving your name and the name of the medical practice. Repeat the information you receive, and be sure to thank the person at the end of the call.

4. Document the conversation in the patient's chart.

✎ *Charting Example*

3/12/07 11:10 a.m. Called pt. with WNL lab results per Dr. Herrera. ID confirmed. Pt had no questions or concerns.
_____ K. Yeremenko, CMA

CHAPTER 9

Legal Concepts

INTRODUCTION

Health care law is complex and multifaceted. Today, patients are more informed and more in control of their health care than in the past. Privacy is a major concern for the medical office, as outlined by the Health Insurance Portability and Accountability Act (HIPAA). It is the medical assistant's duty to maintain patient confidentiality in all aspects of patient care and documentation and to perform within legal and ethical boundaries. One of the medical assistant's primary legal responsibilities is to create and maintain medical records, which are legal records of all care given to patients. These must be kept confidential, whether in electronic or paper form. Another legal responsibility is to maintain accurate knowledge of federal and state health care legislation and regulations, such as OSHA guidelines, CLIA waived tests, and state guidelines regarding immunization administration, IV placement, or phlebotomy. It is critical for medical assistants to understand these areas in order to ensure proper patient care and safety.

PROCEDURES

9-1 Identify and Respond to Issues of Confidentiality

9-2 Perform Within Legal and Ethical Boundaries

9-3 Establish and Maintain the Medical Record

9-4 Document Appropriately

9-5 Demonstrate Knowledge of Federal and State Health Care Legislation and Regulations

Procedure 9-1

Identify and Respond to Issues of Confidentiality

PURPOSE

Maintaining patient confidentiality is of utmost importance, as the latest requirements of the Health Insurance Portability and Accountability Act (HIPAA) indicate. Medical assistants must guard patient confidentiality throughout the day; what is said, implied, written, or inadvertently conveyed must be held to strict confidentiality standards.

EQUIPMENT/SUPPLIES

- patient chart
- telephone
- pen
- lab results

Scenario: Calling a patient with lab results per provider instruction.

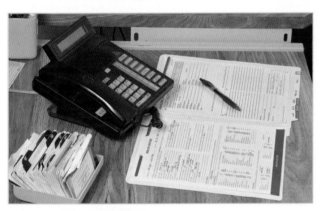

1. Gather all supplies.

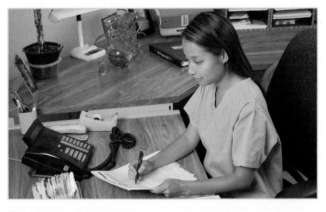

2. Obtain the patient's telephone number from the chart.

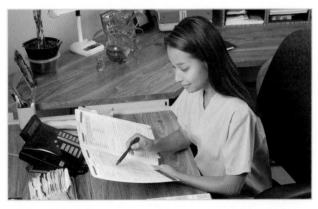

3. Have the lab results in front of you.

ᴡʜʏ❓ *It is important to gather the information you need before you make the call. Preparation allows efficient communication.*

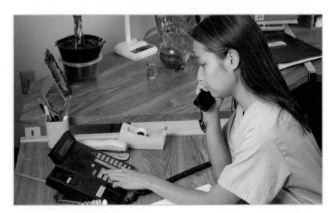

4. Call the patient.

If the patient is home:

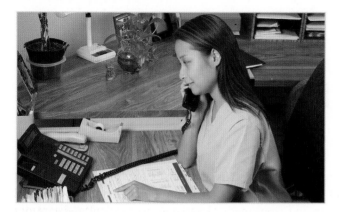

5. Identify the patient by birth date and/or social security number.

WHY? *It is important to ensure proper identification to avoid giving information to an unauthorized individual.*

TIP You may know this patient well and be able to identify the patient by voice; that is acceptable.

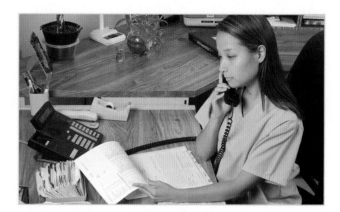

6. Give the patient the lab results and any explanations necessary, or schedule a follow-up appointment if appropriate.

WHY? *This ensures appropriate patient care.*

If the patient is not at home:

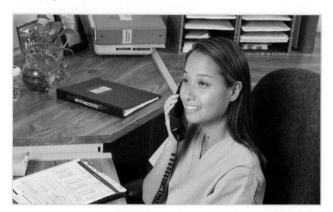

7. Leave an appropriate message while maintaining patient confidentiality. Example: "This is Brett Jones, Dr. Smith's medical assistant, calling for Thomas Peterson. Please call our office at your soonest convenience. Our number is 555-111-2222. Thank you very much."

WHY? *Note that information regarding laboratory results was not left on the message. Only general messages are appropriate unless the patient has documented in the chart that detailed phone messages are permissible.*

LEGAL ALERT! Be aware that under HIPAA regulations, you cannot leave a message that says you are calling from a doctor's office unless the patient has signed a release allowing this.

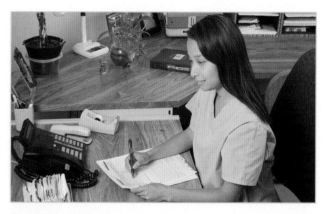

8. Document the conversation.

WHY? *This type of communication with patients must be recorded.*

TIP Other ways medical assistants can protect patient confidentiality include clearing the computer screen, placing charts upside down on counters, and not giving out information without signed consent.

✎ **Charting Examples**

3/08/07 11:30 a.m. Patient called regarding lab results, identified patient, results verbally given, patient scheduled for follow-up on 3/12/07. _____ J. Espinoza, CMA

3/08/07 2:10 p.m. Patient called regarding lab results, patient not home, left message to call clinic.
_____ D. Santini, CMA

Procedure 9-2

Perform Within Legal and Ethical Boundaries

PURPOSE

Because medical assistants are not licensed like physicians and nurses are, they must perform within their legal scope of practice and only perform duties that are delegated to them by the provider. This can vary from state to state and from medical assistant to medical assistant depending on each individual's training. All working medical assistants must be fully aware of their scope of practice in their state, within their own practice, and according to their level of training and expertise.

EQUIPMENT/SUPPLIES

- PPE
- IV supplies
- patient chart
- pen

Scenario: Provider orders medical assistant to start IV of normal saline.

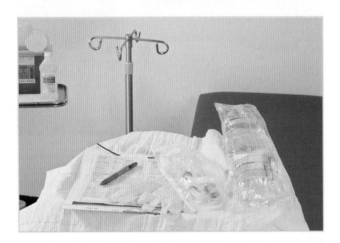

1. Gather all supplies.

If Medical Assistant is allowed per state law and level of education to do so:

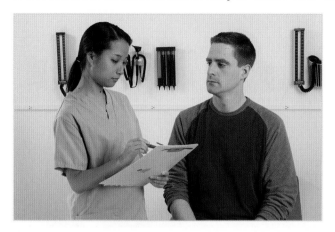

2. Identify the patient.

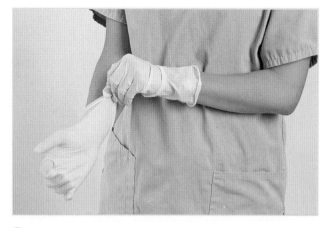

3. Wash your hands and apply PPE.

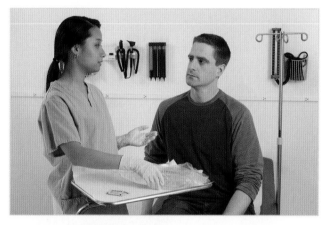

4. Explain the procedure to the patient.

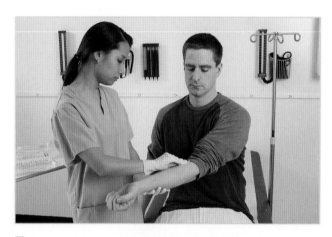

5. Prepare the patient's skin.

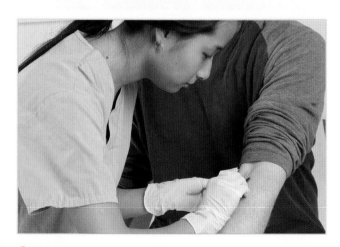

6. Establish an IV (role play only).

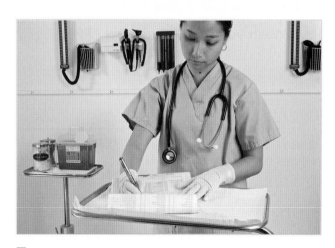

7. Document the procedure.

If Medical Assistant is not allowed per state law to do so:

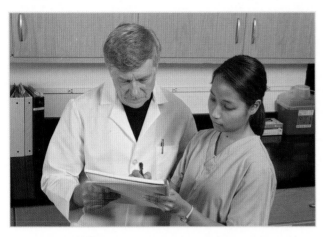

8. Inform the provider that this is not within the scope of practice and/or training.

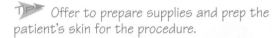 Offer to prepare supplies and prep the patient's skin for the procedure.

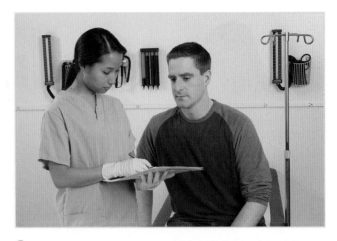

9. Identify the patient.

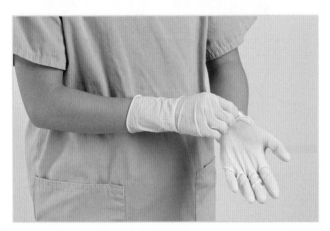

10. Wash your hands and apply PPE.

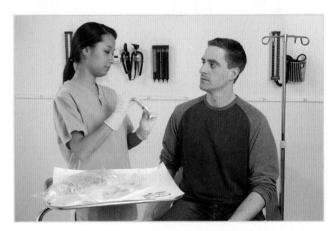

11. Assist the provider as necessary.

 Charting Example

3/12/2007 4:15 p.m. Prepared pt for IV per Dr. Jones. Pt. given verbal education and written f/u instructions to take home. _____ M. Lunde, CMA

Procedure 9-3

Establish and Maintain the Medical Record

PURPOSE

Every patient's personal and medical information is kept in the medical record, whether it is a paper chart or an electronic medical record (EMR). Medical assistants often create new patient records, as well as document in the patient chart and file. Maintaining medical records is an ongoing task; these are legal documents and must be accurate and complete.

EQUIPMENT/SUPPLIES

- blank chart
- dividers
- allergy stickers
- labels
- letter or number tabs
- patient name
- any patient records provided such as past records
- new demographic information sheet and medical history form
- typewriter or computer
- scanner

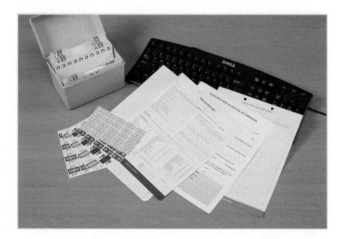

1. Gather all supplies.

For paper charts:

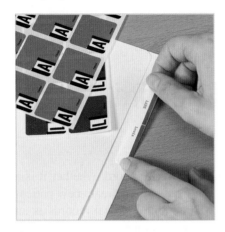

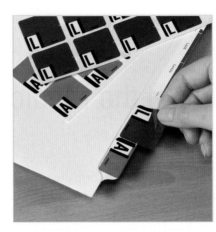

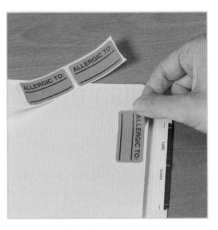

2. Type the patient's name on the label and apply to chart in appropriate place.

WHY? *This identifies the file and prevents filing errors.*

3. Add the correct numerical or alpha tabs.

WHY? *This promotes accuracy and easy retrieval.*

4. Apply an allergy sticker to the outside of the chart per office protocol.

WHY? *A sticker noting drug or other allergies offers a quick and easy reminder for providers.*

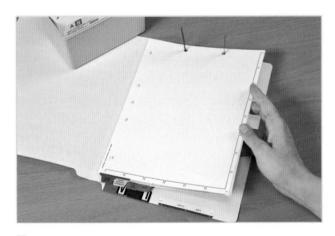

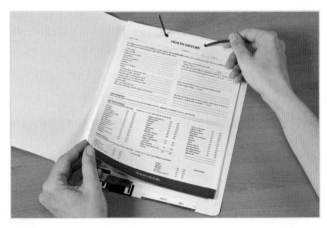

5. Insert the dividers.

6. Insert the patient's paperwork (e.g., demographic forms, history and physical forms, and any past records available) in the correct section and on the correct side, per office protocol.

TIP Every office files papers according to its own protocol. Keep in mind that each office you work in may have a different style.

For electronic charts:

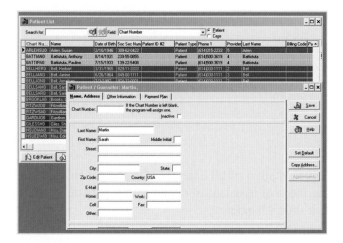

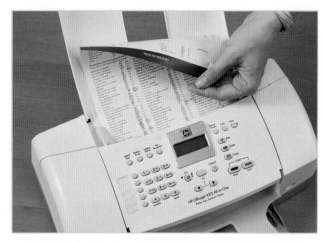

7. Enter patient information into the computer using your office software.

▷ *Electronic medical records (EMR) are numerical; when new patients are added, they are placed in the next sequence automatically.*

8. Scan the patient's old records or forms into the patient's computer file, per office protocol.

▷ *Be sure to maintain confidentiality of this information.*

▷ *While the patient owns the information in the medical record, the practice or physician owns the actual medical record.*

▷ *Medical records include the following: documentation of patient visits and telephone calls, test results, correspondence, physician reports (e.g., operative reports, discharge summaries), medication lists, and missed appointments.*

Procedure 9-4

Document Appropriately

PURPOSE

Because the medical record is the legal representation of all care given to the patient and can be used in a court of law, it is vital for the medical assistant to document all patient care and contact. Legally, if it wasn't documented, it didn't happen.

EQUIPMENT/SUPPLIES

- patient chart
- computer
- pen
- equipment to obtain vital signs

Scenario: **Chart the following patient complaint.**

Patient complaint in laymen's terms: A 27-year-old female has come in complaining of a headache. She states it has been "killing her" for two days and Tylenol just isn't helping at all. She wants to know if she has a brain tumor because her sister died last year of a brain tumor and she had a headache. She wants an MRI today if possible! She explains it feels like the back of her head is going to "blow up" because it feels like pressure, not like the sharp, stabbing pain she gets in her forehead when she has wine. Sleeping, Tylenol, neck massage, cold rags on the neck—nothing has helped, can't the doctor do something to help? She takes no medications and is not allergic to anything.

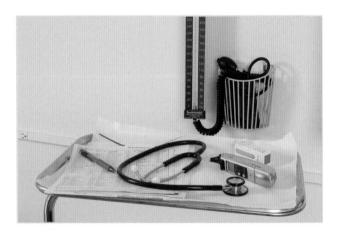

1. Gather all supplies.

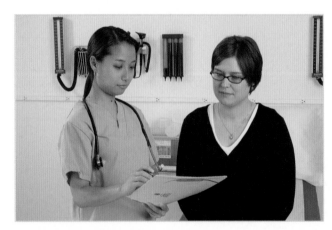

2. Identify the patient.

WHY? *Proper identification prevents errors.*

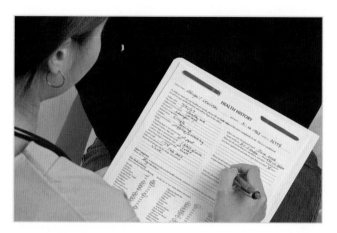

3. Document the date and time per office protocol.

WHY❓ *Date and time is part of correct charting for legal purposes. Charts must be accurate and complete.*

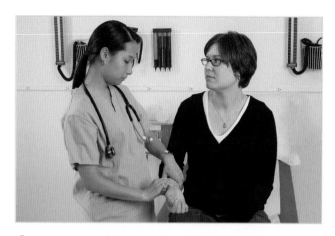

4. Obtain and document vital signs.

WHY❓ *This information is essential for appropriate care.*

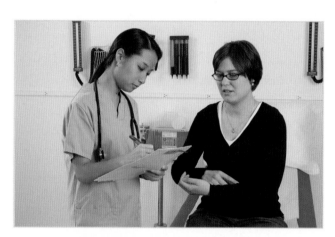

5. Document the patient's problem, making sure to include the following: location, radiation, quality, severity, associated symptoms, aggravating factors, alleviating factors, setting, and timing.

WHY❓ *This information gives the provider a complete overview of the patient's complaint, which is essential for appropriate patient care.*

TIP▶ Chief complaints must be clear, concise, and complete.

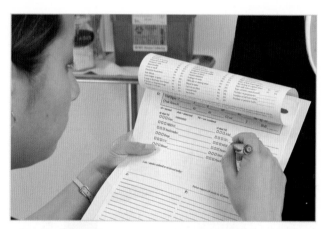

6. Document any medications the patient takes, including over-the-counter (OTC) or herbal supplements.

WHY❓ *OTC medications and herbal supplements can react with other medications or cause certain symptoms. The provider needs this information for accurate diagnosis and treatment of the patient.*

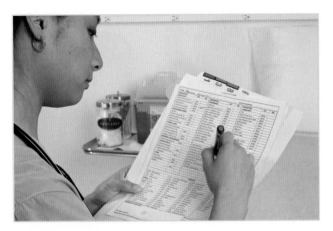

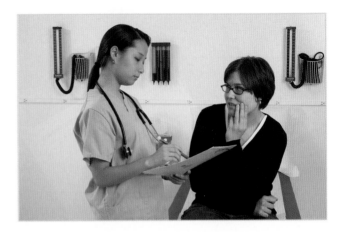

7. Document any medication or other allergies the patient may have.

WHY? *The record of medications taken by the patient, as well as medication allergies, must be kept current.*

8. Document any other problems.

WHY? *Something that the patient may think is unrelated may, indeed, be related to the current complaint.*

TIP If electronic medical records are used, document all information in the correct field in the database.

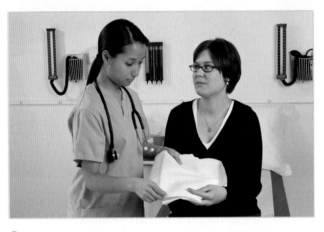

9. Prepare the patient to see the physician.

TIP Anticipate your provider and perform any testing that may be necessary to assist the provider when examining the patient, per office protocol. For example, if the patient has pain with urination, perform a chemical UA; if the patient has asthma symptoms, perform a peak flow.

TIP Care must be taken when using abbreviations. Many abbreviations are no longer allowed due to confusion and/or multiple meanings. Each office should have a list of appropriate abbreviations to use and ones to avoid.

✎ **Charting Example**

10/04/07 10:15 a.m. Ht. 5'6", Wt. 135lbs, T 98.6 F, P 74, R 20, B/P 132/92. CC: 27 y/o female complains of continuous "pressure" HA in back of head x 2d. States pain is "killing her." No other symptoms. Sleep, Tylenol, massage, cold compresses not helping. Family Hx: sister passed away from brain tumor in 2004. Social Hx: drinks wine. Pt. requests MRI. No medication, NKDA.

———————————————— C. Beauregarde, CMA

General Tips for Proper Documentation

Box 9·1

- Use dark ink when writing in paper charts.
- When making corrections in a paper chart, do not use white out. Draw one line through the error and write the correction above it, initial it, and write "corr" or "error" and the date.

General Tips for Proper Documentation, continued

Table 9·1	Prohibited Abbreviations

Note: The following abbreviations should not be used because doing so may cause confusion as a result of handwriting, multiple meanings, etc. This list has been adapted from the Joint Commission on the Accreditation of Healthcare Organizations. Many medical offices have their own such list of abbreviations to use and not use.

ABBREVIATIONS THAT MUST NOT BE USED

Do Not Use	Potential Problem	Use Instead
U (unit)	Mistaken for "0" (zero), the number "4" (four), or "cc"	Write out "unit"
IU (International Unit)	Mistaken for IV (intravenous) or the number 10 (ten)	Write out "international unit"
QD, Q.D., qd, q.d. (daily)	Mistaken for each other	Write out "daily"
QOD, Q.O.D., qod, q.o.d. (every other day)	Period after the Q mistaken for "I" and the "O" mistaken for "I"	Write out "every other day"
Trailing zero (X.0 mg)	Decimal point is missed	Write X mg
Lack of leading zero (.X mg)		Write 0.X mg
MS	Can mean morphine sulfate or magnesium sulfate	Write out "morphine sulfate"
MSO_4 and $MgSO_4$	Confused for one another	Write out "magnesium sulfate"

ABBREVIATIONS THAT SHOULD NOT BE USED

Do Not Use	Potential Problem	Use Instead
> (greater than)	Misinterpreted as the number "7" (seven) or the letter "L"	Write out "greater than"
< (less than)		Write out "less than"
	Confused for one another	
Abbreviations for drug names	Misinterpreted because of similar abbreviations for multiple drugs	Write out drug names in full
Apothecary units	Unfamiliar to many practitioners	Use metric units
	Confused with metric units	
@ (at)	Mistaken for the number "2" (two)	Write out "at"
cc	Mistaken for U (units) when poorly written	Write out "ml" or "milliliters"
µg	Mistaken for mg (milligrams), resulting in 1,000-fold overdose	Use the abbreviation "mcg" or better yet, write out "micrograms"

Table 9·2	Abbreviations Used in Charting

Abbreviation	Meaning	Abbreviation	Meaning	Abbreviation	Meaning
$\bar{a}$	before	Fx	fracture	q.i.d.	four times a day
abd	abdomen	h.s.	bedtime (hour of sleep)	R	right
ant.	anterior	Hx	history	R/O	rule out
AP	anteroposterior	L	left	RLE	right lower extremity
appt	appointment	LLE	left lower extremity	RLQ	right lower quadrant
Ax	axillary	LLQ	left lower quadrant	RUE	right upper extremity
b.i.d.	twice a day	LUE	left upper extremity	RUQ	right upper quadrant
BP	blood pressure	LUQ	left upper quadrant	R/s	rescheduled
$\bar{c}$	with	NKDA	no known drug allergies	$\bar{s}$	without
CC	chief complaint	noct.	nocturnal	SOB	shortness of breath
c/o	complains of	$\bar{p}$	after	spec	specimen
CPE, CPX	complete physical exam	p.c.	after a meal	s/p	after (status post)
Cx	cancelled	PE	physical examination	STAT	immediately
D/C	discontinue	p.r.n.	as needed	t.i.d.	three times a day
F	Fahrenheit	pt.	patient	TPR	temperature, pulse, respiration

Procedure 9-5

Demonstrate Knowledge of Federal and State Health Care Legislation and Regulations

PURPOSE

Medical assistants must be current in their knowledge of federal and state health care legislation and regulations so they can accurately and safely perform their duties within their scope of practice and the law.

EQUIPMENT/SUPPLIES

- controlled substance log
- locked controlled substance cabinet
- keys for cabinet
- expired controlled substance
- pharmacy phone number
- pen
- telephone

Scenario: **Document and dispose of unused controlled substance.**

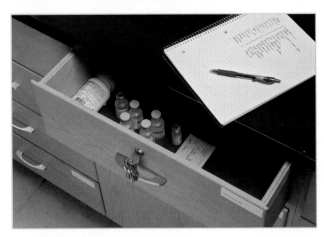

1. Gather all supplies.

ᴡʜʏ❓ *It is important to be prepared, as you cannot leave one person alone with the drug cabinet open.*

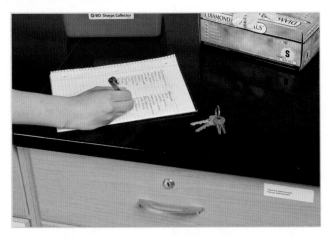

2. Review the controlled substance log to check medication type and quantity on hand.

ᴡʜʏ❓ *An accurate tally of controlled substances is critical for legal purposes.*

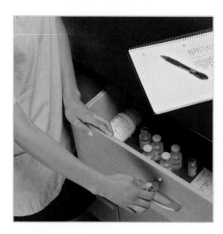

3. Open the controlled medication cabinet.

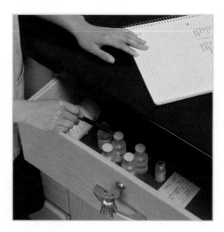

4. Count all of the medications, being sure to check expiration dates.

✓HY❓ *Accuracy in counting is a legal issue. Out-of-date medications must be returned to the pharmacy per DEA law.*

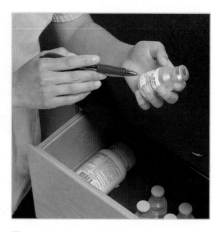

5. Remove expired medication bottle.

✓HY❓ *Expired medications cannot be used.*

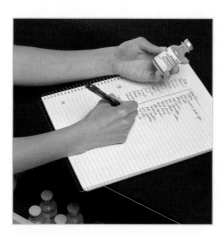

6. Document the current medication count in the log in the appropriate place.

✓HY❓ *Proper documentation is a legal issue.*

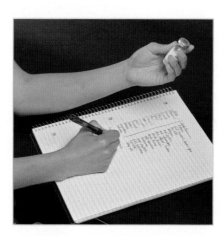

7. Document expired medication in the log in the appropriate place.

✓HY❓ *Proper documentation is a legal issue.*

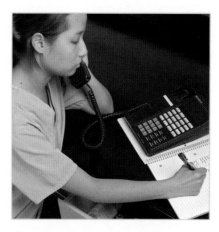

8. Call the pharmacy and arrange for expired medication to be picked up or dropped off and replacement medication to be delivered or picked up, per office policy and legal regulations.

✓HY❓ *The DEA law requires this.*

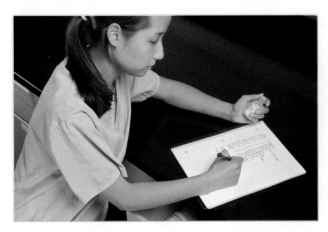

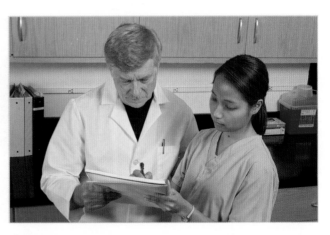

9. Document in the controlled substance log.

WHY? *Proper documentation is a legal issue.*

10. Inform the provider.

WHY? *The provider must be made aware of all controlled substances in the medical office. This is a legal issue and follows proper office protocol. Because the drugs are registered under the provider's name and DEA number, the provider is ultimately responsible for them.*

TIP All controlled substance counts must be done and double checked by at least two persons at all times for backup and legal reasons.

Charting Example

Sample Controlled Substance Log Book

Medication	Count	Exp date	Date counted	Dispensed	Signature
Demerol Tabs, 5mg 30 tabs/bottle	30 tabs	10/06/ 2008	3/12/07	none	B. Jones, CMA/R. James, CMA
Morphine Sulphate 0.2mg/mL, 3mL bottle	3mL	3/07/2008	3/12/07	none	B. Jones, CMA/ R. James, CMA
Fentanyl Patches 100mg/patch 10 patch/box	10 patches	9/05/2008	3/12/07	none	B. Jones, CMA/ R. James, CMA
Norflex 20mg tabs 30tabs/bottle	29 tabs	10/29/2008	3/12/07	1 tab to patient M. Snead d.o.b. 10/13/63 on 3/11/07 per Dr. Smith	B. Jones, CMA/ R. James, CMA
Vicodan 500mg tabs 30 tabs/bottle	30 tabs	1/31/2007	3/12/07	Expired, pharmacy called, returned to pharmacy on 3/12/07	B. Jones, CMA/ R. James, CMA

TIP While medical assistants learn about pertinent laws and regulations in their educational program, once in practice, they must be able to research and keep current with changing legislation or regulations, at both the state and national level.

Patient Instruction

INTRODUCTION

Patient instruction in a wide variety of topics is an important part of the medical assistant's job. The physician determines what the patient needs, but it is the medical assistant who spends time reviewing information and instructions with patients and answering their questions to ensure they understand. This is vital for patient compliance with the doctor's treatment plan. It requires excellent communication and oral speaking skills, as well as psychology and interpersonal relations, and a thorough knowledge of the information that needs to be conveyed. This chapter addresses four key areas in which the medical assistant plays a major role.

PROCEDURES

10-1 Explain General Office Policies

10-2 Instruct Individuals According to Their Needs

10-3 Provide Instruction for Health Maintenance and Disease Prevention

10-4 Identify Community Resources

Procedure **10-1**

Explain General Office Policies

PURPOSE

Explaining general office policies ensures that patients know what the practice has to offer, how it operates, the physicians and staff and their credentials, the hours and location, insurances accepted, and so on. Patients have a right to know all pertinent information about the practice. Plus, clear communication prevents misunderstandings.

EQUIPMENT/SUPPLIES

- office guidelines
- physician/practice brochures
- pad
- pen
- physician business cards
- appropriate patient charting materials, if required by employer

Scenario: **A 48-year-old man comes in to the office. He recently moved to town and needs a doctor who has afternoon appointments.**

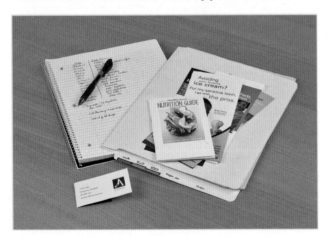

1. Gather needed materials for the patient.

TIP Thoroughly familiarize yourself prior to the patient's arrival with the information you will present, especially when you are not thoroughly familiar with the information you are to explain or teach.

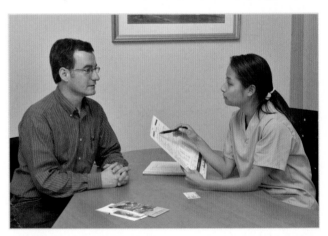

2. Identify the patient.

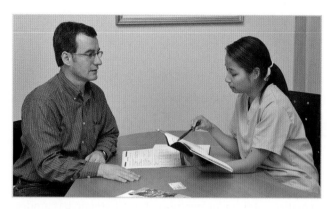

3. Explain the general office guidelines (such as hours, location and directions, and scheduling policies) and provide printed information.

▷ *Prospective patients can be encouraged or discouraged about the practice and physician based on their impression of printed materials and the staff who interact with them initially. Printed information should be clear and concise, and your oral communication should be warm and inviting to instill confidence in excellent care.*

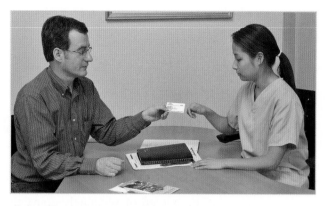

4. Explain the practice, the physicians and staff, services provided, etc. Provide printed material and business cards.

▷ *Printed items are usually available in the reception area and are often mailed to new patients prior to their first visit.*

LEGAL ALERT! *The medical assistant is the "agent" or representative of the physician and must convey information accurately and appropriately as the doctor directs.*

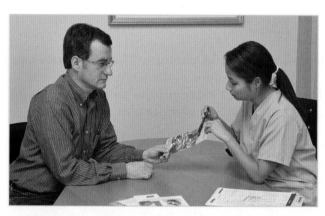

5. Utilize written materials as you explain to further ensure understanding.

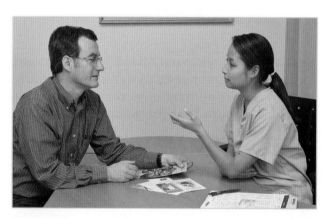

6. Answer questions the patient may have in the appropriate fashion.

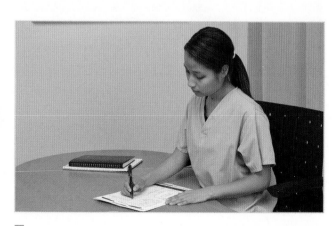

7. Document in the patient chart, if already created.

 Charting Example

3/27/07 2:30 p.m. Visit for potential new patient. Provided verbal and printed information about the practice and the physician. Answered all patient questions. Patient conveyed understanding. Name and demographics in waiting file. He will call with questions and/or appt. _____ J. Lennox, MA

Procedure 10-2

Instruct Individuals According to their Needs

PURPOSE

The burden of accurately conveying information and ensuring the patient-listener has understood is on the healthcare workers and providers. It is vital in communication to adapt your information and style to the individual to foster understanding; this is especially true when dealing with patients with special needs. Some of the possible patient needs to consider include, but are not limited to: age, gender, education, ethnic group, physical challenge, mental challenge, mood or state of being at the time, illness, and medication.

EQUIPMENT/SUPPLIES

- low sodium diet sheet
- sodium and blood pressure handout
- pad
- pen
- patient's chart

Scenario: **A 16-year-old obese female patient appears irritated and anxious. The physician has told her that she needs to eat a low-sodium diet for blood pressure control. As part of your teaching, provide handouts that list low-sodium foods and that explain how salt affects blood pressure. Ensure that the patient understands the diet and why it is important to follow it.**

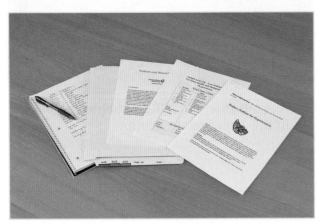

1. Gather the printed information and materials needed for the patient.

TIP Make notes and plan on what and how you will present the information in a concise and logical way. Plan ahead when possible. Being organized will help ensure you convey the information completely and accurately; notes provide a quick reference for patient questions.

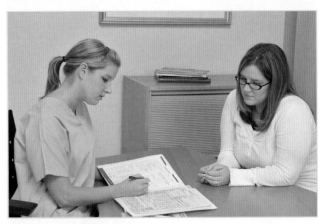

2. Identify patient.

TIP In this scenario, the minor patient would likely have a parent/guardian with her. Identify and speak to the patient but ensure the parent is involved as well.

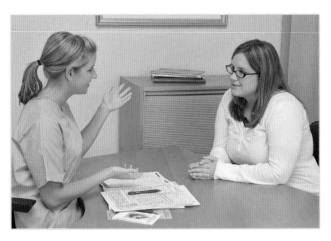

3. Begin by telling the patient what you want to accomplish or teach, and provide an overview of what the patient needs to learn.

WHY? *Patients will understand better if they know what they will be learning ahead of time.*

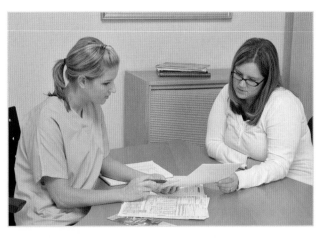

4. Explain why the information is important and why the patient needs to understand it.

WHY? *This is important to ensure that the patient will comply.*

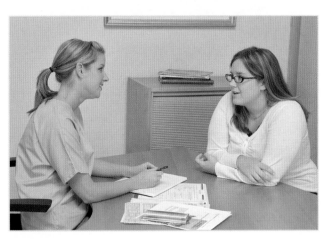

5. Converse with the patient using appropriate general communication techniques.

TIP Speak clearly, use the appropriate level for the patient's understanding without being condescending, use the right body language and gestures for the situation and patient.

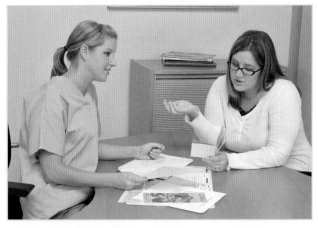

6. Deal appropriately with the challenge of each individual by adapting your communication style, words, and body language, as the patient responds and asks questions.

TIP Communication challenges are innumerable. For example, patients may get angry or they may cry. They may not understand but say they do. They also may become embarrassed or feel put on the spot. Learn to recognize these challenges as they occur, and use the appropriate communication strategies to overcome these barriers.

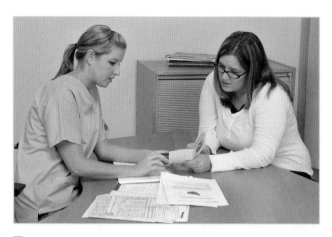

7. Utilize written materials as you explain to further ensure understanding.

TIP If the patient is blind or otherwise visually impaired, utilize other senses or items instead of written materials to help the patient understand.

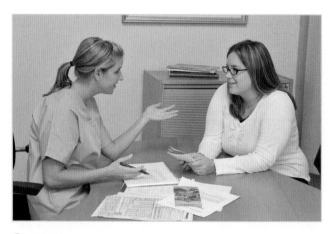

8. Determine understanding by questioning or having the patient repeat back.

TIP This is especially important if the patient's challenge impairs listening or comprehension.

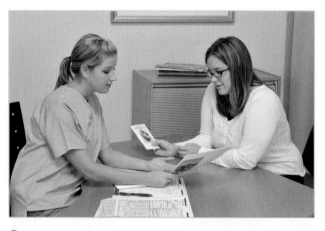

9. Continue explanation using a different approach if necessary (see step #8).

WHY? *It is the medical assistant's responsibility to ensure patient understanding using whatever means are needed for each individual.*

TIP Some patients will need more time and require various approaches.

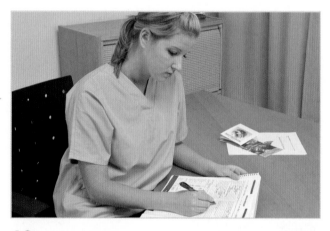

10. Document in the patient's chart.

Charting Example

9/7/07 11:00 a.m. Patient was verbally instructed in a low sodium diet. Printed sheet was given and all questions were answered. Patient indicated understanding by repeating the instructions. _____ G. Hernandez, CMA

Procedure 10-3

Provide Instruction for Health Maintenance and Disease Prevention

PURPOSE

The same basics of communication and understanding apply to all information that is conveyed to patients. As managed care strives to provide quality care while limiting costs, it is important to educate and encourage patients to adopt a healthy lifestyle and diet, and to maintain health and prevent disease.

EQUIPMENT/SUPPLIES

- breast self exam brochure
- article on early diagnosis of breast cancer
- pad
- pen
- patient chart
- breast model

Scenario: **The physician has a standing order that female patients are to be instructed in the breast self-exam during an annual physical exam. Instruct a 35-year-old female patient in performing a breast self-exam. Give the patient a breast exam brochure and a copy of an article on early diagnosis of breast cancer.**

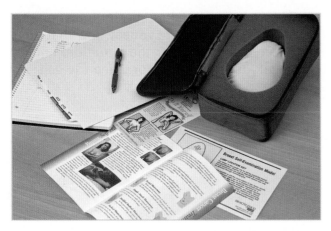

1. Gather materials needed for the patient.

TIP ▶ Thoroughly familiarize yourself prior to the patient's appointment whenever possible. Make notes and plan on what information you will present and how to communicate the information to the patient.

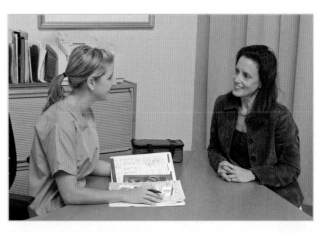

2. Identify the patient.

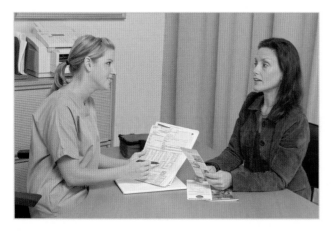

3. Explain what you will cover and the reason why.

WHY? *Patients will typically cooperate when they can be a part of, or at least understand, their care.*

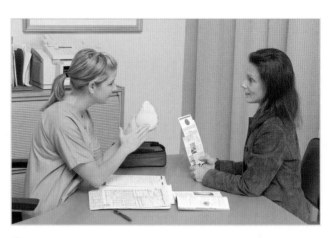

4. Explain the breast self-exam, how it will help the patient, and what to do and when. Guide the patient through a practice on a breast model.

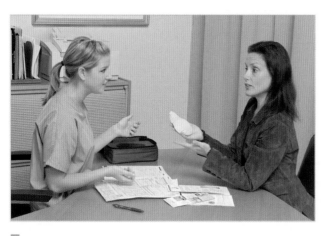

5. Answer questions the patient may have in the appropriate fashion.

TIP Speak at a comprehension level appropriate for each patient. Do not use medical terms the patient may not understand; instead, use layperson's words.

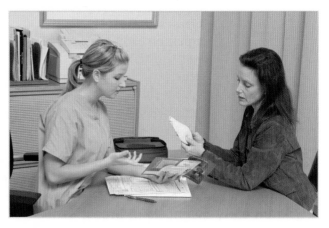

6. Determine understanding by questioning, asking the patient to repeat information, or as appropriate for the situation, and/or observing the patient practice the self-exam on a breast model.

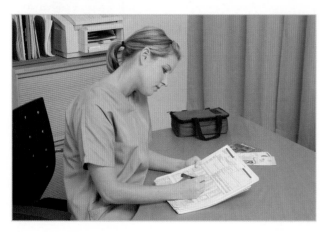

7. Document in the patient chart.

✎ **Charting Example**

7/8/07 10:45 a.m. Patient was given the usual breast self exam brochure, instructed on the breast model, then practiced in exam room. Patient demonstrated correctly on a breast model. Copy of article on early breast cancer diagnosis given and explained. Patient to make mammogram appt. then will return to clinic in six months. _____ P. McClaren, CMA

Procedure 10-4

Identify Community Resources

PURPOSE

The medical assistant needs to provide information for the patient to use. When patients need to do something themselves, give them the tools. This empowers patients in their own care, and by providing them with the resource contact information they need, you will make it more likely they will contact sources of help and be proactive in their health management. Patients typically need both written and verbal information.

EQUIPMENT/SUPPLIES

- list of melanoma resources
- pad
- pen
- patient chart

Scenario: **The patient is a 48-year-old male who has been diagnosed with melanoma by his physician today. The doctor would like the patient to learn more about the disease and to find a local support group to attend. Assist this patient by locating three reputable resources on melanoma such as the American Cancer Society, the American Academy of Dermatology, and the Mayo Clinic. Provide contact information.**

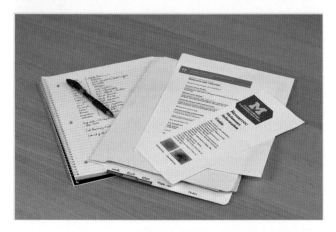

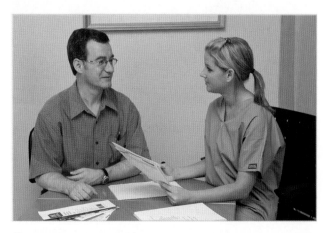

1. Compile the resources needed for the patient.

WHY❓ *The typical medical office already has a list of various resources for patients, although you may have to research resources that are out of the ordinary for the practice.*

TIP When researching resources, compile the list ahead of time whenever possible to avoid making the patient wait. However, this will not always be possible.

2. Identify the patient.

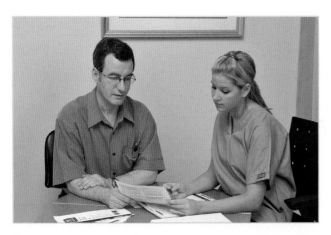

3. Explain to the patient what the resources are for and what the patient is to do with them.

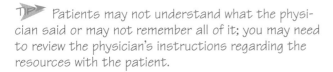 Patients may not understand what the physician said or may not remember all of it; you may need to review the physician's instructions regarding the resources with the patient.

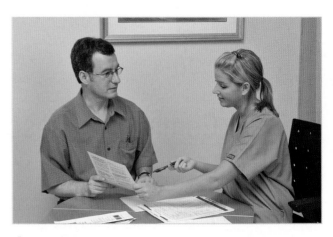

4. Provide a written list or sheet for the patient as well as a verbal explanation.

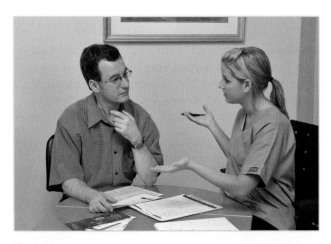

5. Answer any questions the patient may have.

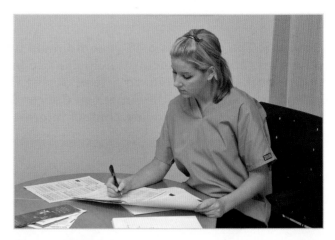

6. Document in the patient's chart.

 Charting Example

8/26/07 9:00 a.m. Patient given contact information on melanoma from American Cancer Society, the American Academy of Dermatology and the Mayo Clinic. Physician's instructions reviewed with patient who indicated understanding. _____ L. Tran, CMA

CHAPTER 11

Operational Functions

INTRODUCTION

Keeping operational functions at peak efficiency is critical for any medical office. This saves time and money by ensuring all equipment is functioning correctly and all supplies are available for use by the healthcare team.

PROCEDURES

11-1 Perform an Inventory of Supplies and Equipment

11-2 Perform Routine Maintenance of Administrative Equipment

11-3 Perform Routine Maintenance of Clinical Equipment

11-4 Utilize Computer Software to Maintain Office Systems: Entering New Patient Information into a Database

11-5 Use Methods of Quality Control

Procedure 11-1

Perform an Inventory of Supplies and Equipment

PURPOSE

A medical practice uses large amounts of varied supplies and costly equipment. By keeping an accurate inventory of these items, the medical assistant helps the practice operate efficiently and ensures that vital materials are always available for administrative and clinical tasks.

EQUIPMENT/SUPPLIES

- inventory form for supplies
- inventory form for equipment
- pen
- clinic equipment
- supply cupboards

- supply catalog
- supply order form
- fax machine
- telephone
- filing cabinet

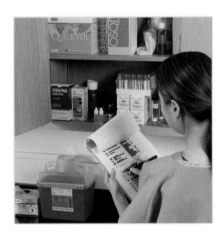

1. Gather all supplies.

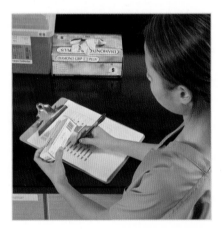

2. Count all supplies in the supply cupboard. Be sure to document the amount, the expiration dates, and any missing items.

LEGAL ALERT! *Be sure to check expiration dates, rotate stock, and never use outdated stock. If a patient were harmed due to use of expired medications, solutions, or materials, the physician and you may be held liable.*

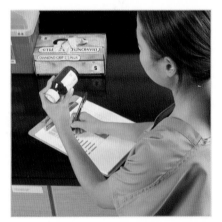

3. Document the count on the inventory form.

TIP *There are many types of inventory forms, some combined with an order form. Follow the employer's instructions to complete the form accurately.*

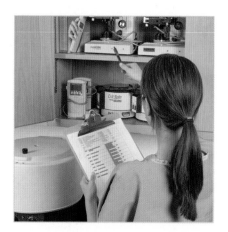

4. Count all equipment used in the office, being sure to check maintenance dates if applicable.

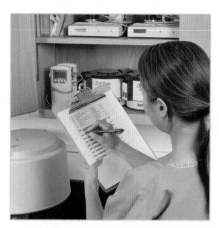

5. Document the count and maintenance dates on the inventory form.

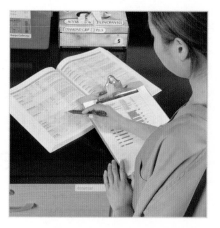

6. For any supplies needing to be restocked, look them up in the supply catalog used by your office and note the item number and amount needed on your office order form.

TIP You may need to check a supply catalog(s) for ordering information. Be sure to use previous order forms as well to find the right information. Some offices use online ordering.

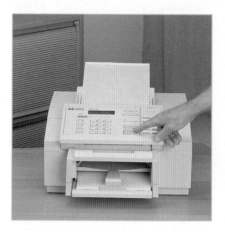

7. Fax or call in the order per office protocol.

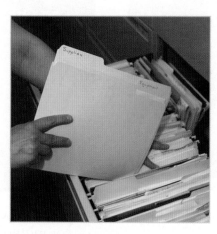

8. File the order form in the correct file.

TIP Document the date you ordered and who you spoke with if ordering by phone.

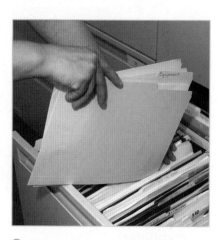

9. If any equipment needs to have a maintenance check, order this per office protocol; otherwise file the equipment inventory in the appropriate file per office policy.

TIP Some offices have a log in which to document the inventory process; sign and date this when you complete the task.

Procedure 11-2

Perform Routine Maintenance of Administrative Equipment

PURPOSE

Healthcare workers rely on office equipment to complete daily tasks in a timely manner. By spending a few minutes to care for and clean administrative equipment, medical assistants can often save money on costly repairs.

EQUIPMENT/SUPPLIES

- computer with software and covers
- disk or CD in the computer
- can of compressed air
- eyeglass or monitor cleaner
- non-static cloth

Scenario: **Perform routine maintenance of a computer and monitor.**

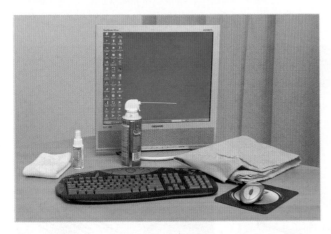

1. Gather cleaning supplies used daily for a computer.

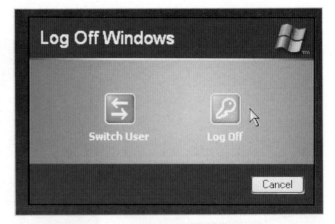

2. Close down all programs and log off computers. Shut down if your employer prefers.

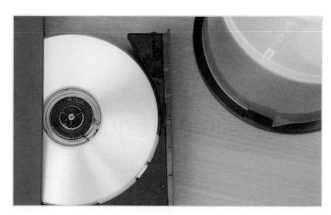

3. Remove any disk or CD in the machine and place it in the appropriate storage case.

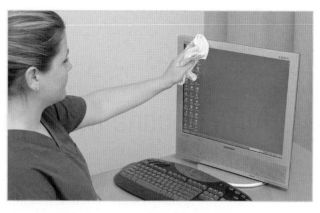

4. Use cleaner and non-static cloth to dust monitor face.

WHY? *Anything that causes static electricity around the equipment might cause a spark, which could damage the CPU.*

TIP Use only the cleaner(s) appropriate for your particular equipment. Read the labels of anything you use.

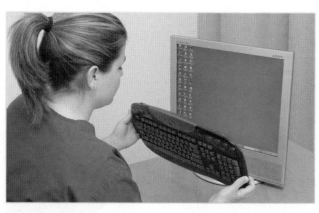

5. Tip the keyboard upside down (if cord allows) to let loose dust and particles fall out. Do not shake or hit. Return it to its place.

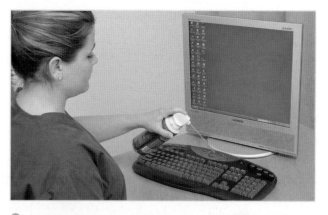
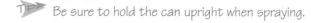

6. Use a can of compressed air to dust the keyboard more thoroughly.

TIP Be sure to hold the can upright when spraying.

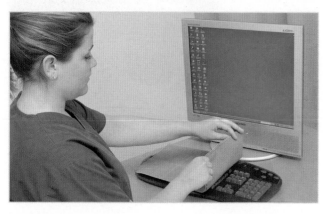

7. Place cover over monitor and/or keyboard per employer's preference.

Procedure 11-3

Perform Routine Maintenance of Clinical Equipment

PURPOSE

Regularly caring for clinical equipment ensures that all items are in proper working order and calibrated correctly, so that tests and treatments will be correct, and the physician and patients are not inconvenienced.

EQUIPMENT/SUPPLIES

- microscope
- slide on the stage
- lens paper and cleaner
- microscope cover
- gloves
- sharps container

STANDARD PRECAUTIONS

Scenario: **Perform routine maintenance of a microscope.**

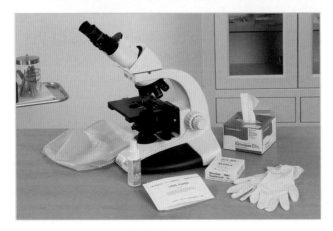

1. Gather cleaning supplies used daily for a microscope and apply PPE.

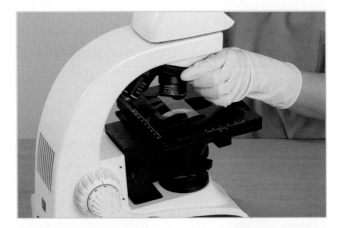

2. Rotate the objectives so that low power is in place.

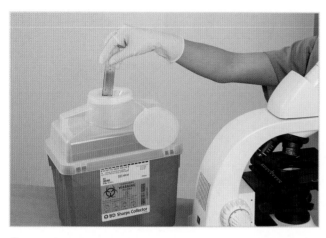

3. Remove the slide from microscope stage and dispose of properly.

Glass slides and cover slips should be disposed of in a sharps container.

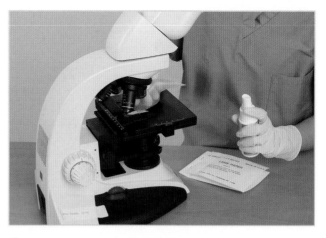

4. Use lens cleaner and lens paper to clean each objective lens.

WHY? *Lens cleaner and lens paper prevent scratching glass surfaces and blocking the view in the visual field.*

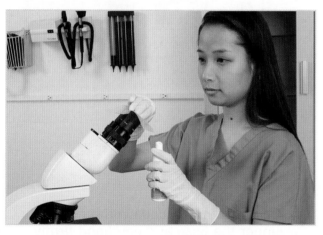

5. Use lens cleaner and lens paper to clean each ocular.

Do not use the same lens paper to clean the lenses and oculars because this could cause the objective lenses to become scratched.

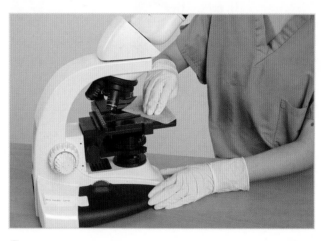

6. Use lens paper or a soft cloth to wipe the stage.

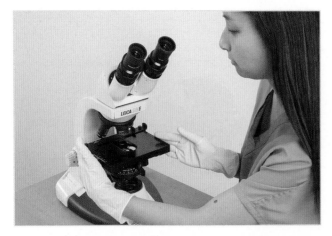

7. Position the stage toward midline to avoid any part protruding while stored.

ᴡʜʏ⁇ *This helps avoid equipment breakage.*

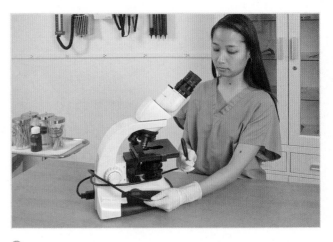

8. Wrap the cord around the base.

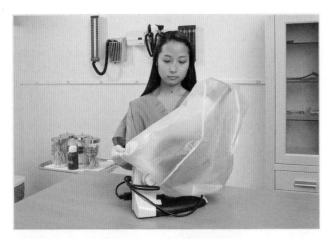

9. Cover the microscope.

ᴛɪᴘ If the microscope in your office or clinic is used often it may never get covered, so it is even more important to clean it to avoid accumulation of dust and particulates that can alter proper function.

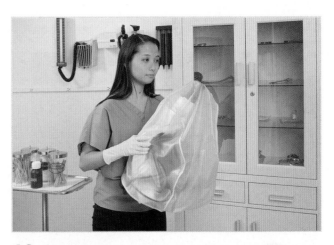

10. Carry the microscope with one hand under the base and one hand firmly gripping the arm, and return it to its storage place.

ᴛɪᴘ Open the storage cabinet door before picking up the microscope so both hands are free to hold it appropriately.

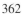

Procedure **11-4**

Utilize Computer Software to Maintain Office Systems: Entering New Patient Information Into a Database

PURPOSE

Technology has greatly impacted the health care system. Many offices use software to chart notes in the patient's medical records, schedule patient appointments, send lab results, order supplies, and maintain financial and billing/coding records. As a result, medical assistants must know how to use computer software to perform a variety of tasks.

EQUIPMENT/SUPPLIES

- computer with patient database
- sample new patient information to use
- patient medical records if available, or patient history/demographic forms
- insurance information

Scenario: **Utilize computer software to establish a new patient record.**

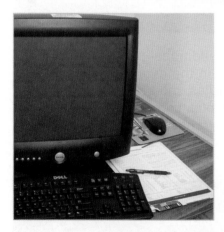

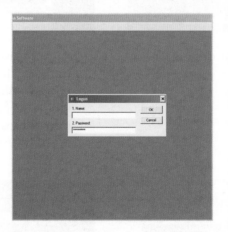

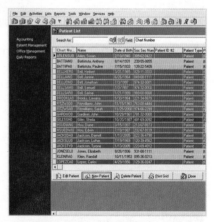

1. Gather supplies needed.

2. Turn on computer and log in as needed.

3. Open the software program and database needed for the task, which is the patient database in this example.

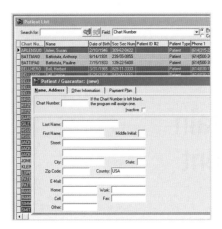

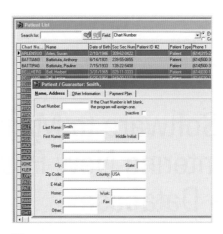

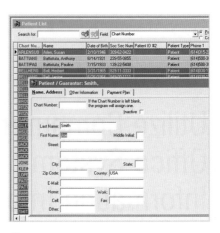

4. Open the screen or window for creating a new patient record.

5. Enter the patient's name, address, and all information required to establish the new record.

6. Save the data when this section is completed.

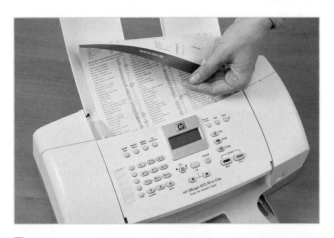

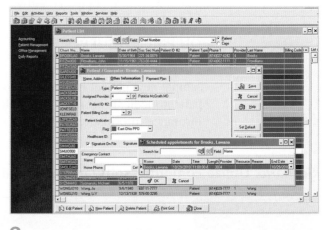

7. Scan in patient history form or any previous records available.

8. If there are additional pages of information needed in the database, such as any known allergies, medications, past medical history, etc., complete all required information to ensure patient record is as complete as possible.

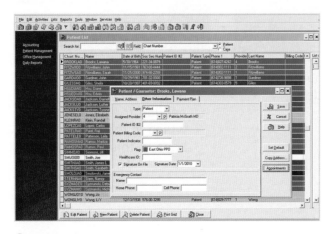

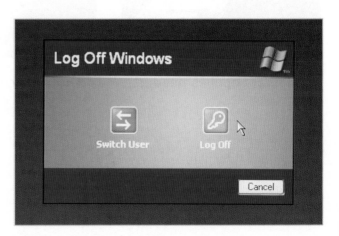

9. Save the data.

10. Close the patient information window(s) for confidentiality.

Procedure **11-5**

Use Methods of Quality Control

PURPOSE

Quality control is a vital function in a physician's office lab (POL) or clinic. By using proper methods of quality control, the medical assistant helps ensure that patient test results are reliably accurate, that diagnostic and therapeutic equipment is properly maintained and calibrated, and that routine tasks are performed correctly.

EQUIPMENT/SUPPLIES

- glucose meter
- correct test strips
- control fluid with expected value
- PPE

- user Instruction Manual
- pen
- quality control log
- biohazard container

STANDARD PRECAUTIONS

Scenario: **Use methods of quality control: Calibrating a blood glucose meter.**

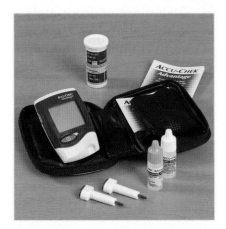

1. Gather supplies and equipment as needed, including the vial of quality control sample.

 Be sure to apply proper PPE.

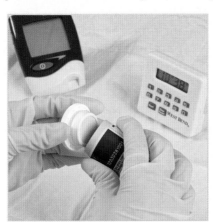

2. Open the vial of test strips for the particular meter being used.

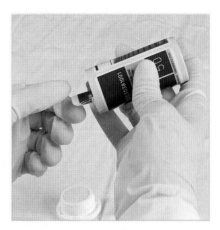

3. Remove one strip without reaching into vial and place on counter.

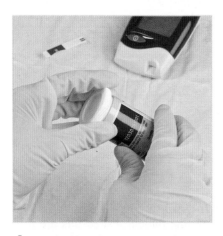

4. Replace cap of the test strip vial.

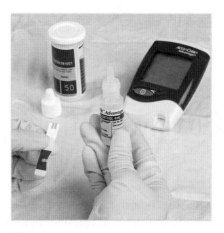

5. Open vial of test control fluid.

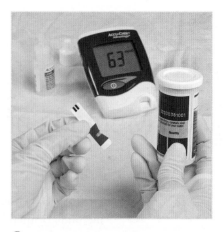

6. Turn on the meter and check the code of the test strips required for the current calibration.

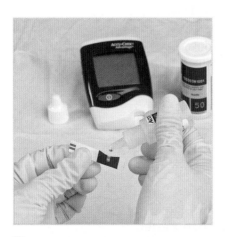

7. Apply control fluid to strip in place of a patient's blood sample and insert into the meter as indicated for the brand of glucose meter being used. Replace cap of control fluid.

▷ Some glucose meters require the strip to be inserted first—follow the manufacturer's instructions for operation.

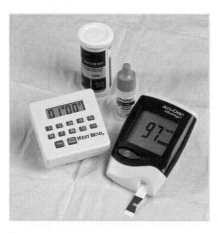

8. Wait the appropriate time for final results and compare to the value stated for the control fluid.

▷ A match of the two numbers indicates the meter is reading and determining the glucose levels correctly, thus ensuring that patient results will be reliable.

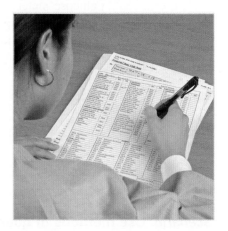

9. Document appropriately in the laboratory quality control maintenance log.

WHY? *Performance of quality control testing requires record keeping.*

▷ Most offices have a log that, at a minimum, requires such information as date, type of test performed, test results, who performed the test, and further action.

▷ QC Log Example: Below is an example of a QC log with two entries. The medical assistant performs this check daily. This type of log often includes many types of equipment and tests.

DATE	NAME	EQUIPMENT	TEST	RESULTS
07/27/07	A. Stewart, CMA	One Touch Glucose Meter	QC accuracy	Expected value obtained -243 mg/dL
07/28/07	A. Stewart, CMA	One Touch Glucose Meter	QC accuracy	Expected value obtained -243 mg/dL

Figure Credits

The anatomical images on pages 106, 114, and 122 have been reprinted with permission from McCall RE, Tankersly MT. *Phlebotomy Essentials.* 3rd ed. Baltimore: Lippincott Williams & Wilkins, 2003.

The anatomical images on pages 131, 279, 284, 289, and 294 have been reprinted with permission from Clay JH, Pounds DM. *Basic Clinical Massage Therapy: Integrating Anatomy and Treatment.* 2nd ed. Baltimore: Lippincott Williams & Wilkins, 2007.

Index